THE GESTALT THEORY AND THE PROBLEM OF CONFIGURATION

Founded by C. K. Ogden

The International Library of Psychology

COGNITIVE PSYCHOLOGY
In 21 Volumes

THE GESTALT THEORY AND THE PROBLEM OF CONFIGURATION

BRUNO PETERMANN

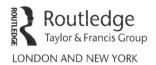

Routledge
Taylor & Francis Group

LONDON AND NEW YORK

First published in 1932 by
Routledge
2 Park Square, Milton Park, Abingdon, Oxfordshire OX14 4RN
711 Third Avenue, New York, NY 10017

First issued in paperback 2014

Routledge is an imprint of the Taylor and Francis Group, an informa business

British Library Cataloguing in Publication Data
A CIP catalogue record for this book
is available from the British Library

The Gestalt Theory and the Problem of Configuration
ISBN 0415-20968-4
Cognitive Psychology: 21 Volumes
ISBN 0415-21126-3
The International Library of Psychology: 204 Volumes
ISBN 0415-19132-7

ISBN 13: 978-1-138-87501-2 (pbk)
ISBN 13: 978-0-415-20968-7 (hbk)

CONTENTS

INTRODUCTION

BOOK ONE

v

BOOK TWO

PART TWO

INTRODUCTION

THE PROBLEM OF CONFIGURATION AND THE GESTALT THEORY

§ 1. *Contemporary psychology and the problem of configuration. Purpose of the present investigation*

Psychology at the present time finds itself in a state of the most widespread conflict over its principles.

During the course of the past decade and a half the conceptions of the problems to be dealt with by psychology, and consequently of its scientific tasks, have changed so much, that one could, and still can, speak of a crisis in psychological research.

The conflict of opinions in psychology has probably never before been as vigorous as it is now. When one considers the individual standpoints at which different investigators arrive in their systematic expositions, one might in actual fact be misled to the conclusion that psychology as a science—in the sense of a system of established knowledge—has no existence. At every turn one opinion stands opposed to another opinion, one statement to another statement, and principle to principle.

Nowhere is this discord within psychology so distinctly evident as in the prominent controversy now current concerning the problem of gestalt [1] ; but on the other hand, nothing reveals more clearly the circumstances out of which such discord was bound to emerge in the present stage of psychology. Here it appears quite definitely as the expression of a decisive phase in its evolution, which every young science has to pass through at one time or another. It signifies nothing less than the endeavour of psychology " to come to itself ", than the struggle to achieve a fundamental orientation which would be adequate to the peculiar nature of psychological data, and which would do justice to the specific methodological and theoretical peculiarity of this field of scientific research.

---

[1] [We propose to use the term " gestalt " throughout the sequel in preference to "configuration ", since it has by now gained universal currency.—Trans.]

The beginnings of the gestalt controversy are, as a matter of fact, still concerned with nothing further than questions of detail. Mach in 1861, G. E. Müller in 1890, Husserl in 1891, von Ehrenfels in 1898 (even in so far as they take their stand, as a matter of course, independently of actual psychological work and more upon logical grounds) still have as their essential objective the further extension of our knowledge of the phenomena. Even if, as with von Ehrenfels, this phenomenological analysis might result in emphasis upon the singularity and irreducibility of the " gestalt " facts, the cardinal significance of this with regard to the systematic conceptions of the psychology of the time as yet receives no attention. The same is true even of the delicate experimental researches of Schumann in 1898, where for the first time a more thorough enquiry into certain fundamental manifestations of the gestalt problem is systematically carried out by means of careful experiments ; or even of the first precisely set out theories, the " Production " theory (cf. e.g. Benussi), or the " Coherence " theory (G. E. Müller).

In its subsequent development, however, a narrowing down of the gestalt problem to questions about underlying principles ensues.

The most far-reaching claims in this direction are made by the school of Wertheimer, Koffka, and Köhler ; to them *the word " gestalt "* has become *the symbol for a basic reorientation.* So much so, that they put forward their theory as a fundamentally " new psychology ", in radical opposition to all other work which has been done in psychology.

Nevertheless, the school of gestalt theory cannot justly claim to have taken the sole, or even the first, step towards an examination of principles. In fact those very principles which are characteristic for the " Total Situation " of to-day had already been emphasized by others independently of the gestalt theory.

In this matter, for one thing, a progressive development which proceeds in succession to von Ehrenfels, through Cornelius (and Lipps) with the clarification of the concept of *Gestalt-quality*, or alternatively *Complex-quality*, up to F. Krueger and H. Volkelt, is worthy of note. Furthermore, the position which Goetz Martius had in any case reached on the basis of his own researches and in the course of reviewing the singularity, from the point of view of scientific theory, of more recent psychological research —a position which he formulated definitively in 1912 in the demand for an "analytical" psychological discipline— is of decisive importance.

Krueger was the first to demonstrate effectually by means of concrete experimental work (1905–6) the "wholeness" characteristic of psychic phenomena ; and Volkelt, in 1912, following Krueger's formulations, published the first clear and precisely expressed description, based on principles, of the concept of " Complex-quality ", as revised in accordance with the orientation towards " wholeness ".

Martius' relation to these problems is not generally known. It was he, in particular, who already quite definitely propounded that line of enquiry in which the probing fcr ultimates has since become established ; and to this latter the current gestalt controversy owes its intrinsic significance. He did this with such exactness and perspicuity, that Jaensch could rightly say that no one had anticipated so early and so thoroughly as Martius the direction of development along which psychology has in the interim moved.

Goetz Martius did not subordinate his psychology to the gestalt problem in the restricted sense. He developed his basic conceptions in much more general studies, orientated by a specific method, viz. in coming to terms with the principles of Wundtian psychology.

Like Krueger, he designated Wundt's an atomistic-synthetic psychology, and demonstrated the inadequacy of the methods borrowed from the natural sciences which he thus characterized. And while calling upon psychology to free itself from them he, in 1912 already, formulated in principle, at least, the *central point of the present gestalt controversy*, viz. the cleavage between the atomistic stand-point of the refuted theory and the characteristic closure, " wholeness," which the phenomena of form-perception manifest.

The " atomistic " psychology, characteristically dependent as it was upon the natural sciences for its method of thinking, tried to conceive the reality of psychic life as built up of Sensations and Feelings, of conscious elements, and set itself the task of carrying through a construction of this sort on *the basis of a study of these very elements with reference to their elementary properties and the laws of their synthesis.*

This old psychology was, of course, aware of the issue at stake in this cleavage; but the way in which a theory thus orientated can cope with such a problem, in terms of its own assumptions only, proves fallible upon critical assessment. The great problem as to how it is possible for a whole to arise out of the elements—that determinate unitariness which distinguishes every individual psychical experience as well as the continuity of experience in its entirety—this problem lies completely outside the scheme of thinking of that psychology. The conceptual equipment provided by the original tenets of this system is in any case deficient in this regard. So when one finds the gaps being closed by simply introducing new special principles, principles of Creative Synthesis, of Creative Resultants, etc., in order to explain the facts in question, one detects, in this itself, the expression of its incompetence really to solve the problem on the basis of its actual system of thought.

While Martius was thus reviewing this state of affairs, he put forward the very point in reference to which the problem of configuration at first quite specially posed, as its experimental and conceptual clarification advanced, was bound of itself to lead up to questions of principles— the point from which the problem of configuration in fact derives its basic significance.

Undoubtedly, the elucidation of fundamental issues is essentially involved in the present-day gestalt controversy —issues which concern psychology in all its lines of enquiry. Each of these issues leads to a different way of viewing the problems, and to a correspondingly different solution of them ; and just in this fashion does that multiplicity and discord within psychology of which we spoke at the outset come into being.

There is only one proper way of surmounting these difficulties, under the circumstances. The more we insist that just in this very problem our concern is, at the present moment, in fact not so much with detailed psychological knowledge, but rather with the ultimate tenets of psychology itself, the sooner will that clarification of the field of enquiry, which is so necessary for the restoration of unity within the detailed work, present itself. It is not so much the multiplication and accumulation of factual data which can lead us any further at the moment. Rather, in the present total confusion of basic concepts a far better prospect of success offers itself in the endeavour to submit the already available material, and the valuations which have been attached to it in its theoretical bearings, to a comprehensive review and elucidation. In this way, the bases of thinking and the standpoints in research which find expression in those currents, can be put to the test as to their conclusiveness and as to their tenability, methodologically and in respect of scientific theory. In this way, through a critically evaluating revision, we may arrive at secure premisses.

With this view, the present enquiry selects in particular, from the great complex of issues outlined, that theoretical solution of the gestalt problem which considers itself the most radical. An attempt is made to break the ground for a critical clarification of the gestalt problem by means of coming to terms with the "Gestalt Theory" in the narrower sense of the word, as it was developed by Wertheimer, Koffka, and Köhler.

Our reasons for particularly choosing the Wertheimer-Koffka-Köhler theory are several. Even the external effects which have accompanied the advent of this theory could decide one upon this. Through it, undoubtedly, the gestalt problem has become so urgent, that at the present time it has come to be the main topic of work in the laboratories, as well as of discussion at congresses.

Furthermore, there can be no doubt that this does represent the most radical attempt to combine the theoretical moments which inhere in the problems of gestalt into an integral system, on the basis of a quite characteristic orientation of principles. This arouses the expectation that here—as with every radical attempt at resolving newly perceived issues in research—the peculiarities of the problem might possibly, through a critical consideration, emerge with special force.

Thirdly, going by the impression one is bound to gain from the writings of the school of gestalt theory, the theoretical apparatus of this theory seems by now to be so far fixed in its outlines that one may hardly expect

B

any further extension of it. For we have here—as will appear from a more thorough analysis—a body of knowledge, rounded off, and rooted in certain uniform tenets, which seems wide enough to embrace the whole of psychology; and one the principles of which are, on the other hand, in their coherence so constituted as not to extend beyond their own framework.

Hence it seems possible and worth while to make an attempt at a comprehensive critical point of view directed primarily towards this theory, so as to evaluate and analyze, in respect to its scientific and theoretical structure, at least one of the paths which are being trodden for the sake of settling the conflict of principles in psychology.

BOOK ONE

THE CONCEPTUAL CONSTITUTION OF THE GESTALT THEORY, DEVELOPED IN ITS GENETIC CONTINUITY

Before we critically join issue with the system of the gestalt theory, we shall have to prefix an account of its conceptual constitution, developed in detail. For there are no works available by the representatives of the gestalt theory themselves, which give a satisfactory construction of the whole system, set forth with systematic completeness, with absolute definiteness of thought, and with clear explication of the internal connections.[1]

The task of *expounding*, in this sense, the content of the gestalt theory is, however, made difficult in a peculiar fashion. It becomes complicated through the fact that an actual development, an actual shifting of standpoints has to be established within the literature of the gestalt theory.

Indeed, throughout the works of the Wertheimer-Koffka-Köhler school the beginning of the "new psychology" is again and again assigned to the year 1912. In fact, they explicitly declare that in the formulations which Wertheimer submitted in that first work of his, *Über das Sehen von Bewegungen*, the essentials in the thinking of the new psychology were already formulated with entire definiteness ; and that all that has followed has, at bottom, in no way proceeded beyond the framework of what was given in 1912, as regards principles. However, when one endeavours to reach an understanding with all that has been published since that time from amongst the ranks of those who acknowledge adherence to the gestalt theory, with the aim of establishing and elaborating this theory, one will soon, nevertheless, have to admit to oneself that it by no means represents

[1] Even the latest account by Koffka, in Dessoir's *Lehrbuch der Philosophie*, which suggests itself most readily here, cannot satisfy these conditions.

7

a permanent body of thought that has remained essentially unaltered and uniform. The literature of the gestalt theory is by no means *homogeneous in its thought*.

Moreover, it cannot be maintained either that in any quite definite place—relatively independent of the previous discussions—the finally conclusive conceptions are to be discovered determinately stated, so that there would be a definitive form upon which, as the most forcible of available formulations, our enquiry could be based. Much rather, the special points in its thinking, which characteristically distinguish the later from the earlier parts, are, in fact, only to be understood in regard to their peculiar significance within the theory, when they are considered *in connection with the historical whole*.

In consequence, the manner of presenting the gestalt theory appropriate for us—in so far as it is planned with an eye to a critical scrutiny—is *the genetic one*. In accordance with this we develop the main conceptions of the theory by following out the process of its internal development, as it emerges in the publications.

Here the singular nature of this development immediately leads to a further peculiarity in our treatment.

We must, it is true, hold to the principle that in an *empirical science* such as psychology indubitably ought to be, the main stress should be placed upon the elaboration of the empirical groundwork and upon the promotion of an understanding of the conceptual generalizations which can be directly derived from the empirical work. Nevertheless, in our genetic study it will be just the doctrinal part which we shall place in the foreground. We shall attempt to build up the contents and the progress of thought from one stage of the theory to the next in as clear-cut a manner as possible. For the way the gestalt theory has developed forces such a *genetic consideration of concepts* upon us, instead of a treatment empirically orientated. We are only adapting ourselves to the special nature of our material when we thus here, in the expository section (and so also later, in the critical part especially) give the *doctrinal content of the theory* the central position.

When we examine the entire literature of the gestalt theory from this point of view, a natural articulation of the material reveals itself to us.

The first writings can merely be regarded, with reference to what is to-day comprehended under the rubric of the " new psychology ", as preliminary steps.[1]

Wertheimer's notion of the ϕ-function lies at the basis of these; but this as we shall very soon show, does not yet deserve to be entitled an expression of the actual gestalt theory's way of thinking.

In a work of Koffka's, 1914, a reorientation of *principles* first comes to clear expression.

The theoretical movement thus inaugurated now proceeds to show transformations, in themselves gradual, but very characteristic. It advances in two ways, which are isolated from each other.

The impulse which found expression in 1914 in Koffka's work was concerned essentially with *formal* moments basic to the theoretical standpoint. The work of the succeeding years, until about 1922, serves to give a *material shape* to the formal methods of thinking which had thus been achieved, inasmuch as the interpretation of known facts—and indeed, even the advancing experimental research as well—is gradually *becoming ever more definitely centred upon the gestalt problem itself*, more especially in the study of perception.[2]

Side by side with these, other efforts occur which, adhering to Wertheimer's basic propositions, have as their object the achievement of *physiological theories*. Such efforts definitively find original expression in the indubitably ambitious study of Köhler, *Über physische Gestalten in Ruhe und im stationären Zustand* (1920). This—frankly emancipated, in its line of approach, from the original endeavour of Wertheimer—*for the first time presents a physiological superstructure really adequate to the formal orientation of 1914;* and this, at the same time, within the framework of that great epistemological enlargement which permits the scope of the gestalt theory to extend beyond the psycho-physical and into the sphere of the physical.

Both lines of thought—they were already constantly intercrossing, while in process of development— eventually merge (this has, of course, occasionally been

[1] Wertheimer, 1912 ; Köhler, 1913 ; Koffka, 1913.
[2] As this receives a conclusive formulation of a sort in Koffka's " Perception ", 1922.

accomplished before, as e.g. by Köhler in 1920) in the last step in its thinking which is still wanting for the construction of a finished gestalt theory. *The notion of gestalt becomes a genuine " principle for a system "*, when the point is reached where *characteristic and specific " Gestalt laws "* are erected (Wertheimer, 1923; Köhler 1920; Koffka 1922).

Thus there emerges the *final form* of the gestalt theory, as this has received a more or less conclusive exposition as the " new psychology " by Wertheimer in 1925 in his Kant lecture, as well as by Koffka in his textbook account. We shall pursue this line in more exact detail, with the object of grasping as adequately as possible the content of the theory.[1]

CHAPTER I

THE THEORY OF THE ϕ-PROCESS—SIMPLY A PRELIMINARY STEP TO THE ACTUAL GESTALT THEORY

We must commence our study with Wertheimer's work of 1912, to which the inception of the development of the gestalt theory's thinking is traced. Through this work, *Über das Sehen von Bewegungen*, there runs in a characteristic fashion a duality of problems, side by side. The first, the *theory of the seeing of movement*, which, in consonance with his theme, occupies the central place in the work, is followed to a certain degree as a special matter, by the consideration of that theoretical problem which actually concerns us here, *the theory of the seeing of gestalt*. Correspondingly, we shall, to begin with, develop the various crucial points which are linked together in the theory of the seeing of movement, in Wertheimer's work.

---

[1] We thus *by no means*, be it noted, intend to give anything in the way of a complete *history of the conceptions propounded in regard to the gestalt problem in general*, or even to the particular theory we are concerned with. To that end, cf. e.g. Krueger, *Neue Psychol. Stud.* I, Introduction, 1926.

§ 2. *The seeing of movement : The thesis of the sensation-equivalence of the seeing of movement, and the theory of the directed φ-process*

The central point in Wertheimer's treatment of the problem of movement is to be found in his definition of *the general character of the experiences of movement*, which forms the basis, from the phenomenological side, for Wertheimer's further ideas.

This is summarized in a sentence which we set down here as the *thesis of the sensation-equivalence of the experience of movement* : " When two optical stimuli succeed each other, then, within a certain range of the speed of sequence (viz. in the range of the so-called Optimal Interval) the experience of uniform movement is bound to them in just as *ordered* and (*physically*) *immediate* a manner, as a corresponding sensation to the action of a single stimulus." (Wertheimer, 1912, p. 136.)

The equivalence of the experience of movement to the sensory process, which is expressed in this sentence, appears more closely defined in two directions : According to the formulation of the sentence, it consists, in the first place, in the *ordered*, i.e. relatively *unequivocal determination by the stimulus*, in exactly the sense in which this was always postulated in the theory of sensation (in accordance with the formula, " the stimulus decides the sensation ") ; and secondly, it is defined by the *denial* of any *psychical mediation* of whatever nature—i.e. in a positive way, by the assumption of an *immediate co-ordination between phenomenon and physiological correlate*.

In these two conceptions, the notion of the unequivocal determination by the stimulus and the notion of the immediacy of the physiological correlate, the substance of the thesis of the sensation-equivalence of the seeing of movement is fully comprised. And in fact, these two definitions are interdependent in a quite specific way : The idea of the immediacy of the physiological correlate is a special form of the idea of the unequivocal determination by the stimulus, but does not as a matter of course necessarily involve it ; while conversely, from the unequivocal determination by the stimulus would follow the immediacy of the physiological correlate.

In this connection the notion of the determination by

the stimulus stands in the forefront for Wertheimer.
Or, to put it otherwise, the finer logical distinctions we
have just raised play no part in 1912. This appears quite
clearly from the sentence quoted above, as well as from
the whole tendency of Wertheimer's work, its general
orientation in terms of correspondence to stimulus.[1]

This is confirmed, too, by the way in which, starting
with the generalized formal presentation of the framework
for the formation of concepts set out in the above fundamental statement, the development of the ideas proceeds ;
how the concrete, detailed statements which constitute
the positive contribution of the " Wertheimer theory "
of 1912, the statements toward the *closer definition of the
required physiological correlate*, are achieved.

Formally the process of thought is of the nature of a
simple inference by analogy. "When a sensation comes into
existence as a result of the action of a single " stimulus ",
this occurs because of a mode of excitation within the
sensorium corresponding to, and characteristic of, the
sensation. However, according to the thesis mentioned
above, the experienced phenomenon of movement depends
in quite corresponding fashion upon the stimulus-sequence,
comes into existence on account of it ; so, quite
correspondingly, an excitation is assigned to this occurrence
of the impression of movement, which is specifically
co-ordinated with, and peculiar to, the experience of
movement.

This *requirement of an unequivocal physiological process
co-ordinated with, and characteristic of, the experience of
movement, the ϕ-phenomenon*, was already in its fundamentals doctrinally embodied in the thesis of the
equivalence to sensation. It finds its factual realization
in Wertheimer's construction of a somatic process of this
nature on the basis of the objective stimulus-conditions
present in his experiments.

The theorem for the construction of this so-called
ϕ-*process* reads as follows : " Given, are certain conditions
of interdependence (by Thesis I, regular and unequivocal)
between variations of stimulus-complexes ; required, is

[1] Wertheimer's standpoint of 1912, as we are reconstructing it here,
finds clear and cogent expression in Koffka's (1913) " Introduction "
to the *Beiträge zur Psychologie des Gestalt und Bewegungssehens*, which
he issued in continuation of Wertheimer's investigation.

an occurrence in the brain, so constituted that these regular facts should be inferrable from it." [1]

The solution to this problem is achieved by means of two postulates about somatic functioning in general, namely, the postulate of the action of the field, and the postulate of the short circuit.

The assumption is that the somatic processes in the nervous apparatus *do not* consist in " single excitations " which are exactly circumscribed, and spatio-temporally directly co-ordinated with the place and duration of the action of the stimuli in a *detailed fashion, but* that

(1) To every *single stimulus*, besides the geometrically consequent direct excitation, there corresponds in addition a *field-action*, which proceeds from that basic excitation and spreads over the surrounding parts, at the same time waxing and waning as a temporal process ; and it is assumed that

(2) When *two stimuli* at two places (*a* and *b*) *succeed each other*, because of this, something novel in nature appears, which takes form as a *resultant* based on the field-excitations, " a kind of physiological short-circuit from *a* to *b*."

This physiological concatenation in the seeing of movement is expressed more precisely as follows :—

One may conceive that " in the space between the two places (*a* and *b*) a specific transition of excitation is occurring. If the intensity of the field-action of *a*, for example, has reached the maximum point of its curve of development, and if now field-action arises from *b*, then excitation will flow over—a physiologically specific event the direction of which will be determined by the fact that *a*, and the field-action about *a*, is first present there ".

Thus, the fact of the spatially and temporally interposed " ϕ-phenomenon " " between " the sensations *a* and *b* (Wertheimer's schema *a* ϕ *b*) is physiologically represented by the " *between* " *process* ; and the fact of the sequence-condition in the movement-transition from *a* to *b*, finds expression in the assertion that the " between " process arrived at on the basis of the above-mentioned postulates is a " directed " one. The somatic basis of the ϕ-phenomenon, the " ϕ-function ", is affirmed to be a *directed physiological short-circuit*.

[1] Koffka, 1919, p. 257.

§ 3. *The seeing of " gestalt " : Its derivation from the seeing of movement, and the theory of the simultaneous φ-process*

The theory of the "physiological short-circuit" is concerned, to begin with, only with manifestations of the *experience of movement.* However, further characteristic experimental findings lead beyond this to an analogous treatment of the seeing of *simultaneous gestalten.*

According to Wertheimer's findings, it is possible, under the very same conditions of stimulation and merely by means of varying the speed of succession, to bring about the appearance of the new impression of a stationary identical object, of a simultaneous configuration in fact, instead of the impression of movement : The " optimum " interval " changes into the " simultaneous interval ".

These observations upon the relation between optimum interval and simultaneous interval [1] find theoretical application in the further course of the train of reasoning, in a manner which we reduce to a definite formula as the *thesis of the equivalence of seeing gestalt and seeing movement.*

The seen *gestalt* of the simultaneous interval is the psychical correlate of the same physiological processes which serve to explain the *movement* seen in the successive interval, and indeed in such a way that the peculiar nature of this simultaneous impression must be deducible in a direct manner from the purely quantitative changes in the stimulus event.

If this thesis is applied to the physiological schema offered, there emerges the starting-point of Wertheimer's line of thought towards his concrete *theory of the perception of configuration.*

If the interval between the stimuli becomes smaller and smaller with reference to the stimuli, then, of course, the field-actions and short circuit processes accompanying them would by no means entirely vanish as a result of this. They now, in fact, appear as a simple sort of " physiological connectedness, indeed, as a *unitary total process resulting, as a whole, out of the single excitations* ",[2] upon the elimination of the time factor.

---

[1] Which, we may note, Linke had already (1912) published, though indeed in a different terminology.

[2] Koffka, 1913, p. 288. The meaning of this conception can perhaps be made clear by comparing it with the more familiar concept of an interference process in physics.

Thus arises the concept of the *simultaneous ϕ-process*, upon which Wertheimer's *gestalt* theory of 1912 takes its stand, a concept which, of course, subsumes all the defining statements which we were able to set forth when we discussed the *successive ϕ-process*.

When we recapitulate these defining statements, the following emerge as established :—

(1) The fundamental idea of Wertheimer's gestalt theory of 1912 is that of the unequivocal determination of the gestalt experience by the stimulus—corresponding exactly to the relation " stimulus—sensation " at that time still held by Wertheimer to be thoroughly unequivocal.

(2) The physiological process " ϕ ", which can in accordance with this be deduced from the stimulus conditions, and which in addition expresses the peculiar character of the gestalt experience, is developed (*vide* accompanying diagram) :—

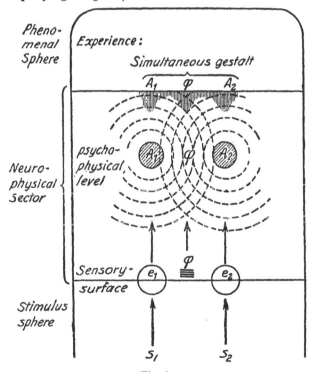

Fig. 1.

(*a*) On the foundation of the *individual excitations* $e_1 e_2$ evoked by the stimuli $S_1 S_2$.

(*b*) Through the occurrence of a peculiar *concatenation of action* assumed " between " these, which

(α) " Results from " the single excitations—*being made possible as a concatenation* by the occurrence of the *field-actions* of those single excitations in a common *intermediate area* (cross-process)—and which

(β) is specifically characterized as the *short circuit process*.

§ 4. *The principles inherent in Wertheimer's contentions of 1912, and the actual gestalt theory*

In accordance with our thesis that Wertheimer's theory of 1912 is to be regarded merely as a preliminary step to the later actual gestalt theory, it becomes necessary, in the first place, to enquire whether in those formulations a far-reaching general transformation of thinking, in contrast to the then customary ways of thinking, is really given positive expression. The question is whether it emerges definitely and clearly therefrom that the formulations concerned ought to be looked upon as the expression of a " fundamental reorientation ", or whether such wide claims cannot be admitted within the framework of what was then at hand.

To this end it is necessary to analyze the conceptual material of the Wertheimer theory presented in the foregoing exposition, with reference to the *principles inherent in it*.

In this connection it will, of course, not serve us sufficiently to keep to the words themselves, but the sense of these words can only be deemed to be satisfactorily defined, when we carefully take into consideration the context of thought in which they appear.[1]

But when we take our stand upon such a criterion, the frequently advanced claim (especially by Koffka) that here already, in 1912, a decisive turning point is revealed, appears to be by no means incontestable. The basis

---

[1] Thus we lay down a standard such as Wertheimer himself, in subsequent controversy, emphasizes as essential, when he says, in 1922: One ought to examine not so much the " general doctrines ", but how a person uses them; how the argument is carried on in concrete problems, and *what concrete positive significance lies behind the terms applied* (Wertheimer, p. 51, 1922).

provided by Wertheimer's work for this claim lies in the term " total process " which also occurs instead of " simultaneous φ-process ".

But what does this term represent in the thought context of Wertheimer's work ?

When we analyze how the genesis of this " total process " is conceived, an unequivocal discovery emerges.

These " total processes " are as a matter of fact not considered, as their nature requires, in themselves, in detachment from the elementalist standpoint ; they are derived from the single excitations which lie behind them, from which they *result* by the " short circuiting " of the " field-actions "

Hence, the criterion which the later gestalt theory is wont to proclaim as decisive for its new orientation, namely its emancipation from the elementalist standpoint, is by no means satisfied by these concepts of Wertheimer, in 1912.

In fact, Wertheimer, while explicitly distinguishing between the actual " reception of stimulus " and the " unitary transition process " arising besides this, states that the "specific cross-functions" are only "built up (!) in a characteristic fashion upon the foundation of the single excitations (!) ". Here the description of the process as " unitary " clearly has only the significance of an elucidatory epithet for just that remarkable " transition of excitation "—in contrast to the " directedness " in the case of the seeing of movement.

This interpretation of Wertheimer's formulations finds welcome support in the fact that twenty years before Wertheimer exactly the same trends of thought and formulations already occur with Exner—in his case, however, with explicit reference to the true logical import of such views. Exner, writing in 1894, says (p. 201) :—

" The total impression produced by a picture which flashes across the retina is compounded of the excitations of innumerable and functionally dissimilar fibres. That we, in spite of this, receive a unitary impression, in which the partial sensations are wont to go unrecognized, is due to what I would call the principle of *Central Confluence*."

A number of excitations passing up to the cortex " flow together " to a unity whose constituents we can separate only with uncertainty and after practice, or even not at all. A "total impression" then results; and this for the reason that a sum of excitations in the cortex, involving a variety of paths, acts like a unitary "excitation process".

Here then Wertheimer's " total process " is anticipated in the " unitary excitation process " of Exner, and his principle of the "short circuit" in the "confluence principle". Their methods of arriving at these concepts are in no way different, hardly even in terminology.

At the same time, however, Exner makes a further statement as to the conceptual import of this singular " unitary excitation process ". He explicitly affirms that this unitary excitation process—corresponding to the principle of confluence which is fundamental to his deductions—in spite of its "unitariness" is still "for all that *determined* in its character by the *single* excitations of the fibres ".

Exner thus explicitly draws attention, with apt emphasis on the special assumptions underlying his formulation of concepts, to the " synthetic character " of these concepts. It is incomprehensible, therefore, how anyone in complete agreement with their conceptual structure, should be able to extract anything so different from Wertheimer's conceptions.

Originally, indeed, nothing more than this was read into Wertheimer's conclusions of 1912, as appears plainly from the account Koffka gave of them, in the "Introduction" to *Beiträge zur Psychologie des Sehens von Bewegungen,* which he issued in continuation of Wertheimer's research.

In this exposition Koffka attempts to formulate the upshot of Wertheimer's research programmatically. His aim is to elaborate the particular reading of the problem which would define the scope of the succeeding individual contributions. It is, accordingly, entirely designed to present what the author, orientating himself concretely by Wertheimer (and surely in agreement with Wertheimer's own interpretation) at that time considered to be essential in that investigation.

From Koffka's exposition this, at any rate, is plainly evident : That at that time (1913) the material content of the physiological theory propounded was regarded as the *essential* point, and not, perchance, any more far-reaching, more general conception of principles as to an orientation in formulating psychological theories in general. This seems to demonstrate effectually that the achievement of the actual gestalt-theoretical orientation can certainly not be wholly referred back to Wertheimer's work of 1912. This is borne out when the relation of the Wertheimer gestalt theory of 1912 to the treatment of the gestalt problem before then is examined.

One observes immediately that, conceptually, Wertheimer's point of view does not, in its general purport —that is, setting aside its physiological vestment—in any way directly transcend the standpoint which von Ehrenfels, in *his* attempt at solving it, had already taken up with the first and more rigorous formulation of the gestalt problem. The basic notion in Ehrenfels' interpretation, the hypothesis of special " gestalt qualities " which accrue to the " sensations ", has been entirely retained. In fact it is perhaps put forward in a more substantial manner ; for one finds that with Wertheimer these new qualities have been given their own correlate on the physiological side, in the form of definite " cross-functions " and " short circuit processes " corresponding to them.

Really this is nothing but a translation of Ehrenfels' line of thought into physiological terms with this single peculiarity : that—in virtue of the facilities for more detailed derivation afforded by the physiological mechanism hypothetically introduced—this additional total process itself permits of being built up, in a definite way, " out of the single excitations." [1]

On the whole then, one can only conclude that at that time there existed very few definite statements going towards the establishment of the present gestalt-theoretical orientation. To resume them positively, once more : They would seem to be fully comprehended in the fundamental

---

[1] In accordance with this, the polemical alignment, as it was at that time vigorously adopted, in adherence to Wertheimer, e.g. in Koffka's *Beiträge*, towards Benussi's theory (derived in the last resort from von Ehrenfels through Meinong), refers only to one definite aspect of the scheme of thought. This was the presentation of von Ehrenfels' conceptions in the form of the distinction between founding and founded contents, which, as exemplar of a so-called " psychological theory ", naturally must conflict with the notion of an unmediated physiological correlate.

tendency towards a *physiological theory*, which is already avowed in the theorem of sensation-equivalence, and in the· thesis of the *correspondence of the seeing of gestalt and the seeing of movement*. Moreover—and this, too, is not inessential for appraising the situation of that time— in the investigation as a whole, the gestalt problem does not by any means yet become particularly prominent.

In fact, as far as the actual conceptual scope of the theoretical construction drawn up for it is concerned, it is by no means even clearly enough posed as a problem. Ultimately, only the theory of the optimal interval is fully worked out physiologically. As for the simultaneous interval, the gestalt phenomenon, the question is really obscured. The singularity of the phenomenal experience present in this case, the unitariness, is believed to be indicated in that a " total process " is referred to on the physiological side ; and this concept is thought to include, somehow, an analogous definition, which is supposed to correspond directly to that phenomenal unitariness (see p. 60 below).

Before these circumstances are cleared up, there is still a long way to go, and the goal is only gradually reached —through altogether different considerations, freed from the bondage of the physiological theory, and in the frame-work of a revision of principles arising out of the general doctrine of perception.

CHAPTER II

THE ACHIEVEMENT OF THE ORIENTATION IN THE PROBLEM, WHICH IS CHARACTERISTIC OF THE ACTUAL " GESTALT THEORY "

I. THE PROPOSAL TO TRANSFORM THE STANDPOINT OF PSYCHOLOGICAL THINKING IN ITS PRINCIPLES

The proposal for a revision of principles, in the direction of the modern gestalt-theoretical way of regarding the problems of psychology, definitely occurs for the first time with Koffka, 1914.

Indeed, Köhler had already, in 1913, prepared the way for this noteworthy line of thought—through a keen critique of certain habits of thinking of the refuted psychological theory, in his treatise *Über unbemerkte Empfindungen und Urteilstäuschungen.* In 1914, however, in Koffka's "Report on Research" (*Forschungsbericht*) "Psychologie der Wahrnehmung," there is added a definite indication of positive points of view in regard to a reorientation.

In connection with this, Köhler's submissions are to be valued merely as a critical preliminary, but, as such, they are of great significance ; the more so since they are still made use of in the same spirit, e.g. in Koffka's exposition of 1925.

§ 5. *The first critical considerations opposing the " old " psychology : Köhler, 1913*

Köhler's criticism of the refuted way of thinking in psychology makes a central issue of impugning a basic assumption which serves, to a certain extent, as a " limiting-law " in the traditional psychology—the so-called *Constancy Hypothesis.* This is the notion of the " rigorous determination of our sensations by the stimulus ". To compress it into a brief statement, it affirms that to a definite stimulus there corresponds one and only one quite definite sensation, which is always the same, and remains identical throughout different instances, as well as under varying circumstances, in accordance with the theorem : " The stimulus decides what is given in sensation."

The aim of Köhler's discussion is to demonstrate the untenability of this point of view.

Köhler orientates his animadversions by the view that this doctrine is irrefutable as a principle, but at the same time, naturally, also unprovable [1] as a principle.

He accordingly sees only a single standpoint from which a fruitful discussion is possible in this connection : The doctrine of sensation must be appraised *according to its " applicability in scientific technique "*—and, moreover, according to its *characteristic and unavoidable auxiliary assumptions.*

---

[1] In this he follows Stumpf, who had already previously, in his attempt to defend the sensation theory, taken up the standpoint that it should rank as a *working hypothesis*—and certainly of immeasurable value as such, according to Stumpf.

Köhler endeavours, very acutely, to dissect these auxiliary assumptions out. He comes to the following conclusions, after an analysis of what may be called the "*meaning theory*" :—

"(1) Besides the sensations about which we make statements, there are also sensations for which this is in principle impossible, which are on an entirely equal footing with the others as regards their reality, but which remain 'unnoticed'.

"(2) Even when we are concerned with observed sensations, these are not the direct point of departure of the investigation, but really only the judgment uttered about them; and this (the effect of a special 'meaning' factor) has to be strictly distinguished from the sensations. This judgment may be false, may involve an illusion as to the true character of the sensation.

"(3) Since in many cases nothing can be established either in regard to a judgment, or in regard to a sensation to which it might refer, this leads to the amplification that there are also 'unconscious judgments' and also judgments of this sort about 'unconscious sensations'."[1]

The consequence to which a test of the applicability of these assumptions in scientific technique leads, is very definitely of a negative order :—

"The two auxiliary assumptions of the unobserved sensations and unobserved illusions of judgment prove, from the nature of the matter, to be general and also irrefutable in the majority of concrete instances. This is the first reason for which these assumptions do not commend themselves from the point of view of scientific technique; and I do not hesitate to say that it is a sort of scientific instinct which seems to forbid me to make assumptions about which nothing can be determinately stated. Secondly, for a particular instance there proves to exist no independent criteria as to when one has to have recourse to these assumptions, and further, when one must admit an observation which represents an exception from the basic hypothesis (that of the rigorous determination of our sensations by the stimulus). This opens the door to arbitrariness. Thirdly, there proves to be an imminent danger that, in virtue of these assumptions, entire groups of phenomena may be debarred from

[1] Quoted from Koffka's account (1914, p. 712).

research, and opportunities for progress thus left unutilized ; and finally, it appears that the auxiliary assumptions, in accordance with their nature, undermine our reliance upon observation, and consequently, upon the facts of psychology, and therefore cripple the pleasure in observation, the impulse towards progress."

These are weighty *negative contentions* among which the *demand for fundamental determinability* is pre-eminently germane.

Köhler is not content with this only. He indicates a quite definite remedy, and therefore also enunciates the *positive standpoint he then held* (loc. cit., p. 79). He says :—

" In accordance with the observations, we . . . assume that, in general, in the genesis of sensory data, besides the stimuli and the hitherto known peripheral conditions, an additional *set of factors,* above all of a *central kind,* is of essential importance ; that those very simple relationships between stimulus and sensation, which the basic hypothesis sets up as absolute in the highest degree, represent extreme instances, achieved by means of isolation. In these cases, the influence of the stimuli and of the peripheral conditions can be entirely decisive, because the remaining factors, which otherwise have effect upon processes of sensation, either fall away or are invariable, and hence become relatively indifferent as far as these laws are concerned.".

(See attached diagram in which I have summarized these ideas.)

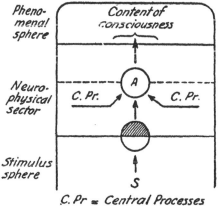

C. Pr = *Central Processes*

Fig. 2.

Two points are theoretically critical in these formulations :—

(1) Köhler protests against the importation of special psychical processes, and assumes instead a *direct physiological representation of the phenomenal perceptual datum in its entirety.*

(2) He establishes the special nature of the physiological process implied in this, by the hypothesis that *special central factors accrue* to the occurrences set up in response to the stimulus, of such a kind that his first requirement is fulfilled. He sets up a *theory of Central Induction.*

If we are correct in summing up the positive outcome of Köhler's considerations of 1913 in these two points, there can be no doubt about our decision as to their significance for the course of development of the gestalt theory.

In its conceptual structure, this new proposal of Köhler's is by no means very different in its essentials from the tenets of the sensation doctrine. Köhler merely substitutes for the " psychical induction ", the " unconscious inferences ", a different and in other respects just as little controllable induction of a central sort. But the " single excitations " continue unaltered as the foundation for this induction.

Köhler's proposal therefore still persists entirely within the framework of the synthetic way of thinking, which remained to be overcome later.

At any rate, in one point Köhler already proceeds beyond Wertheimer. Hereafter, the relationship " stimulus—sensation " can no longer be discussed after the fashion in which Wertheimer still unhesitatingly makes use of it. If we recall, once more, the general conceptions which could be demonstrated in Wertheimer's basic thesis of the " sensation-equivalence of the experiences of movement and of gestalt ", we see that the notion of the unequivocal determination by the stimulus, indeed *the stimulus as starting point*, which occupies the foreground with Wertheimer, is now *discredited.*

It can be stated otherwise, thus: Köhler's notion, which could be characterized as one of central representation, signifies *a whittling down of the Wertheimer thesis of the sensation-equivalence* of the gestalt experience, in the sense that henceforth only one of the conceptions comprised in that thesis should be taken into account, namely, that of the unmediated psycho-physical correlate (this being nothing other than Köhler's requirement of the assumption of an unmediated physiological representation).

This step beyond Wertheimer is, however, not of direct importance in regard to the further development on the side of *principles*, even though it still appears influential subsequently.

Köhler's work can, therefore, essentially claim only a negative importance in the progressive total development of the gestalt theory.

Formulations which definitively lead to a reorientation of the point of view in matters of principle, opposed to the traditional way of thinking, occur for the first time in the literature of the gestalt theory with Koffka, in 1914.

§ 6. *The achievement of an antisynthetic standpoint as positive manifestation of a transformation of principles*

Starting from the concept of *perception*, which is conceived *as contrasting with the concept of " sensation "*, Koffka broaches the same problem as occupied Köhler, but reaches conclusions having a far wider bearing.

By way of describing the " old " theory of perception, he establishes that " perception meant . . . as opposed to sensation, the more complex, the higher, the later. The sensations were *elements* out of which the perceptions *built themselves up*, and belonged, owing to their close relation to the stimuli, almost to the pre-psychological. With this was associated the fact that in the doctrine of sensation phenomena were studied which were as far removed as possible from the natural facts of the matter, laboratory artefacts, in which the pure regularity of the sensations, their determination by the stimulus, were most clearly revealed. A further consequence of this was that all sorts of hypotheses had to be resorted to, in order to ' build up ' the perceptions by means of these sensations. Thus the study of perception was not approached impartially, but by way of the sensation. The bare description of what was given receded, even fell under the suspicion of failing to cope with the intrinsic

facts of perception, as it was exposed to numerous
' illusions of judgment ' " (p. 136).

By contrast to this, there " has during recent years come
to pass a *reaction*. . . . The point of view has been
reversed : the *immediately present perceptual datum is
acknowledged as such* and is *described* as exactly and as
appropriately as possible. This description serves as the
point of departure for the formation of a theory. In the
extreme event, there follows from this that the endeavour
is no longer to obtain an understanding of the *perceptions
from the sensations*, but to obtain an understanding of
the *sensations from the perceptions* " (p. 136).

It is plain how, in comparison with Köhler, this reveals
a more far-reaching conception of the implications of
the problem. Köhler's considerations are throughout
orientated by the relation of stimulus to sensation, and
attempt to prove the inadequacy of the refuted point of
view in this connection.[1] Koffka's researches are orientated
by a different antithesis, that which is conceived to hold
between " sensation " and " perception ".

Even if Köhler, following Krueger, describes the standpoint he attacks as " psychological atomism ", in his
actual research he hardly follows out this problem of
" atomism ". Nay, instead of taking his stand upon such
a formulated problem of method, he does so, actually,
upon one of theoretical import. Koffka, on the other
hand, here sketches as incisively as possible, a picture of

---

[1] This is not controverted by the fact that, in continuation of the
remarks cited above (p. 23), Köhler (1913) wrote : " In accordance
with the observations, we further maintain that (especially in the cases
where " complexes " are present) a *description of what is given in sensation
must remain incomplete, and untrue to the reality, so long as the familiar
variables of our sensory psychology are deemed to be adequate for the purpose* ;
that, moreover, in the customary descriptions, a large and important
part of the properties of perception is neglected. This actually retires
to the background in the extreme instances achieved by isolation ;
but from the point of view of the psychology of perception is often
more important than the current moments of sensation, as soon as, in
addition to the peripheral conditions, the remaining factors also exercise
their influence : namely, in the psychical correlate of *manifolds of
stimuli*, especially in the *perception of things*, as in ordinary life "
(pp. 79–80).

Köhler, indeed, here perceived the problem which occupies Koffka ;
but this problem by no means stands in the forefront of his discussion.
Köhler's *main interest*, as also that of Wertheimer, centres on the problems
of *physiological representation*.

an *antithesis of method*, which is supposed to have formed itself and emerged in the research of the time. He talks of a *change of the point of view in research*, which he wishes to explain in his communication.

Herewith Koffka's posing of the problem becomes concerned with principles in quite a different sense.

The characteristics Koffka ascribes to the two opposing views, in this connection, are altogether precise.

The impugned point of view is specified as being one according to which perceptions are "built up" out of sensations, i.e. as being "synthetic"; and the *remedy* is considered to lie in an orientation which starts from the immediately present perceptual datum as such, *which no longer derives perceptions from sensations, but derives sensations from perceptions.*

We may describe this orientation as an *antisynthetic* one—but only in a negative manner, since a definite characterization of the positive theory was not within the scope of Koffka's contentions at that time. Rather does he, where it is necessary for him to adopt any decisive statements of this nature, always turn to the works of Wertheimer and Koffka discussed above.

In spite of the fact that Koffka's work rests upon these other works, as far as its matter is concerned, one observes forthwith, that here the discussion is shifted to another level, the direct approach to which does not lie in the works of Wertheimer and Köhler.

This is already apparent from the fact that Koffka relies upon a far more extensive field of psychological investigation for illustration or substantiation of his opinions about the true nature of psychological work. He makes use of the investigations of Hofmann, Jaensch, Katz, etc., in which the change of front he calls for is supposed to have become manifest in research already.

Only in the light of these considerations does the true position of this work of Koffka in the development of the literature of the gestalt theory, define itself. Its actual theme, its nuclear conception, is the *proclamation of the anti-synthetic standpoint of totality.* Its positive outcome for the complete elaboration of the gestalt theory lies in the expansion of this totality standpoint into a general principle of method, especially within the study of perception.

Only then does the movement inaugurated by Wertheimer, Koffka, and Köhler become a matter of principles. Before 1914 it cannot be considered as such.[1]

Hence it is the more noteworthy that in 1912 already exactly the same ideas were expressed elsewhere, in Goetz Martius' address " On Synthetic and Analytical Psychology ", as grounds for the abandoning of the refuted psychology.

In this address Goetz Martius for the first time brought forward in public, in a comprehensive manner, the problem of principles in psychology which had already occupied his attention for a long time. He brought it forward as he saw it in the light of his own scientific development and in the light of the forms of actual research which had meanwhile arisen.

It is not essential for us to note the positive solution which Martius calls for. Only his attitude to the " old psychology " need concern us here. There can be no doubt, at any rate, that he is avowedly opposed to a psychology "which has to resolve the manifestations of mental life *into their elements and derive them from these elements* ".

By demonstrating the consequences of this point of view which, as he puts it, aims at accomplishing " a *synthetic* derivation of intricate psychological manifestations, including even those of community life, from psychical elements ", Martius reaches this conclusion : That the evolution of psychology in fact compels one to a different conception of the meaning of psychological research, to a conception which takes as its *starting point* " *the complete sensible reality*, Fechner's work-a-day world ". This conception he endeavours to characterize more precisely in its methodological bearing, in that he calls for an " analytical " advance in psychological research.

In brief, both the antisynthetic point of view, and the complete sensible perception as starting point, were already

---

[1] In this we do not suggest that the earlier works of Wertheimer and Köhler are altogether without significance for the development of the gestalt theory. In fact, they enter into Koffka's work unavoidably to a certain extent, in that they can rank a₀ *concrete* embodiments of the very principle which has here risen to be fundamental. However, we maintain that, as regards the *orientation of principles*, they represent merely preliminary steps and no more.

propounded by Martius at that time. That is to say, the very two points from which Koffka also started, when formulating his ideas upon principles, in 1914.

Here we must not omit to note that Martius' submissions were not unknown to Koffka. He quotes this work of Martius' as far back as 1912.

2. THE FIRST DELINEATION OF ACTUAL "GESTALT THINKING"

With the demand for an antisynthetic orientation of principles, the decisive break with the traditional "psychology of elements" is accomplished in a definite sense. The further development depends directly· upon its elaboration. This entails—once a general demonstration had been achieved in reference to the principles involved in the standpoint of research only—the further factual working out of the point of view, in the direction of the more precise interpretation of the concept of *gestalt* which is thus made possible.

§ 7. *The establishment of the specific significance of the gestalt concept*

From this angle, too, Koffka comes to the forefront in 1915 in connection with his " Auseinandersetzung mit Vittorio Benussi ".

Koffka discusses the reasons why he considers it necessary to transcend the elementalist standpoint in principle, with reference to three matters, viz. the descriptive, the functional, and the physiological definitions of the facts of perception.[1]

According to him, the following appear to be essential :—

(1) " Descriptive : The typical form of experiences as given (simultaneous and successive) is *not the summative one, consisting of true elements and divisible into such elements*, but the elements as a rule form " a definitely characterized togetherness, i.e. bounded units, frequently

---

[1] In the course of this Koffka makes use of a number of points from Wertheimer's work of 1912, but especially of later statements of his, which were published by a student of Wertheimer's, G. v. Wartensleben, *Die christliche Persönlichkeit in Idealbild*, 1914. (Wa.)

apprehended in reference to a centre . . . to which the other parts of the unit are co-ordinated in an hierarchical system.   Such units are to be entitled gestalten, in the precise sense (v. Wartensleben, 1st and 2nd note).   These gestalten are in no wise less original than their parts. " Frequently the whole is apprehended before the parts come to consciousness at all " (v. Wartensleben, loc. cit.).

Hence pure description of experience *can no longer be orientated by the concept of sensation* (in its descriptive form).   It will have to commence with the gestalt and its properties.

(2) Functional : The typical form of the combination stimulus—experience is no longer the sensation (psycho-physical definition of this concept).   The gestalten too are descriptively no less original.   *The endeavour to derive the whole from its parts or to erect it above its parts, has very often failed.   The whole does not arise from the compounding of the parts,* but has to be regarded as a datum of experience, the authentic correlate of the stimulus datum, in as direct a fashion as has hitherto been customary with the sensations only.   Alterations of a summative nature in the stimulus may produce qualitative alterations of the experience.   Hence nothing can be known as to how the experience will eventuate merely from information about the stimulus.   Finally, the relationship stimulus—experience is further complicated in that the state of the entire nervous system is involved in it.

This *total state* influences both the quality of the experience occurring, and its " unitariness ".

(3) Physiological : The typical form of the cerebral process correlated with the experience *is no longer the single excitation* of a locality of the brain plus *association,* but total processes, above all their wholeness (not summational) characteristics, and these must be employed in the propounding of further hypotheses.

It is not sums of single excitations which are involved but characteristic total events.

A fundamental shifting of the centre of gravity of the line of thought is plainly discernible in these formulations. Though many of Wertheimer's declarations of 1912 appear again here, this shows itself particularly clearly when the above exposition of Koffka's is compared with his previously published one (1913).   The change expresses itself in the distinct prominence given to the difference between the summative conceptions of the old viewpoint and the conceptions held by the new viewpoint, thinking in terms of wholes.

It is true that even here a nuance in the definition of the gestalt problem essential for its concrete import is still lacking. This emerges most clearly in Köhler's expository summary (1924), " Gestaltprobleme und die Anfänge der Gestalttheorie." The real crux of the gestalt theory's task now appears in a new formula, that of " the problem of natural units " in the perceptual world.

Köhler develops this formula on the basis of a critique of the " old " way of looking at the matter. This sought to explain the figural organization of perceptual reality, as well as the fact that this perceptual reality conformed to the reality of the stimuli, by *the hypothesis of point-by-point stimulation and isolated conduction to the central organ.* He emphasizes that " *the hypothesis of anatomical mechanical organization of elements* does not accomplish what it should. It would only explain why the retinally ordered, adjacent, minimal areas of stimulation do not become mixed up, as it were, or something like that, *en route* in higher somatic fields " (p. 516).

" But no attention is paid to the problem present in the fact of the *intrinsic articulation of the visual field* " We say " the inkpot is imaged in the eye ", but do not in any way reflect that the demarcation of the inkpot-process thus tacitly assumed is not really founded in the theory. For between the " inkpot elements " and the " surrounding elements " exactly the same real relations exist as among the " inkpot elements " *inter se*—that is, none at all. " That natural whole vanishes, since we apply the hypothesis in such a manner that these wholes cannot ensue from it alone " (p. 517).

It is incumbent, therefore, to investigate these " natural wholes " which manifest themselves in the " intrinsic ", that is " non-anatomical articulation " of the field of vision. In these the *problem* of gestalt becomes most definitely apprehended.

The subsequent works are devoted to providing proof that the discovery of what such " natural wholes " are, positively exhausts the entire domain of psychical manifestations in an adequate degree. They show how the "gestalt conception" must be accredited in all branches of psychology.

§ 8. *The extension of the "gestalt way of thinking" to the different special provinces of psychology*

The decisive subordination of, primarily, the entire facts of *perception* to the gestalt concept (in the sense of "natural wholes") culminates, at first, essentially in the attempt to re-interpret the experimental material already known, in accordance with the formulated principles that had been achieved.

This part of the task has been comprehensively dealt with by Koffka in particular in his article " Perception. An Introduction to Gestalt Psychology ", 1922. In this a really systematic construction, at least of the "*new doctrine of perception*", is presented, such that the gestalt point of view is in fact brought to bear everywhere.

It is characteristic that here, in particular, an *enlargement of the range of what is included under perception* has come about, since the phenomena of "comparing" are especially subsumed under it as well. The consideration of comparing connects up, firstly, with Koffka's own previous studies on the difference threshold (1917), and secondly, makes use of Köhler's work on the analysis of the behaviour of the chimpanzee, and the formulations arising out of it (1915–19). However, it is just these works of Köhler which lead to a great deal more. To begin with, it is true, the specific features of a gestalt-theoretical approach are hardly revealed in them. In his first studies (1915), as also in the *Intelligenzprüfungen* (*Mentality of Apes*)[1] (1917), no such note is actually present. Hence one must either take it that Köhler was at that time not so thoroughgoing a "gestalt theorist", or that he at any rate deliberately refrained, at that time, from any decisive affirmations in regard to our problem. Even though the word "gestalt" (and with it the name of Wertheimer) occurs (p. 225), there is no mention of any possibility of laying down theoretical conclusions in connection with it. These works can fairly be looked upon as in essence purely empirical.

In 1918, however, we find a concept put forward by Köhler, in connection with this work, which becomes of

---

[1] [References are to the English edition. Trans.]

immediate importance to the gestalt theory, and is adopted by it at once. This is the *concept of " structure-function "* or, alternatively, of *" structure-process "* which he propounds. Köhler here talks of " structure " not only when " gestalten " in the restricted, actual sense of the word are in question. He also applies the concept to the " mutual relatedness of colours " as this is supposed to be present in the comparison or even simple apprehension of two different colours. He talks of *colour gestalten* and of " structures in general " and co-ordinates them, on the physiological side, directly with " structure processes " which, determined by the stimulus, are supposed directly to represent them (see below §§ 49–53).

The significance of the concept thus propounded is important, firstly, because herewith the phenomena of comparison are in actual fact brought directly within the system of " perpetual gestalten " ; and secondly, because the concept leads to a theory of reactions, which can be given a gestalt-theory nomenclature and which is characterized by Köhler's key-word " structural reaction ".

The achievement that this key-word represents—so the facts of the matter reveal themselves to be subsequently, in its further elaboration—is that volitional phenomena in the last resort appear to require no new principle, as opposed to the principles which were developed in the study of perception. Just as the phenomenal gestalt in perception—in conformity with the principle of direct physiological representation—signifies the simple " structural reaction " of the perceptive system in reference to the " stimulus structure ", so does the *concrete activity, the " behaviour ",* develop in the sensori-motor system as a " structural reaction " to the stimulus situation objectively given at the time (see below, § 63 f.).

Furthermore, the fact that such " behaviour " can be meaningful with reference to the stimulus-situation, that both man and animal react " with insight ", according to the concept thus formed calls for no new theoretical viewpoints. *The concept of insight* ultimately stands for nothing more than *the fact of a direct coupling of stimulus-structure and reaction, with the presupposition that the identity of the structure is maintained.*

The significance of the concept of structure-function in the framework of the further elaboration of the theory becomes particularly evident in Koffka's *Growth of the Mind*, 1921. In this, the entire treatment of the problem really rests upon that concept. Koffka himself, at the end of his book, in a brief statement summing up the tendency of his line of thought, expressly describes the essence of psychical development as an " arousal and perfection of configuration structures ". Indeed the entire contents of his two chief chapters on the " special features of mental growth " are devoted to the task of bringing comprehensively into application the notion of structure (in Köhler's sense)—partly following closely Köhler's own groupings of problems, and the critical repercussions of these in the literature.

Nevertheless, there is still a long way to go before the theory is actually pushed, along these lines, to the stage of definite principles. We have already been anticipating this, in describing the consequences of Köhler's proposals.

In truth, we are only at the beginning of tracing the stages by which the different conceptual concatenations, represented to-day by the caption " gestalt theory ", genetically unfolded themselves. To trace how an actual system coalesced out of the tendencies hitherto discussed requires a much more thorough analysis. Only thus will it become clear what the empirical tenets which we have briefly indicated signify in relation to the system.

CHAPTER III

THE CONSOLIDATION OF THE ACTUAL SYSTEM OF THE GESTALT THEORY

The prosecution of the " gestalt " *tendencies* in the direction of their coalescence into a specific *completed system* takes place along two lines. Köhler develops a new approach towards the *founding* of a system of gestalt theory. This approach, planned in a characteristically rigorous theoretical, and straightforwardly hypothetical way, is concerned with a direct *proof* for the hitherto developed *assertions about the significance of the gestalt concept*. And Wertheimer discovers concrete principles for the elaboration of the gestalt system, for the elaboration of the standpoint into a body of thought derived directly and specifically *from the gestalt concept*.

I. THE PSYCHOPHYSICAL-DEDUCTIVE FOUNDING OF THE BASIC PRINCIPLES OF THE GESTALT DOCTRINE BY KÖHLER

Köhler's achievement advances the gestalt conception in a most astonishing fashion. In his book of 1920, Köhler provides, on the basis of an epistemological analysis of certain structures in physics, a fundamentally new case for the acknowledgment of the primary significance of the gestalt category for scientific theory. Beginning with this, he develops a deductive theory of psycho-physical events "from the starting point of physics", in the shape of a positive hypothesis in substantiation of the Wertheimer theorem of the immediate physiological representation of phenomenal gestalten. And he rounds off this scheme of thought finally, in 1924, by demon-strating its validity in general for the entire range of the problems of wholeness which have become significant for scientific theory, including even the problems of general biology (the vitalist controversy).

Thus Köhler creates an entirely new position for the gestalt concept in scientific theory.

§ 9. *Köhler's epistemological extension of the "gestalt thinking" to physical domains*

The starting point of Köhler's enquiry is the general task of providing an assured status for the gestalt concept in itself. In solving his problem, he directs his attention to those sciences which have the highest standing in scientific theory, namely physics and physical chemistry. Working from this basis, he endeavours to obtain scientific citizenship for the concept of " gestalt ". He emphasizes the value of this method not only for the conversion of opponents, but also for strengthening the adherents of the theory, for he admits : " Indeed, even those who are already accustomed to working with the concept of the gestalt, as that of some physically perfect reality, some-times become aware of a slight obstruction in their procedure. This signifies that constructs are being handled which are only empirically legitimated, and have no theoretical foundation at all, as yet." He infers from this the urgent necessity " to enquire about gestalten, or at any rate what may be similar to them, for once not among the fleeting uncertainties of observed experiences, but among the fixed forms of inorganic natural events ; and wherever possible to utilize, for the benefit of the gestalt theory, that clearness and definiteness to which man has attained in observation and thinking in physical matters so much earlier than in psychology ".

In order to produce proof that " gestalten " are also to be found in inorganic physical events, Köhler in the first place formulates the concept of the " gestalt " quite precisely. He does it in full accord with Koffka's antisynthetic approach, and by the *criterion* that its " characteristic properties and effects cannot be put together out of the properties and effects of a like sort of its so-called parts " (p. ix) (cf. already Cornelius).

With this as his starting point, he believes that it is easy to prove that a gestalt phenomenon is present in e.g. *systems of electrolytic solutions*. Theory and experiment teach us that when two electrolytic solutions are in osmotic communication a *difference of potential* arises at the common boundary surface, whereas before contact neither solution appeared to be electrically charged. There arises, therefore, " with the osmotic connection of the two solutions . . . a new *property of the system as a whole*."

Herewith the nature of this fact, from the point of view of scientific theory, is disposed of, as far as Köhler is concerned. " The gestalt theory insists, without introducing marked limiting conditions to begin with, only that structures of the type envisaged by it have more properties than would arise as resultants from properties of a like sort of so-called parts. It leaves the closer definition of the concept of ' part ' open, in this case, as is indicated by the epithet ; but in the above example, it would without hesitation designate the two solutions as the ' so-called parts '. Accordingly, the *communicating system of solutions has gestalt characteristics* " (p. 34).

Köhler reduces the question of the status of the *gestalt criteria* given by von Ehrenfels, to the same conclusion.

Of the two gestalt criteria given by von Ehrenfels, the first amounts, in a certain sense, to Köhler's definition of gestalt. It states :—

" If we allow the stimuli (tones, lights, etc., in the physical sense) which when acting upon one person in combination (e.g. as a melody) evoke a phenomenal spatial gestalt, etc., to act, not upon the single individual, but upon as many individuals as they (the stimuli) number, then the sum of the experiences of these many people is poorer than the experience of the single person. What the manifold of stimuli evokes in the single consciousness over and above the total effects of the separate stimuli upon the sum of the different individuals—this constitutes the specific gestalt properties of the experience " (pp. 35–6).

But this criterion can only claim limited validity. Köhler says—with justice—" I am not convinced that this criterion, suitable as a first rough indication, can be held to be intrinsically sufficient. It almost seems to suggest that some sort of new phenomena (gestalt qualities) are in a single person simply added to a sum of sensations which are nevertheless exactly determined by the separate stimuli. This would be a conception through which the radical significance, and, I believe, the essential value of the new category would be greatly impaired. The criterion requires somewhat too little of its objects " (p. 36).

" On the other hand, it is true that every instance of a gestalt perception also fulfills this condition " (p. 36). That is, the first Ehrenfels criterion gives a necessary but not sufficient condition for the gestalt character of a phenomenon.

The *second* Ehrenfels criterion, that of *transposability*, states that it is characteristic of gestalten " that they are maintained in their specific properties when the absolute data upon which they depend undergo displacements of a definite nature " (p. 37).

This criterion too, which, as Köhler shows, would be a sufficient but by no means necessary indication of the presence of gestalten, is satisfied by the systems of electrolytic solutions described, just as the first one is.

Köhler maintains, on the ground of these considerations, that it is entirely safe to assume that such systems of

D

solutions present a paradigm which justifies speaking of gestalten in physics as well.

Not satisfied with this, Köhler also points to other, far more extensive departments of physics, which are likewise supposed to be amenable to the gestalt conception ; all those departments, namely, where "problems of distribution" are concerned.

In contrast to the "distributions" of "things" known to the "naïve" person, in which—in *purely additive juxtaposition*—every individual thing is independent of every other, and is not noticeably influenced by alteration of the distribution, spatial order, or the removal of one or several things (e.g. distribution of the furniture in a room) in contrast to these additive distributions of things, Köhler considers distributions as they occur in *physical systems*. There are physical systems "which in general *do not remain indifferent to any displacements or alterations of state at one point*, but immediately react markedly to any interference of this sort". In these, according to Köhler, we have "*more than merely additive groupings*".

A study of such phenomena obviously promises to throw a great deal of light upon gestalt problems. Köhler therefore searches them out, and in their most precise forms to boot.

"Extreme instances of such behaviour will be found not where (as in gases) even at short range, an effect arises only after an appreciable time, but where every point of the system lies in a field of force of the remaining points of the system, and where a displacement at one point leads to extensive general displacement practically instantaneously. If one attempts to alter the charge of an insulated electric conductor at one point, the charge on the whole system is immediately displaced."

In the distribution of the electrical charge on a conductor, we have therefore, according to Köhler, a new instance exemplifying gestalten in physics.

A large number of other, quite similar examples can be ranged with this. Distributions of thermodynamical equilibrium, distributions of thermal energy, distributions of electrical potential in a field, distributions of stationary currents, either of diffusion currents or of electric or hydrodynamic or heat currents ; and so on.

He asserts as a principle, that "something of the nature

of gestalt ", in the sense of the criteria assembled above, is present here. And he sets out to prove that these physical phenomena do in fact present *something epistemologically altogether singular.* Köhler attempts to verify this in experimental as well as theoretical methodology.

All in all, a foundation thus emerges for the thesis that genuine " gestalten " occur in physics. The gestalt category is therefore taken to have been proved to be a conceptual form primary for the sphere of physics as well, and urgently requiring recognition of its singularity.

§ 10.　*Köhler's constructional solution of the psychophysical problem*

An *entirely new basis* for the *psychological* or *psychophysical gestalt problem* is created by this extension of the gestalt concept to the sphere of physics, which Köhler puts forward. The notion of a *specific physiological correlate*, as this represented itself to Wertheimer as a solution of the gestalt problem, can only now receive a material form which is adequate to the consequences of the gestalt orientation of principles sketched above. The hitherto dominant, synthetically propounded theory of Wertheimer can now be discarded, and a serious effort made, from the antisynthetic standpoint, in the physiological enquiries as well.

The basic conception of the new physiological theory is very simple :—

Since it has been shown that there are in point of fact physical gestalten, we may assume that such gestalt processes are also specially developed in the nervous system. They arise, for example, as configured processes even in the retinal periphery. Hence isolated stimuli upon which the other processes could be built up are no longer present there. And they extend from there through the entire " longitudinal section " of the " optic sector " as far as the central zones, in such a manner that *the whole optic sector* presents a *unitary region of excitation which is configured throughout its extent*—in the same sense as an electrical field may be said to be so, according to Köhler.

This region of excitation is determined in regard to its

particular form of excitation—it is to a certain extent
" controlled "—by the spatial distribution of the activations from without, which arises on the basis of the
stimulus distribution.

In a particular part of this sector, which we were
previously accustomed to isolate as the central part, it is
distinguished by the fact that a configural psychic process
now corresponds to it, of such a kind that "*what is without
is within*".

We have summarized briefly in a diagram the system
of activations and parallels, which, according to this,
constitutes the process of perception, in order to present
clearly the contrast between this viewpoint and that of
Wertheimer (Fig. 3).

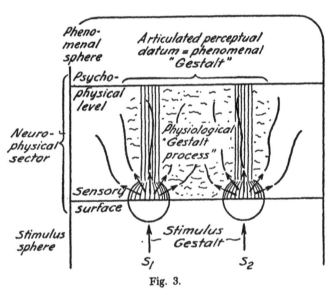

Fig. 3.

Just as Köhler's general schema departs from that of
Wertheimer, so does his concrete embodiment of it.

The feasibility of the attempt to demonstrate concretely
the presence of such "gestalt processes" in the physiological
sphere, fits into an entirely different frame from that of
the former " physiology " of Wertheimer. In the last
resort, its frame is the *most general of all ways of thinking
in modern physical chemistry*.

The actual proposal Köhler makes harks back in substance to certain considerations of G. E. Müller. Müller, in connection with his psychophysical theory of colour perception, had so defined the nature of the excitations, by elaborating Hering's less definite concepts of assimilation and dissimilation, that the *two mutually opposed directions of a reversible chemical transformation* seemed to be involved. Köhler accordingly takes the retinal system, or alternatively, the system of the complete optic sector from the retina to the psychophysical region, as being from the physical point of view simply a chemical *system of interacting electrolytic solutions*, whose chemical behaviour is considered to be " controlled " by the action of the stimulus.

Inasmuch as the stimulus conditions may be taken to be constant, at least over certain periods of time, in optical gestalt-perception, and hence the chemical process to be, correspondingly, stationary or at any rate quasi-stationary, the basic hypothesis emerges as follows :— " Excitations of somatic fields, when external conditions are constant, are *quasi-stationary chemical reactions in dilute solutions* " (p. 13).

The detailed propositions to which Köhler then proceeds are essentially only explications of this basic principle. These appear to bear out completely Köhler's claim that it is possible to determine the physiological events by direct deduction " from physics as the starting point " ; and this to a degree where—as Köhler maintains—the phenomenal datum appears immediately comprehensible from the physiological starting point.

In this connection, therefore, Köhler's discussion leads straight to the conclusion that the " Wertheimer problem ", the question of the immediate physiological representation of phenomenal gestalten, appears to be completely solved.

§ 11. *Köhler's logical incorporation of all problems of wholeness in his physical-physiological gestalt doctrine*

In still another respect does Köhler's discussion lead to consequences of apparently extraordinary significance. It is carried through to a conclusion of comprehensive import for scientific theory.

The whole physical-epistemological discussion of 1920 was primarily directed only toward the goal of displaying the psychological phenomenon in a characteristic context. But in 1924 Köhler—after further conceptual exploration of his contentions—stretched the bounds of his conceptions substantially further. He sees with great penetration that the problem which the gestalt theory treats as the central one in psychology, exists in exactly the same way also in the sphere of general biology ; that, indeed, it is there the very ancient problem which comes to the fore in the dispute between vitalism and mechanism. And he notices, furthermore, that a resolution of this vitalist dispute of a distinctly special kind is contained in his hypotheses.

The point of the dispute, and Köhler's own position, is most clearly distinguishable, according to him, from the results of the more recent investigations of experimental biology upon " morphogenetic adjustments " in germ development which has been somehow disturbed.

The result of these researches is well known to be as follows : A lesion of the germ, or of single cells of it, is in the course of development " smoothed out " in a characteristic manner. The end form of the organism as it unfolds itself from the normal germ still appears, with exactly the same constitution, even when single cells are at certain stages of development either dissolved out or severed from the cell-complex then present by appropriate chemical or mechanical means. Hence in such obstructed development the single cells which remain give rise to something quite other than in normal morphogenesis.

This fact entails great difficulties for a mechanistic explanation in biology. For the very " mechanism " in the single cells appears in some incomprehensible way to alter, " adapt," " regulate " itself somehow according to the circumstances, although, naturally, it actually " knows " nothing about these circumstances. The vitalistic solution of the dilemma, assuming definite super-mechanical, truly vitalistic powers, entelechies, and so forth, is also not satisfactory.

Köhler then re-interprets the matter characteristically. The difficulty in both the mechanistic and the vitalistic treatment lies in the question as to how the " purposiveness " is to be understood.

Köhler eliminates this question. He regards the normal, as well as the obstructed development of the germ in its various stages, not in terms of its final goal, but simply in terms of the constitution of each of the stages in itself. He looks upon it " as a *spontaneous self-articulation* . . . of the processes through their own physico-chemical properties and forces ", in exactly the same sense as an electrical field regulates itself as a " gestalt " through such self-articulation.

Hence it is understandable why every cell does not react only in the sense of a wholly definite " mechanism ", in a " machine-like " fashion. Patently, in Köhler's contention, " the separate parts (must) *each time carry out different functions, just according to the altered total structure* which is set up by the interference and within which the parts lie " (p. 514). Single reactions ensue in a manner as if " local occurrences ordinarily take their course ordered and organized according to the needs and condition of the whole organism (as this is constituted from time to time) ".

Köhler's general propositions about the peculiarity of "physical gestalten " completely cover the biological set of problems. Basing himself on these, Köhler raises the claim of having advanced the problem beyond both mechanism and vitalism. Vitalism has no place in this, since nothing unusual is involved but only a set of facts thoroughly known, and indeed of an exact natural-scientific character. Mechanism is relinquished, inasmuch as it is no longer a question of "machine theory " but only of gestalt processes.

Thus Köhler's gestalt standpoint here apparently reveals its force in one of the most profound of meta-physical problems. Going by it, he presents in a most consistent form the logical or ontological position of the entire range of all possible problems of wholeness which scientific reflection encounters. The whole extent of these questions—from psychology and physiology to general biology—without exception, in principle fits in with Köhler's idea of the " physical gestalt ".

Complementarily to the conspicuous rigorousness which, as our above review has shown, seems to be distinctive of Köhler's argument, here it undoubtedly shows itself to have an especially *imposing range of applicability*.

No matter whether, in critically coming to terms with it, one accepts or rejects this theory as it stands, one will not be able entirely to resist the impression that it represents an undeniably imposing body of thinking in natural philosophy.

2. THE PSYCHOLOGICAL REFINEMENT OF THE GESTALT CONCEPT INTO A PRINCIPLE FOUNDING A POSITIVE SYSTEM

Alongside of Köhler's enquiries there appear, much more modestly and making fewer claims, the newer works of Wertheimer himself. In these—after a long pause (1912–21)—he adds his quota to the foundation and profounder clarification of the gestalt doctrine.

Nevertheless, these works are undoubtedly of no less importance for the complete shaping of an actual gestalt *theory*. It is possible, indeed, that, as far as the after effects upon scientific technique are concerned, they contain the more pregnant conceptions.

The special mark of these works consists in the fact that in them the *phenomenal psychological gestalten* once more appear, *being treated much more independently* ; and this in such a manner as at the same time to express tangibly the coalescence of the psychology of gestalten into a complete system.

Independently of gestalt physics and gestalt physiology, here other considerations are advanced, orientated much more by the phenomenal gestalten and empirical psychology. The consequence of these is in essence that as a result of the analysis of phenomenal function, too, the gestalt concept receives a new focussing, in fact one which is, when all is said and done, essential for a substantive consolidation of the system of the gestalt theory, in the narrower sense, in psychology.

The preliminary step to this is the renewed and keener elaboration of its contrast with the elementalist standpoint (1921).

§ 12. *The primacy of the whole over the part in psychical events*

Wertheimer elaborates *de novo* the import of the anti-synthetic viewpoint, pursuing Köhler's distinction of

" summative " from " super-summative " thinking—but with a new, and extremly significant, shade of emphasis.

The summative way of thinking, which Wertheimer considers to be specifically expressed in the two central theses of the refuted psychology, the " bundle thesis " and the " association thesis ", builds up its aggregation " like a mosaic " " by means of simple additive juxtaposition ", in typical " plus-summation ", " determined according to mechanical, arbitrary, and intrinsically chance moments ".

However, it cannot be accepted as equal to the psychical facts. For—as Wertheimer emphasizes—" only seldom, only under definite, characteristic conditions, only within very narrow limits, and perhaps altogether only in approximations, is a state of plus-summation really to be found. It would seem to be not sufficient to take this limiting case as the typical basis of the happening."

Positively considered, this event proves rather to be as follows : " What is given is *in itself* ' configured ' in different degrees." It presents itself exclusively in " graded stages of *presentation* ' *by main features* ' (in respect to comprehensive whole properties) in varied delineation, up to the precisely, wholly configured datum in respect to all ' sub-wholes ' and ' parts '—in fact ' *gestalten* ' *as primary.*" And, developed more exactly : " Given, are more or less wholly configured, more or less defined wholes or whole processes, with multifarious very concrete whole properties with *inner conformance to laws,* characteristic *whole-tendencies,* with *whole conditionalities* for its parts."

At first glance not much that is new seems to be given in this, over and above Koffka's formulations of 1915. (See above, pp. 29–30.) But the new accents which appear must not be overlooked, accents which become decisive for the coalescence of the gestalt theory into a system.

These consist in the stressing of the *characteristic whole-conditionalities,* in the *special notion of psychical conformance to laws in general,* which is added here.

In description of this conformance to laws, Wertheimer speaks—still rather vaguely, it is true, as is excusable in a programmatic context, but nevertheless plainly enough—of primary " states of whole-adjustedness ", of " autochthonous wholes ", in which the parts are first largely " conditioned as a result of concrete gestalt laws ",

" defined by inner necessity " " evoked by intrinsic whole-conditions ".

The gestalt- or structure-process as such, as a whole, is therefore supposed to be " functionally " " *inwardly* " *active*, in such a way that the " parts " are conceived to be defined in terms of it—on the basis of *primary* " *tendencies towards defined, conspicuous gestalt* ".

There can be no doubt that in what is offered here, further precision is given to what the gestalt concept connotes in the gestalt theory. Henceforth the extremely *far-reaching idea* that *the " whole " determines the " parts " retroactively*, or to put it in a better way, that the " parts " are dependent upon the " whole " in their " so-being ", is explicitly given the central position.

Empirically, this superordination of the whole clearly emerges in many examples among those Köhler compiled in 1924 (pp. 521–2). It is revealed in the way in which, within the gestalt-totality, the properties of the parts are not determined in their own right, but " adjust themselves in accordance with their situation in the whole unit "; for example, in optical illusions, or in the observations of Gelb and Granit, according to which the difference threshold depends upon the figure-character or ground-character of the surface being studied[1]; or in certain researches on simultaneous contrast, according to which the local colour appears to be determined according to the position of the spot in question, or otherwise by the way in which it belongs to a large, whole area.[2] It is thought to be shown also in the way " in which gestalten segregate themselves out of the total field of vision ". " It is not the fact of a definite field-surface being, for instance, homogeneously coloured, which makes it palpably a gestalt in itself, but only when the surroundings are otherwise configured in a suitable manner does that surface spring forward as independently formed "[3]; and so on.

The meaning of the advance in conceptual determinateness which is now manifest, becomes quite clear when one compares what, for example, Koffka said in 1915 in respect of the functional description of the Wertheimer gestalt process. On the negative side, the issue, at that time, was still the possibility of managing with the single

[1] See below, p. 180 ff.   [2] See below, p. 173 ff.   [3] See below, p. 140 ff.

stimuli ; and on the positive side, the point of view was that the whole does " not arise out of the combination of the parts, but is to be understood as the experiential situation specifically correlated to the stimulus situation, in as direct a manner as has hitherto been customary only with the sensations ". But the whole is not taken to be autonomous in the sense that the question of whether it has any retroactive relation to the parts deserves consideration.

It is just this which Wertheimer contributes, namely, a pronouncement as to the *relation of the " whole " to its " parts "* . The " whole ", the " structure ", is conceived as having a peculiar, *material* relation to a part of itself. The description of this relationship by the proposition " the whole is more than its parts " is no longer sufficient. Now it must read " the whole is prior to its parts ", i.e. it is *logically as well as materially superordinate* to them.

Thus Wertheimer himself formulates negatively : The parts are therefore not to be rated primarily as the " prius ", as foundation in plus-combination, and with conditions of their occurrence which are in principle indifferent ; they exist largely as parts resulting from their wholes under intrinsic conditionalities, are to be regarded " as part " in reference to these wholes.[1]   Herewith he gives expression to a fundamental conception, one which is crucial for distinguishing the significance of his position from the point of view of scientific theory. We designate this, in its positive application, as the *principle of the primacy of the whole over the part*.

Only this fundamental conception enables the gestalt concept to progress still farther towards a distinct, practical, scientific meaning.

§ 13. *The notion of the conformance to laws of the gestalt, as formal presupposition for the conceptual tenets of a specific gestalt " theory "*

The principle of the primacy of the whole over the part provides the framework for a further development, in

---

[1] Thus is explicitly formulated, in psychological terms, a principle which is already present in the background of Köhler's physics. Since it does not there stand out in a way which allows of as clear isolation as here, we have, for reasons of exposition, relegated its elucidation to the present context.

which the *gestalt concept* comes to the fore as a *specific explanatory concept*.

This development takes shape in the effort to refine the notion of the specific conformance to laws of gestalt, and in the effort to erect absolutely circumscribed, concrete " gestalt laws ".

The pre-occupation with this task dates back earlier than this. Köhler had already announced, in 1920, that Wertheimer had discovered a characteristic constant condition, in regard to structures of phenomenal events, the " tendency towards precision of the gestalt ". According to this, "phenomenal spatial gestalten [tend], under the most varied circumstances, such that only a certain weakness of the conditioning stimulus-factors is common to them . . . to pass over into particularly simple and precise structures, which are thus marked out from any sort of irregular units ".

Wertheimer himself, in 1923, develops a series of formal principles—i.e. principles related to the structure as such —which are said to determine the manner in which " parts " (separate points) coalesce into a " whole ", a gestalt. (These are purely descriptive, being based on definite observations upon series of point-constellations of the most varied sorts, and generalizing these findings.) They are the factor of *nearness*, the factor of *likeness*, the factor of the *common destiny*, the factor of the *good gestalt*, and the factor of *closure*.[1] These are designed to make manifest the *inner conformance to laws of the gestalten*, especially, as is evident, in the " tendencies " to " good " and to " precise gestalt ".

And at the basis obviously lies the view that in these gestalt factors we are concerned with *absolutely primary manifestations*, with the *most primordial moments of action*, by which all phenomena, as far as these can be reduced to the factors, are *explained* with entire adequacy.

The discovery of this conformance to laws opens up new perspectives for the propounding of theories in psychology. One need only think of Koffka's treatment of the array of problems in the psychology of thinking,

---

[1] For greater detail, see below, p. 148 ff. We must not omit to mention that the discovery of these factors, or at least of analogous ones, must be dated back as far as 1902, and must, in fact, be placed to the credit of G. E. Müller.

in 1925. Having declared that the " gestalten " which are present in thinking, have to be designated " thought gestalten ", he simply continues in the following words (p. 574) : " Since gestalten are at issue here, all previously derived gestalt laws are valid . . ."—and with this the problem of the psychology of thinking is apparently solved, at least in principle !

This example shows how far one can go with the gestalt laws or factors.

The gestalt concept has herewith acquired a new rôle in the gestalt theory, one which is of the utmost importance for the characterization of the theory.

In all the discussions of gestalt theoreticians hitherto examined by us, the gestalt problem is this : We are concerned, in its phenomenal aspect, with the accurate description of the gestalt fact ; in its functional aspect, with giving a detailed account, in the most definite way possible, of its conditions and its inner coherence ; and finally, with constructing a substructure for it, on the physiological side. In the prosecution of these three lines of enquiry from the point of view given by the general orientation, the gestalt concept is thus precisely fixed and theoretically elaborated, primarily as a problem and as a task for the gestalt theory.

But now the methodological situation takes an entirely new turn. The *gestalt concept ceases to be in any way considered as a problem. Rather has it become the explanatory principle* from which, as a primary given fact, the phenomena may be deduced.

Reflection readily shows how the import of the gestalt idea has here, at the same time, become markedly more specific.

To be able to proceed in this way " in scientific technique " a certain presupposition has to be implicitly acknowledged, which can be briefly formulated as the *postulate of the autarchy of the conformance to law of the gestalt*. By this we mean that tacit assumption at the back of every such " explanatory method ", which affirms that we *neither require, nor are able*, to *trace back* the laws governing gestalt to simpler manifestations ; but that we have in them *ultimate facts*, facts so *entirely universal in character* as to be *fully* valid *in virtue of themselves only*.

In fact, there can be no doubt, that only by the acceptance of this assumption is justification provided for the attitude adopted by gestalt theoreticians (e.g. especially Koffka and Fuchs) in practical research. At any rate, if this assumption is repudiated, the application of the gestalt concept as an explanatory concept in the exact sense here in question becomes impossible.

In the consolidation of the gestalt theory as a psychological system, this assumption has, as may be expected, an extraordinary importance. It alone enables the gestalt concept of itself to become a principle of a system, on the basis of which everything else is theoretically conquered.

Herewith the gestalt concept receives its final specific delineation. This is the culmination, the final consequence, of that line of thought which led to the precise fixing of the gestalt concept in the significance of the primacy of the whole over the part. Thus is expressed, in the most clear-cut manner, the fact that gestalten cannot really be understood " from beneath ", but must be considered in their entirety.

Herewith, also, the *possibility of advancing beyond the study of perception* comes to fruition. (See above, p. 33.) Gestalt laws do not only regulate the inter-articulation of presentations which, as in perception, occur as self-sufficient " gestalten ", under conditions which remain unchanged (at least during a certain period of time). They are held to be equally operative— especially the " tendency towards precision "—when, starting with a definite initial situation, a " progression ", a " dynamical process " in the direction of a quite definite " solution ", an " end situation ", takes place in the psychical sphere (e.g. in experiments in the psychology of thinking).

In principle, the *gestalt dynamics* which has to be brought to bear here is throughout aligned with the *gestalt statics* (taking for granted the conformance to law of the gestalt) as this was developed in regard to the perception of e.g. stationary objects. But this for the first time clears the way for an *application of the gestalt theory to the manifestations of processes of thinking and of volition.*

Hence the erection of concrete gestalt laws is a task

crucial in all respects for the perfection of the system of gestalt theory. The conception of the primacy of the whole over the part, which is at the back of it, viewed in the light of the *autarchy* of the conformance to laws of the wholes, is the true formal nucleus for the tenets of the system.

§ 14. *The notion of the "gestalt disposition" as material presupposition for the empirical feasibility of a specific gestalt "theory"*

Through the clear-cut fixation of the gestalt concept in the significance of the priority of the whole over the part, and its interpretation in accordance with the acknowledgment of an *autarchy* of the conformance to laws of the gestalt, it is possible to put forward a system of gestalt theory in the specific sense of the word.

However, a new, not unimportant extension of the conceptual apparatus is still possible, for the *accomplishment* of this. For as yet, this sort of gestalt theory has made no provision for empirical findings which make it impossible to disprove the dependence of the modes of occurrence of gestalten upon *internal conditions*. This dependence upon internal conditions is what is meant in the "old psychology" when the influence of "attention", or "apprehension", is mentioned.

Originally this dependence is hardly taken account of by the gestalt theory. Right up to the present time, it is still in part passed over in utter silence, in accounts of the gestalt theory. Or if it is given any attention, as e.g. by Köhler, 1920, it still appears wholly as a matter which should best be treated incidentally. For originally the gestalt theory is orientated solely in accordance with the stimulus, and builds up the physiological and then the phenomenal gestalten upon that basis, as we have seen.[1]

The positive organization of the facts in question only

---

[1] Köhler admits, in 1920, that the "changing circumstances" of the receptor system, as "conditioning topography", can also play a rôle, in addition to that of the stimulus constellation, in constituting the gestalt process in the neurophysical sector. However, this does not give a convincing and concretely particularized gestalt-theoretical interpretation of our problem. All that is stated is that these facts, as such, are not excluded, and that they cannot, therefore, be immediately claimed to be incompatible with the theory.

comes to pass later, as I can see it, fundamentally only in 1924–5, both with Köhler and with Koffka—and this through the concept of the gestalt disposition.

Previous to this, to be sure, another concept, the concept of " attitude ", had already appeared, brought forward to explain the phenomenal structures in those cases in which constellations of stimuli and gestalt processes did not adequately correspond to one another.

Wertheimer already makes use of this concept. In that case, however, and later too, it is in the main not actually connected with gestalt ideas in its import. And above all, in the form in which it was introduced at that time, it does not do justice to the full implications of the problem we are here concerned with.

Wertheimer is, in fact, aware of this problem, in 1912— and it was still exactly the same in 1921—only within a specific limitation, one which enables him, in accordance with his realistic, stimulus-physiological orientation, to speak of a factor of " *objective* attitude ".

It is because he introduces it in an altogether special connection, that Wertheimer arrives at the view that this " attitude " factor may be understood in the sense of an objective moment of action ; one which is regulated by the circumstances of the stimulus, and not in any way by the subject.

The experiment upon which he bases himself is indeed remarkably one-sided. By means of the stroboscope he presented in repeated succession a first phase consisting of a sloping line, and a second phase consisting of a horizontal line. These were so arranged, that upon simultaneous presentation the sloping line appeared below the horizontal line, and at an angle of about 45° to the right, from its centre. What was observed in every case was a swinging downwards of the sloping line to the horizontal position, with a movement of revolution to the right—conformably with the smallest distance (cf. the factor of nearness, p. 148). These trials are reckoned as a preliminary experiment. He then immediately carries out another similar one, in which the arrangement of stimuli is such that in the first phase the sloping line runs to the left above, and revolution to the right again appears.[1]

---

[1] Cf. Linke and Biener already.

According to his paramount thesis of the direct and unequivocal determination by the stimulus, in the second experiment revolution should actually have ensued leftwards—again conformably to the least distance. Thus this thesis seems to be violated.

However, it may be rescued. Wertheimer assumes that, purely as a result of the course of events in the preliminary experiment, a definite after-effect remains, of such a sort, that in the main experiment the physiological apparatus is prepared in a special manner, is in fact " set ". Just as a motor can, by being put in an appropriate circuit, be " set " for a quite definite motion, so here too, as a result of a definite " placing in circuit " (a kind of " facilitation ") a corresponding " set " of the physiological " apparatus " ensues. More clearly, a definite *state of being set* results in this apparatus, and determines the course, the " motion ", in the main experiment. And, moreover, this " state of being set " appears simply as a consequence of the action of the stimuli in the preliminary experiment. It is " *objective* " *in nature*.

Such a concept of a " state of being set " has, naturally, only a limited connection with what is otherwise meant by " attitude " in psychology,[1] and still less connection with the general problem arising out of the influence of subjective factors, on the whole. Wertheimer is not even aware of this general problem ! And his way of arriving at concepts is certainly not adapted to the problem, even though his term " attitude " is often construed as if it could cover something of the sort. But no approach to it is possible from Wertheimer's concept of " attitude ", or better, " state of being set ". In this matter one must also not be led astray, when Wertheimer himself at times roundly asserts that he has met the general problem in propounding this concept.

Koffka (1922) was the first to encounter the necessity of envisaging the problem much more generally. With him the question arises of how the ambiguity of the gestalt in certain drawings, the reversal of figure and ground, is to be explained. Koffka's solution is to introduce a somewhat far too vague concept, that of the " figure-attitude ". He believes it to be intelligible, by reason of such a figure-attitude, why in one case the inner

[1] Cf. G. E. Müller, int. al.

field, and in another the outer field, acquires figure-character (cf. p. 165). Conceptual definiteness is only attained in a still later phase of development, when Koffka endeavours (1925) to elucidate the concept of " attitude " theoretically, in a characteristic manner, in fact in the direction of the concept of disposition.

We shall follow Koffka's line of argument in his inter-pretation of the question. How can it be explained that in simultaneous size comparison the " mutual relatedness " of the two compared lengths is not unequivocally effective ; but that on the contrary, within a certain liminal range, the judgment can as readily be $a > b$ as $a < b$, upon repeated presentation of the same stimulus situation a, b.

In the first place, of course—conformably to the general orientation of the gestalt theory set forth above—the judgment is normally in all respects always " the expression of a phenomenal state of affairs, of the constitu-tion of what is given " ; or better, it is the immediate consequence of the " mutual relatedness " in the physio-logical total happening—without any sort of importation of " higher functions " and such-like.

Nevertheless, unequivocal determination by the stimulus conditions does not take place, and for this a special circumstance comes into question.   " The relational phenomenon, especially in the case of smaller differences, depends not only upon the stimulus constellation, but also upon the *instruction*.   This is only a special case of the dependence upon internal conditions.   The observer who awaits the presentation of two stimuli which have to be compared, under a definite instruction, is *no longer indifferent* towards these stimuli, but is ' set ' *in such a manner* that the possible reactions to the stimuli are not all equivalent.   *Because of the attitude certain reactions are favoured* and others are prejudiced . . ." (p. 537).

But what does this attitude consist in ?   It consists in a gestalt *disposition*.   " Before the stimuli act no gestalt is present, but certainly (as . . .) we cannot help concluding a gestalt disposition is, and this leads to a gestalt process when the stimuli act upon the person . . ." (p. 537).   " If a specific gestalt-attitude exists, then a gestalt phenomenon corresponding to it will arise, even though the stimulus situation would evoke a different phenomenon in the ' indifferent ' individual " (p. 537).

The hitherto indefinite concept of attitude is equated with the concept of gestalt disposition and thus receives a very precise connotation. At the same time Koffka covers the whole compass of our general problem by this means; for it is possible to do justice to all special cases of the "general dependence upon internal conditions" without exception, by inserting the appropriate "disposition ".

And in the last resort it is most closely consistent with the general system-principle of the theory. For what comes into question here is a "*gestalt disposition*"; and Koffka believes this to be established by the fact that such a disposition can also be phenomenally experienced, in which event it appears veridically as a genuine gestalt phenomenon. (Koffka observes, for example, that in the comparison of two lengths with the, so to speak, "expectation", established by the instruction, that the lower one is smaller, even before the presentation of the stimuli a "trapeze gestalt" may set in, and this may then on occasion, upon presentation of the stimuli, prevail in experience as a false judgment.)

These gestalt dispositions, like the phenomenal gestalten, are, moreover, as a matter of course conceived to be founded physiologically, in the gestalt processes.

In this manner Koffka arrives at the conclusion : " The phenomenal gestalten, the gestalt processes, and the gestalt dispositions belong together in the closest fashion. The creation of the first concept necessarily entails that of the others." And furthermore : " The essential properties which we have observed in the phenomenal gestalten we should likewise ascribe to the gestalt dispositions and processes we have deduced " (p. 538).

Conversely, by the assumption of these gestalt dispositions, a final, integrating explanatory principle is introduced into the gestalt theory. This principle rounds off the system as a whole, in that it invests the central principle of the system with the elasticity chiefly lacking to it, as regards its conformity to the facts.

CHAPTER IV

THE ARCHITECTONICS OF THE FINAL BODY OF DOCTRINE OF THE GESTALT THEORY

To give a final conspectus of the total system of the gestalt theory, as it now presents itself, viewed as a whole, we briefly summarize the essentials once more. We shall consider in succession the following, and so round off finally what has already been set forth.

(1) The extent of the gestalt theory's systematic field in general.

(2) The principles of construction of the system of gestalt psychology.

(3) The organization of the gestalt-psychological system in its integrality.

§ 15. *The extent of the gestalt theory's systematic field in general*

(1) The systematic field of the gestalt theory is not confined to psychology. Gestalt theory is a way of considering things, necessary for general biology and physics as well.

(2) In physics, there are exact specimens of "structures", which seem valuable as supporting the new category of gestalt.

(3) In biology, the introduction of the gestalt theory signifies nothing less than the resolution of the controversy between vitalism and mechanism.

(4) In psychology, the introduction of the gestalt theory signifies the possibility of deriving the entire range of psychical phenomena from one unitary and determinate basal doctrine, in the form of a "unitary theory".[1] Taking cognizance of the corresponding physical-physiological notions, it signifies the possibility of concretely establishing psychophysical parallelism—by following up the Wertheimer problem.

§ 16. *The principles of construction of the system of gestalt psychology*

(1) The building up of the system of gestalt psychology is accomplished with characteristic dual prominence of

---

[1] Cf. Spearman, 1925.

two lines of thought : that of the psychophysical gestalt theory, and that of the psychological gestalt theory.

(2) The *psychophysical* conception in the gestalt theory is bound up with the elaboration of the gestalt theory in physics and physiology. It leads—in virtue of the presupposition that structure is preserved throughout all stages of the psychophysical apparatus—from the physically real world of things to the phenomenally given, and to a derivation of the phenomenal in the last resort from the stimulus as starting point, conformably to the general concept of the " structural reaction ".

(3) The *psychological* conception in the gestalt theory has its foundation independently of physical speculations in a descriptive, as well as functional analysis of the phenomenally given. It has its roots in the general notion of the *autarchy* of the conformance to law of the gestalt ; and its concrete embodiment is the erection of fundamental gestalt laws in detail, above all, the principle of the precision of the gestalt. More especially, its field extends to everything in which adherence to the objective stimulus is either impossible or difficult.

§ 17. *The organization of the gestalt-psychological system in its integrality*

(1) The unitary character of the theoretical standpoint leads gestalt psychology to abandon the refuted ways of organizing psychological facts, in especial, to give up the old distinction between sensory processes and higher processes.

(2) Instead of this, a new organization emerges in the gestalt doctrine, and this is a direct expression of the general principles of the gestalt theory. Psychology as gestalt theory is organized—by analogy with the constitution of physics—into the provinces of gestalt statics and gestalt dynamics.

(3) *Gestalt statics*, apparent in physics wherever static or stationary processes of a gestalt character are concerned, evidences itself in psychology whenever an " event independent of the time dimension " is given, that is to say, whenever—as for instance in the perception of resting objects—an integration lasting for a certain time, a " structure " of what is optically given, persists.

Gestalt statics includes e.g. the processes of perception, but over and above these also e.g. the processes of comparing, and the presence of colour-structures (see above, p. 33). These characteristically evince a strict determination of the " total gestalt " by the conditions, above all those of the stimulus situation.

(4) *Gestalt dynamics* is always in evidence when conditions are at issue which do not in themselves already fully settle the gestalt character. Upon insufficient or " weak " stimulation by the stimulus situation, the final gestalt structure is of its own accord produced from within outwards, in accordance with the peculiar conformance to laws of the gestalt. The processes activated by the stimuli have the " tendency ", in their own right, to actualize definite gestalt moments.

(5) The entire field of psychological facts is exhausted in this duality of gestalt statics and gestalt dynamics. In particular, the introduction of any sort of special principles in order to " explain " the so-called higher psychical processes becomes superfluous, by reason of the specific laws which receive formulation in gestalt dynamics. (Cf. p. 50.)

BOOK TWO

TOWARDS A CRITICISM OF THE GESTALT THEORY

To enquire into the tenability of the gestalt theory's hypotheses, it is necessary to follow up more exactly the details which form the concrete support for the convictions of its adherents.

Here we need not concern ourselves further with the precursor of the gestalt theory, the derivation of gestalten from *field excitations* and *short circuit processes*, as Wertheimer represented these in 1912.[1] We have already shown above (p. 17 ff.) that this derivation proceeds from a wholly synthetic-atomistic angle, since it conceives a " total process " ("simultaneous ϕ ") as arising out of primarily basal elementary excitations through definite " cross processes ". Hence it is at once evident that this mode of explanation does not accomplish what must be demanded of it on the basis of the special standards since then laid down by the gestalt theoreticians themselves. According to Köhler's disquisition of 1924, the being configured, the "intrinsic articulation " of our perceptual data, can only be admitted to be explained if, firstly, it has been deduced that in general certain inner coherences can arise physiologically within the primarily basal aggregate of single excitations ; and secondly, if over and above this it is also made evident, that such coalescences appear just in this very manner, that is, directed towards intrinsic articulation. The second requirement can certainly not be coped with on the basis of Wertheimer's theorems. For if a coalescence were at all comprehensible for the physiological elementary processes on the basis of the hypothesized field-excitations, it would have to be a coalescence " of all with all ". A *selective* coalescence,

---

[1] Since only the gestalt problem is germane to us, we do not, for reasons of space, discuss the theory of successive ϕ and its tenability as an explanation of the seeing of movement.

such as the facts demand, such that the various gestalt units delimit themselves within the field of vision over against one another, cannot be envisaged by Wertheimer. And the assertion that Wertheimer's " simultaneous ϕ " at all events explains the fact of coalescence occurring at all, is equally unproven. Wertheimer himself can say nothing more about this ϕ process than that it presents a " *kind of physiological connectedness*, indeed a unitary *total process* resulting *as a whole* out of the single physiological excitations ". Thus he simply hypostasizes what has to be explained without making the attempt to show the connection directly " from the starting point of physics ", that is, from the starting point of the physiologically known properties of the excitation processes which can be presumed. If one attempts to fill in these gaps by Wertheimer's means of thinking, one arrives back at the points Exner established (see above, p. 17). However the genesis of the so-called " total excitations " may be conceived, physiologically nothing more is present than a multiplicity of states of excitation of single cells, in reciprocal action, it is true, in virtue of the so-called " short circuits ". The situation is by no means improved by this introduction of a " short circuit " effect as the principle of the reciprocal action—apart from the fact that the vagueness of the whole position is only increased thereby. " Just as the optic nerve excitations cannot become whole processes by reason of their antagonistic induction, so this cannot ensue for them by reason of any other sort of reciprocal action." (G. E. Müller, 1923, p. 99.) We must thus conclude, with G. E. Müller : " It is therefore an evasion to designate a collection of excitations a unitary total process because of the circumstance that they mutually influence one another through crossfunctions." Wertheimer gives us nothing more than a *bare verbal solution* of the problem.

Hence our critical discussion need no longer delay over it. We shall therefore turn immediately to the final form of the gestalt theory, as this presents itself to-day, and we shall attempt to test how well it is founded.

What is most impressive here is that Köhler seems to have been successful in extending the gestalt principle to the territory of physics, which is held to be so secure, in scientific theory, and then providing an *hypothetical* psychophysical substructure for the psychological gestalt theory.

These considerations of his are so impressive for the reason that, to a certain extent, they present a " transcendental " deduction of the gestalt *category* in general, and, at the same time, a physico-physiological deduction of the gestalt *psychology*, in particular.   Accordingly, we shall have to come thoroughly to terms with them.

Not till our second book shall we take up the detailed investigations of the *empirical research* which has been instituted from the viewpoint of the gestalt theory's position, for the purpose of verifying, or establishing and elaborating it.   We shall have to put these empirical findings to the proof as to their true scope, on the basis of immanent criticism, as well as by comparison and contrast with other observations.

PART ONE

TOWARDS AN APPRAISEMENT OF THE CONSTRUCTIONAL FOUNDATION OF THE GESTALT THEORY

The possibility of building up the system of gestalt psychology in a really constructional manner is due, as we have seen, to Köhler's grounding of the gestalt theory upon physical considerations, and the physiological elaboration of these.

It has its roots in Köhler's fundamental thesis that even in physics there are provinces subject to the gestalt category. And it is accomplished in Köhler's attempt so to construct the neurophysical happening (on the basis of this insight into the logical structure of certain provinces of physics, and with the concrete approach of " physics as the starting point ") that the phenomenal gestalten appear to be explained.

Criticism of the hypothetical foundation of gestalt psychology will therefore have to concern itself firstly with Köhler's gestalt physics, and secondly with Köhler's gestalt physiology.

CHAPTER I

KÖHLER'S EVIDENCE TO DEMONSTRATE A GESTALT-THEORETICAL PROVINCE IN THE SYSTEM OF PHYSICS

An analysis of Köhler's gestalt physics must extend to two, in themselves well delimited, parts of physics, the theory of electrolytic solutions, and the theory of physical " distribution systems ".

The peculiar nature of these two spheres, Köhler considers, justifies one in speaking of a gestalt-theoretical province in the system of physics. For the dominant significance of specific gestalt-theoretical categories is supposed to be discoverable in them, through the closer epistemological clarification of their conceptual structure. Let us consider the first of these spheres.

I. KÖHLER'S "DEMONSTRATION OF A FIRST PHYSICAL GESTALT FACTOR"

§ 18. *Köhler's line of argument in proof of the gestalt character of systems of electrolytic solutions*

The proof Köhler adduces as warrant for his view that systems of electrolytic solutions have gestalt character, appears to be very simple. The facts to which Köhler refers can readily be reviewed. Let us, to bring a concrete example in support immediately, consider two solutions, one of HCl and one of LiBr, separated, to begin with, by an impermeable partition. Now imagine instead of this isolating partition another one introduced which allows the diffusion of the two solutions; or in fact imagine the partition removed. An extraordinary phenomenon now occurs in this whole. At the surface of contact of the two electrolytes—which of course were previously in nowise electrically charged—there arises an electrical difference of potential. That is to say, the whole made up of the two solutions reveals a characteristic electrical property. And this property, this difference of potential at the boundary surface, was certainly not present before contact of the two solutions was produced, while the solutions together did not yet constitute a whole ; for the solutions were previously electrically "neutral".

Is it therefore not true that in very fact "the characteristic properties . . . of the whole do not [allow] of being put together from properties of the parts of a like sort"? Is Köhler correct in affirming that this must indeed be looked upon as a " first physical gestalt factor " ?

The question is, whether in fact a new sort of relationship, one that has hitherto escaped epistemological analysis, is revealed in the quoted example; whether in fact the relationships here under discussion "have not hitherto adequately occurred to the philosopher, as a philosophical problem, in the course of his physical enquiries". To settle the point, we shall follow out more clearly, how the *physical facts of the matter* and the *logical interpretation* must be confronted with each other. We believe that the philosophical elucidation of the physical facts of the matter demands *not only this logical orientation*, but far more *a correct physical interpretation*. With Köhler this very physical interpretation appears at one place, but this the crucial one, to be inappropriate.

What does "part" of the whole mean in a solution system ? Does the physicist actually view the relationship in a manner which makes it permissible to treat the two single solutions, as such, as "parts"? If Köhler himself speaks of the physically "real character" of the whole, and sees in this the justification for alleging physical gestalten in general, one may, conversely, with at least equal if not greater justice, insist that the concept of "part", too, should have meaning only in so far as a "physical reality" is actually connoted by it.

Now what are the "physical realities" which, as "parts" of the solution system, constitute the system of reactions according to physical theory ? In the view of physical theory, they are, as is well known, the ions of the solutions concerned.[1] It is well known, too, that physics explains the fact of the occurrence of a difference of potential at the surface of contact also in terms of the ions. It appears as a consequence of diffusion taking place. Before osmotic communication, the pairs of ions of the two solutions are arranged in two groups (e.g. Solution 1, H^+ and Cl^- ; Solution 2, Li^+ and Br^-) so that each group appears superficially to be electrically neutral. Then diffusion takes place, the distribution of the ions within the whole alters. The ions travel at varying velocities corresponding to the ionic concentration in the two solutions. The varying velocity of the ions causes the difference in electrical potential. This, therefore, explains Köhler's phenomenon. But the explanation—quite contrary to Köhler's belief—is obviously directly in terms of the interaction of the parts.

The relevant property of the whole seems to be wholly derivable from "properties of the parts of a like sort". The ions have a characteristic electrical charge in their own right. And even if something special can be demonstrated to hold superficially for the solution system of charges in the form of the potential difference, this by

---

[1] A point the significance of which has already been discussed by Becher. (See below, p. 66.)

no means signifies the appearance of a phenomenon which was not present in the components.

Thus, in following up a line of thought which insists that the concept " part " must be applied in a narrower fashion, one adapted to the physical facts of the matter, the conclusion soon emerges that Köhler's argument collapses at all points. The remarkable logical fact he alleges to have discovered vanishes.

Even if Köhler is not willing to grant our demand that the facts be held to in applying the concept " part " to be a just one, the position is still untenable for him, once we have penetrated somewhat more deeply into the physical facts. Our argument can be adapted to this, too.

We may safely concede to Köhler that it is possible to say that the two components can be regarded as " parts " of the electrolytical system of solutions, in the true sense. Are the properties in question then really not " present " in forms " of a like sort " in these parts ? Of course, they are not apparent as potential differences, superficially distinguishable. But such properties, alike in kind to subsequently arising potential differences, are nevertheless " present " !

It is true, one does not take note of these when one thinks of what one is dealing with as a " solution ", as defined simply in its *pre-scientific* sense ; but only when one takes into account, that the moment one speaks of the *physical* state of affairs, the "electrolytic solution", everything is implied which belongs essentially to this solution, in any way, as a physical property of it ; that is, above all that property which is directly characteristic of it, the state of ionization which alone makes the solution an " electrolytic " one.

When this fact is taken into account, viz. that definite electrical properties are already specific for the physical character of those " parts " from the outset, even setting aside the consideration that they are parts of the whole osmotic system, the antithesis which seduced Köhler to his far-reaching inferences disappears. It exists, in fact, solely for a conception of the data which stands suspiciously near to a *pre-physical* way of thinking. In an analysis which probes the physical constructs in the totality of their properties, these difficulties, on the contrary, vanish completely.

Probably this last form of our argument, at all events, should be acknowledged as effective even by Köhler. For indeed, the same idea lies at the basis of his own exposition, in the place where he disavows the attempt to propose chemical compounds as examples of super-summative structures in the sphere of natural science. It is true that in these compounds the " whole " does actually possess properties quite different from those of the " parts " ; and it is true that in the present stage of theoretical interpretation the properties of the whole cannot be deduced from those of the parts. Yet he does not in any way accept such chemical compounds as evidence in proof of the true occurrence of gestalt phenomena in nature. For " after so many marvels of discovery in natural science, it is possible, too, that the apparent new formation currently acknowledged by the as yet hardly a century old chemistry, may some day be reduced to basic physical conceptions, as physics and physical chemistry progress ".

Exactly similar is the line of argument we have carried through in opposition to Köhler's pre-scientifically conceived concept of " solution ". For we have established that the only concept of electrolytical solution relevant to the discussion is the one authentic to, and really elaborated in detail by, natural science ; and we have then observed that the singular facts fundamental for Köhler do actually vanish on this view.

§ 19. *Becher's version of Köhler's line of argument*

The outcome of our criticism up to this point would justify us in rejecting Köhler's claims that gestalten are involved in an electrolytic system, if Becher had not meanwhile given a new turn to Köhler's arguments. Becher, in his exposition of Köhler's theory, has explicitly incorporated our counter-argument into his commentary, and has sought to prove that it cannot pass as a valid refutation of Köhler.

He admits the correctness of the view that " the electromotive force does indeed [appear] as a summation phenomenon, produced by very small electrical charges, which are present also in the single solutions when these are not in osmotic contact ". But he does not grant the conclusion we have drawn from this.

He is of opinion that Köhler's assertion that there is more in the properties of the whole than in the properties of the parts is in no respect invalid. " The combination of solutions nevertheless does exhibit something that is entirely absent as long as the part solutions do not come into osmotic contact . . . i.e., the forces between A particles (from the HCl solution) and B particles (from the LiBr solution) ". The specific " whole-property " is thus supposed to lie in these forces, and hence justifies speaking of a " gestalt phenomenon " in this connection. This counter-argument of Becher's must be more closely investigated.

In the first place, we can satisfy ourselves that here an entirely new argument is really being brought to bear. Becher has in no way defended Köhler's former argument by prosecuting the clarification of the above critical interpretation, with reference to the facts, to a point where Köhler's view would be shown to be still the correct one. Instead, even though he comes forward as a defender of Köhler's conclusions, he plainly admits, without cavil, that the line of argument adopted by Köhler is not quite unimpeachable. In the second place, Becher attempts to bring forward a new sub-stantiation of his own for Köhler's conclusions, in the place of Köhler's line of argument ; but in this case, too, the physical analysis of the facts of the matter does not seem to us to be adequate to the material and logical circumstances.

Becher bases his line of argument on the electrical forces which are supposed to arise between the particles of the different solutions and which are ostensibly not present before the osmotic contact. To this one must reply, firstly, that such forces are certainly present even before the osmotic relationship is set up, even though they are quantitatively perhaps different. But one must specially emphasize that even if Köhler were correct in saying " that these forces are not effective, to begin with ", yet, physically these forces are not of significance for the process critical after production of the osmotic contact. The genesis of the difference of electrical potential which, macroscopically considered, must in any case be taken to be the crucial phenomenon of this contact, is in no way connected with these electrostatic forces.[1] On the contrary, this difference of potential ensues simply as a result of the free mobility of the ions, in the sense of statistical mechanics—as a result of their specific differences of velocity—along exactly the same lines as, for instance, in the theory of gases, the phenomenon of diffusion likewise ensues simply in virtue of the statistical-mechanical propositions about the mobility of gas atoms. The identity of the laws of electrolytic solutions and those of ideal gases, shows that for elucidating the phenomena occuring in the diffusion of the solutions in a solution system, we need actually not take into account the electrostatic conditions, as long as we are concerned with the diffusion process as such; and this apart from the fact that the electrical field which appears and gradually forms itself in the progress of the diffusion process, naturally has a retroactive arresting influence on the diffusion process (cf. the theory of galvanic chains). Becher's opinion that what is peculiar of the whole osmotic system is to be found in these electrostatic forces does not meet the case.

Hence Becher's interpretation, too, cannot compass what it should. Proof that the gestalt category must be acknowledged as a fundamental category of physics can thus in no way be derived from the phenomena present in electrolytic solutions. At all events, these phenomena do not compel such a conclusion. The next question is, to what result an enquiry into the other branches of physics, from which Köhler also draws confirmation for his assertion would lead.

2. KÖHLER'S DOCTRINE OF THE GESTALT CHARACTER OF " DISTRIBUTION SYSTEMS "

§ 20. *The distribution systems of physics and Köhler's interpretation of them*

Distribution systems are all those physical constructs in which " every point of the system lies (more or less)

---

[1] But mark : The genesis! The *existence* of the difference of potential, or its operation, is of course definitely identical with these electrostatic elementary forces and their effects. But *the fact that a difference of potential* should primarily even *arise at all*, is due to altogether different factors.

in a field of force of the remaining points of the system "
—whether it be a field of potential, or one of charge, or
one of current (cf. the examples quoted by us, p. 38,
above).

Constructs of this sort have a special character, in that
the distributions of current or of charge, of energy or of
potential, present a peculiar state of closure, by reason
of the fact that "a displacement at one point leads to
extensive general displacement practically instantaneously".
Köhler believes he has proved that in all physical constructs
of this sort something typically "gestalt-like" is to be
found.

He believes it possible to extract this result from a
simple, so to speak "phenomenological" clarification of
the scientific situation, as this *de facto* presents itself in
the investigation and theoretical reduction of these
structures in actual physical research ; that is, merely
by separating the theoretical facet out of the practical
business of the science. How he sets about it, and what
arguments are advanced in the course of it, must now be
followed up in detail.

We shall content ourselves with one pregnant example,
in placing Köhler's ideas before us; and we shall choose
the example which Köhler treats first of all and most
thoroughly—the distribution of a quantity of electrical
charge on a conductor.

Taking first the physical facts :—

Physics teaches us that this quantity of charge
"arranges itself" in a manner determined according to
the geometrical conditions of the conductor ; that is,
the elements of electricity arrange themselves in a
momentarily quite definite "density" at the separate
points of the surface of the conductor. When further
quantities of electricity are added—that is new "parts"
—a new total distribution sets in, which is indeed
distinguished from the former one in the absolute value
of the amount of the charge, but not in the relative
distribution of the charges at the separate points. For
every periodically selected total charge *a distribution alike
in every case, as regards "structure"*, arises.

In this, the distribution of electricities is *entirely
dependent upon the form, upon the "topography" of* the
conductor. And in accordance with this Köhler says that

F

a *specific "proper structure"* of the distribution of electricity is set up periodically on a given conductor. Köhler forthwith regards this situation, *the fact of proper structure*, that is, *as the expression of a real gestalt.*

As a matter of fact, the *gestalt criteria* laid down by him (see above, p. 36) are perfectly satisfied in this case. In detail, the following hold (cf. Köhler, p. 79) :—

. (1) The proper structure does not allow itself either to be " partitioned " or " compounded " actually ; for the " moments " of structure [1] carry one another (each one carries the whole remaining structure, and this in turn carries each moment) ; and furthermore, " a local interference upsets the structure as a whole."

(2) The structure is dependent upon the given physical form (more generally, physical " topography ") and this *in its entirety* and *as a whole.*

(3) The structure is independent of the material of the conductor, of the kind and of the total amount of the charge ; that is, is transposable in respect to quantity.

(4) It is " spatially transposable " in that it depends only upon the relative dimensions of the physical form and not upon the absolute scale of these (second Ehrenfels criterion for gestalten).

(5) It always exists as a structure only in the physical whole, which coheres electrostatically ; it presents itself, therefore, as a circumscribed unity (corresponding to the first Ehrenfels criterion for gestalten).

Thus far what Köhler establishes. His inference that electrostatic distributions have gestalt character is based on these points.

But what does it all come to ? Köhler has demonstrated that " electrical distributions " (and analogously, the distribution systems further discussed by him) can be designated " gestalten " in the sense of this concept as fixed by the above-mentioned criteria. Has he thus proved that there is a gestalt-theoretical province in physics ? Is it a fact that peculiar logical relationships are present in this division of physics ?

The answer to this question calls for a more probing enquiry.

---

[1] That is, in this case, the quantities of electrical charge, in general the " parts ", which are intended to be distinguished as non-autonomous by the word " moment ".

§ 21. *A direct testing of Köhler's contention by means of a model distribution system which can be envisaged in its entirety*

To enable us to analyze in closer detail the problems emerging at this point, we shall commence from a definite example in physics, one which can be more simply envisaged than the examples Köhler treats. In this case it will be easier to decide the question of whether anything logically peculiar arises in the " structures " which he, too, is able to invoke.

Let us construct a model of a " distribution system " which can be particularly well envisaged.

Imagine a simple experiment: Let a series of any number of completely and equally magnetized steel needles serve as material for it. For the purpose of the experiment each is provided with a small cork disc which suffices to keep the needle floating straight. Imagine now, to begin with, two such needles, with similarly orientated poles (say north pole upwards) floating upon an adequately large surface of water, and thus freely mobile. Then imagine another magnet fixed at any particular height over the centre of the water surface with the south pole downwards. What happens ? Physically, quite definite interacting forces exist here, which are expressed in a movement of the floating poles, and lead to the result that the two floating magnets assort themselves in a position of rest at a quite definite distance from each other and from the controlling magnet.

If we add a third, a fourth, a fifth floating needle, then in every case, as a result of the action of these forces, a quite definite distribution, a quite definite configuration of the needles (regular triangle, rectangle, pentagon, etc.[1]) forms itself.

It seems as if a " gestalt " has been achieved. Actually, Köhler's gestalt criteria are satisfied by this magnetic system.

Transposability, in the sense of the second Ehrenfels criterion, pertains to them. One has only to apportion two needles instead of one to each cork float, thus

---

[1] Cf. as a companion picture the quite corresponding " distributions " which are ascribed, in the theory of the atom, to the electrons constituting the atom pattern.

doubling the magnetic polar strength at every place, or one has only to treat the fixed magnet in a corresponding manner, and one immediately obtains a configuration geometrically perfectly analogous to the first one, and unaltered in essentials. Similarly, it always exists as something unitary only in the *whole*, as this coheres magnetostatically, conformably to the first Ehrenfels criterion. Furthermore, as soon as one removes a part from the whole ("local interference") the structural situation as a whole does indeed appear to be upset, the equilibrium ceases to exist ; instead, the parts that are now left assort themselves into a new and different structure. As for the possibility of compounding, this is out of the question here.

It could be objected that nevertheless the case is different here, as compared with the conditions of distributions of electrostatic charge which Köhler revealed in his theory of distribution systems. One difference still remains. In this case we cannot actually talk of "proper structure ". If a needle is removed or added, everything in the entire field is indeed disturbed, but the "same gestalt does not form itself anew " from within outwards.

However, if we make it clear why this is so, a simple modification of the model can easily be introduced, in such a manner as to obtain a wholly exact picture of the conditions which were essential for Köhler in his electrostatic phenomenon.

Proper structure could not be ascribed to the quoted model, since "proper structure " must always be related to a definite "topography ".

Thus, the difference between our magnetostatic construct and the constructs of electrostatics, consists in the fact that what appears in the case of electrostatic gestalten as "conditioning topography " is not represented in our magnetic example. From the physical point of view, be it noted, the fact that the magnetic rods can shift about only on the surface of the expanse of water which serves as supporting medium corresponds to the action of a conditioning topography. However, as regards the different "distributions " which actually arise, this topography seems too remote to be quite clear in its efficacy. But we can easily introduce such a conditioning topography in a very tangible manner into our experiment.

We need only limit the surface of water at the disposal of the magnets for their free mobility by means of " screens ", and then our experiment will correspond in all respects to Köhler's conditions.

Let us assume, for instance, that the free surface of water available for the movement of the magnet poles is bounded off in the shape of a narrow elliptical ring. Thus the self-regulation, the spontaneous reinstatement of the original gestalt after disturbing influences, may be made clear very tangibly.

In the first instance, it is true, difficulties still persist. If, for example, we take six magnets (all with their magnetic north poles uppermost), and bring them into the field of movement somehow, a distribution spontaneously forms itself—the formation being, as is immediately clear, a " quasi-regular " hexagon. If we now disturb the structure by removing part of the magnets, say two of them, it appears that the conditions are in this case different all along from those present in Köhler's electro-static model. The distribution gestalt which now arises, the quasi-regular rectangle, is actually, as Köhler would put it, an entirely new gestalt, which has nothing to do with the previous one ; but the fact that in the electro-static example a " proper structure " of the topography could be spoken of, purports that upon such removal, or alternatively, addition of " quantities of charge ", the same " structure " is still seen to reinstate itself spontaneously, in spite of the altered total content of charge. It seems, therefore, as if a special factor, over and above the topography, is present in the electrostatic example, one which we have not included in our model.

However, in this respect, too, congruity can readily be obtained. If we imagine not six or four magnetic poles but 6,000 or 4,000, the picture, as seen from the standpoint of the gestalt theory, immediately appears different. In the case of the first " quantity of charge " the poles form an elliptical or curvital gestalt, and in the case of the second " quantity of charge ", the very same ; and this with equal distribution of relative " density " in both cases.

When we consider this result, the fact of the proper structure of the conductor appears to be reducible to two features : to the " conditioning topography " and to the fact that in electrical charges—speaking in terms of the electron theory—we are always concerned with " infinitely numerous ", single, small parts of electricity, within the characteristic, topographically conditioned distribution of which the " gestalt " is engendered.

Our magnetostatic model, amplified in this direction, does indeed present all the pertinent " gestalt phenomena ". Moreover, we may note that, looked at it in this way, the gestalt problem emerges in a perhaps still more precise manner in our model than with Köhler's; for in a certain sense (that is, in so far as we wish to consider only two-dimensional gestalten) we can dispense entirely with the conditioning topography.

The gestalten which appear here arise in a perfectly free, topographically unconfined manner. They are therefore apparently a more pregnant example of the fact that physical gestalten form themselves in spontaneous " self organization " out of the simple modes of physical action.

For our purposes this model has still more extensive advantages. It permits of making abundant use of the possibility of investigating first of all the most simple instances, and of advancing steadily to more complicated conditions of distribution thereafter.

Let us consider, firstly, the simplest case, a "system" consisting of only two movable components. The conformance to gestalt, in this combination, consists in the fact that for given polar strengths, under these conditions, the two floating magnets spontaneously assort themselves to a definite distance from each other.

But to comprehend this "gestalt manifestation", if one desires to apply this term here at all, one certainly does not require any method of thinking exceptional in physics. In principle this is a case where two points are given, in connection with which certain forces of attraction and repulsion are present, determined for the time being by their relative distance; thus an equilibrium of the combination is only possible when the distance is continually altered until attraction and repulsion reciprocally combine to a resultant of zero value. There can be no question of any sort of special methods of thinking, or of any special problems to be considered.

Or is it possible to see in the union of two forces to

produce a resultant anything that transcends the so-called additive ? We may be at rest on this point, for Köhler cannot attack our line of argument on this score. Köhler has explicitly elucidated the extent to which genuine summation is supposed to play a rôle in physics. He emphasizes that the definition of what is summative is not given in so clear-cut a manner as to allow one to discover non-summative structures in physics with little trouble. And the warrant he brings for this is that the basic constructs dominating physics, namely the scalar ones (mass, electrical charge, energy, potential) as well as the vectors (thus the forces in particular) all remain " summative " in character, even according to his inter-pretation. Thus, if we have shown, in reference to our magnetic system, that its configuration permits of being understood, to the last detail, on the basis of the simplest principles of force, in terms of the interdependence of action of the fixed and the movable magnet poles, then Köhler too must concur in the conclusion that here it is at no point necessary to invoke the gestalt concept in any way whatsoever as a new physical category.[1]

Let us now, as we proceed to more complicated instances, consider the enlargement of our magnetic pair into a magnetic trio. Once more the very simplest combinations of the actions of forces ensue. On the basis of these, the three movable needles now present separate from one another as much as possible, while the fixed guiding magnet attracts them to itself. The consequence will of necessity be interpreted without any gestalt reflection, purely in terms of the interrelationships of the actions of the different forces and what results from them ; again purely on the basis of considerations which, as Köhler

---

[1] If Köhler desired to speak of a gestalt process in this connection, he would, to be consistent, have to allow it in the entire sphere of physics, wheresoever states of equilibrium, etc., appear at all. To choose a directly " machine-like " example : He would likewise have to say that the position of equilibrium, in which the pendulums of a centrifugal governor upon a rotating axle at a given velocity of rotation arrange themselves, is to be designated a " gestalt phenomenon ". But since Köhler in fact deprecates, with a strong sense of his purpose (bearing in mind his solution of the vitalist problem) the confounding of gestalt-like with machine-like, we believe we are not mistaken in assuming that for the above example the answer would read : " Not gestalt " ! Yet the same state of affairs occurs in the magnetic example. We have merely a combination of a definite number of forces, fixed by the distance or the position of the media—just as in the centrifugal example.

himself says, have nothing to do with conformance to gestalt.

In principle the situation has to be envisaged in the very same way when we proceed to four, five, or more movable components. Here, too, the constellation, which geometrically-dynamically undoubtedly has a gestalt character, in principle ensues in every detail from the simplest reflection upon the equilibrium of forces, without the importation of other categories.

Hence in these simpler examples we are unable anywhere to discover anything peculiar, beyond the usual—that is, according to Köhler, transcending the "summative" level of physics. But what follows from this for the assessment of the logical situation in Köhler's own example, the "electrostatic gestalt structures"? We managed to "copy" Köhler's electrostatic example perfectly in our magnetostatic model by introducing—

(1) A conditioning topography
(2) The multiplication of the components to an "infinitely"[1] numerous number.

In our systems of few components no means of explanation transcending the usual apparatus of physical thinking was found necessary. Hence we must now enquire whether, on account of these two alterations, something new in principle in any way enters into consideration.

If, to begin with, we consider the *significance of the conditioning topography*, we find that the total character of the *physical* approach is in the main not changed as a result of this, at any rate. The logical meaning of this influence of a conditioning topography can already be recognized, in a simple manner, in the most primitive physical situations—e.g. in the actions of forces upon a point the degree of freedom of which is limited by fixing its mobility, e.g. by means of guiding rails, etc. The simplest reflection suffices to show that these guiding rails stand for nothing other than the introduction of certain further conditions of force, which can be immediately

---

[1] In this connection, the number is, of course, in the view of the physicist to be regarded as in the last resort nevertheless finite, and can accordingly only be held to be "very great". The term "infinite" must therefore be interpreted in the sense of a limiting process. (See below.)

discerned in the pressure requirements these guiding rails are liable to, under the influence of the forces of the system, and the amounts of which can readily be established on the principle of the parallelogram of forces (e.g. movement on a sloping plane).

Hence conceptually new features are not introduced through the conditioning topography, with limitation to a small number of components, to begin with; even though what Köhler believes he can observe to be conformable to gestalt in "physical structures" is certainly determined, as to its so-being, in a directly critical way by reason of that topography.

What of the influence of multiplying the components? When we consider the situation from the purely *physical* point of view, it is clear that in this case, too, no alteration of the logical relationships can arise. It is always the interrelated actions of the forces pertaining to the constellation which remain responsible.

It is true that the *mathematical interpretation* of these combinations becomes extraordinary difficult with · increasing numbers of components. Where two or three components are concerned the case is simple, as in the example discussed above, because from the outset the argument can take into account the fact that the two or three needles are sure to arrange themselves in a definite symmetrical distribution, in the position of equilibrium. But let us take no more than four or, say, five components, and ignore the fact that we are inclined, on the grounds of symmetry, to take the distribution into a triangle or rectangle as the given one. Which mathematical propositions enable us to discover the distinctive distribution of the components which corresponds to the position of equilibrium? Clearly, the issue here is to try out, mathematically, all possible distributions up to a point, and to select from among these manifold, infinitely numerous, different possibilities that constellation which *de facto* manifests the conditions of equilibrium. We have in physics, in addition to the previously mentioned direct analysis of the action of force, a simple means of discovering the position of equilibrium, namely by carrying out a determination of the energy content, and utilizing the minimum of energy as a principle of selection.

Accordingly, there are two possibilities. Firstly, the

direct method of calculating the relationships of force, and secondly, this method of energy balances just stated. Both, however, naturally become more and more difficult mathematically the higher the number of the components rises. Stating it purely as a point of principle, we can say that in the limiting case of the " infinitely " numerous components which corresponds to Köhler's electrostatic example, the mathematical situation is distinguished by the fact that the solution has to be sought for a system of *infinitely numerous equations with infinitely numerous unknowns*.

Regarded in this context, the mathematical aspect of the question appears throughout to parallel the progressive complication of the problem. But new logical peculiarities do not, it is clear, arise.

Thus a direct logical analysis of the physical conditions in distribution systems, as these present themselves in the light of the model constructed by us, leads to the conclusion that no place can be indicated, as far as they are concerned, where it would be necessary to go beyond the framework of the usual means of thinking in physics. The hypothesis of special gestalt-like principles has no place in the physics of distribution systems.

§ 22. *Critical analysis of Köhler's detailed arguments for the gestalt character of distribution systems*

Having reached this result by our *direct testing* of Köhler's idea of a gestalt physics, we shall now have to resolve the question of how it is possible—in more immanent criticism—to come to terms with Köhler's *detailed arguments*, those which are essential in the substantiation he offers for the hypothesis of a gestalt character of distribution systems.

Three different lines of thought can be isolated in Köhler's discussion, as lines of argument independent of one another. Two of these derive from the ostensibly demonstrable *peculiarity of the methodology* in this sphere of physics, and the third can be described as an *ontological* one.

To begin with, Köhler is of opinion that he can verify his point of view by pointing to the fact that, as regards *theoretical methodology*, entirely new forms of handling the problems, forms immediately peculiar to this very sphere of problems, are here required.

In all the cases which Köhler puts forward as examples of physical gestalten, the mathematical point at issue is the solution of the Laplace differential equation. Now, it has become apparent that the solution of this differential equation is, mathematically, a problem of a quite special sort. To master it unusual efforts are needed. It has exercised mathematicians from the time of Dirichlet and Neumann; and only Fredholm and Hilbert have at length succeeded in indicating a more comprehensive method in the theory of *Integral Equations*, a means for the constructional representation of the concrete solutions which is at any rate in principle always feasible.

Köhler then draws this conclusion: If the problem of the Laplace differential equation, which can be taken to be an adequate mathematical representation of the physical state of affairs in " distribution systems ", if this problem calls for a methodology so singular as that of integral equations, then something quite singular must also be present in the physical " distribution systems ", something which distinguishes these prominently from the rest of physical phenomena; and this special factor is their gestalt character.

However, this line of reasoning cannot pass as sound, for actually, upon closer consideration, the Fredholm technique of integral equations ought not to be so completely contrasted with the methodology (a more " primitive " one, it is true) applied in " non-gestalt " physical problems. It is really impossible to overlook the connection between the two, when one has once made clear to oneself the mathematically crucial step of Fredholm-Hilbert which leads to the mastery of the problem. This consists in the important discovery that the theory of integral equations can be brought into direct relation with the theory of simultaneous algebraic equations. It is even possible to derive the methods *for the solution* of integral equations directly from the computation of systems of algebraic equations, through a limiting transition. Thus the problem of the integral equation appears to be identical with the problem of the solution of a system of infinitely numerous simultaneous algebraic equations with infinitely many unknowns.[1] The logical side of the matter is particularly illuminated, when one discovers that Fredholm arrived . at his new theory from the starting point of these very systems of equations; and that, therefore, not only logical equivalence, but also historical-heuristic priority can be claimed for these systems of equations.

We may now apply to these facts Köhler's idea that the logical character of the physical problem is reflected in the content of the mathematical relationships requisite for its theoretical solution. If we start from this basis now, our thesis of the homogeneousness of the logical structure of physical problems throughout the entire sphere of physics, which we have opposed to the standpoint of Köhler, merely receives further substantiation.

If Köhler could reach such opposed results, the reason is only that he has viewed the mathematical-physical situation in a purely one-sided manner. In his logical enquiries he did not bear in mind everything that he himself knew of the physics or of the mathematical physics of the matter.

The case is exactly the same with Köhler's attempt at a *verification* by way of the *experimental methodology*. Here, too, the peculiarities which Köhler stresses are distinguished only in degree from the conditions in other spheres, described as not conforming to gestalt. The experimental investigation of distributions (which, moreover, as Köhler also admits, *de facto* possesses no significance at all in physical research), the methodology of tapping the field in order to establish the value of the charge or potential at the separate points with the aid of a probe (touch-balls, etc.), has characteristic difficulties, as is well known. The probe begins to distort the field of the conductor being investigated, and thus also its charge structure, as soon as it is introduced into the field.

But to see in this difficulty, which according to Köhler occurs nowhere else in physics, evidence that quite novel relationships are here present, does not seem permissible. For in principle—despite Köhler—the same difficulty

[1] Cf. the latest exposition by Toeplitz and Hellinger in the *Enzyklopaedie der mathematischen Wissenschaften*, which summarizes, and, especially, sets out clearly the stages of development of these conceptions.

exists elsewhere in physics too, to some extent even in the simplest weighings where, at bottom, a measured total action of forces would have to be reduced with reference to the combined disturbing influences of the environment. This becomes of itself on occasion the nucleus of a positive experimental task—consider Jolly's experiments to measure the gravitation constant.

The position is no different either with a third contention, which Köhler touches upon at the outset of his " verification by way of the theoretical methodology ", but which we would rather separate from the arguments from theoretical and experimental methodology, and contrast with them as a special one—namely, the *ontological argument*.[1]

Köhler believes that he has been able to indicate, by a simple consideration, the *quite special ontological dignity of these very structures* in physics, and this in support of his gestalt theoretical interpretation of distribution systems.

These structures show a remarkable singularity. If the Coulomb-Cavendish law, or the equivalent Laplace differential equation, is alone granted—no further presuppositions that have to be empirically admitted are necessary—then the solution is rigorously determinable without further trial, if it is at all feasible, directly from the given physical form of the surface of the conductor. Köhler's opinion is that " the structure on a conductor and on its surrounding field thus almost makes the impression of a unit to be defined ' a priori ' ".

Indeed, it is " *in some sense more than a mere empirical finding*, one which might also have been able to prove arbitrarily different in its intrinsic nature ", it is an *expression*—to use Köhler's term—of a " *law of being* " in *Nature*, a state of affairs of peculiar existential reality. Furthermore, all this is valid *independently of all specific* " *hypotheses about material*, that is the majority of all auxiliary assumptions in physics, which remain

---

[1] We are disposed to treat this line of thought as an independent argument, in spite of its not occurring as such with Köhler, who uses it only as an introduction to his statements about theoretical methodology. Yet this is quite in line with the gestalt-theoretical manner of thinking ; and at the present stage of our criticism of Köhler's gestalt physics, can only be regarded as a reinforcement of Köhler's position.

without decisive significance for the gestalt problems ".
It is *to be referred solely to the " structure " as such*. In
other words the " gestalt " as such is more profoundly
existential than the " material " upon which it erects
itself ; to the " gestalt " belongs an individual reality—
likewise *independent of the " material "* ; it appears as
an autonomous ontological reality, as a *primary* actuality,
which must needs also be understood in terms of itself—
quite in keeping with the basic thesis of the gestalt theory.

The development of this argument is apparently very
simple. The special ontological dignity of " gestalten "
is inferred from the fact that gestalten spring from
" existential uniformities " of nature, independently of
assumptions about material. But this fact is supposed
to be substantiated by reason of the quasi-aprioristic
character of the units in question.

In order to criticize this ontological argument we
should really have to take up a position in regard to a
variety of questions. We should have to enquire : (1)
What is the meaning of quasi-apriori character, what does
the existentiality of a law signify ? How can one infer
existentiality from the quasi-apriori character ?   (2)
What does the " structure's " specific independence of its
material signify ? And what follows from this ?

It will be sufficient, however, not to cast our discussion
in a form as comprehensive as would be unavoidable if
we wished to go into the actual problems in Köhler's
ontology; for the *criterion* of the existentiality of gestalten,
their " quasi-apriori character ", can be put directly under
scrutiny.

Hereupon it at once emerges how the whole line of
argument turns back upon itself. Apart from the fact
that the nomenclature " quasi-apriori " must be admitted
to be hardly happy, whence does this " quasi-apriori
character " of the units derive ? From the uniformity
of conformance to laws, and this, be it noted, clearly the
conformance to laws *on the part of elements* !

If the fact that such a great multiplicity of physical
problems can be comprehended under *one form* of this
kind, apparently *everywhere homogeneous*, aroused Köhler's
amazement, he should really have settled, by profounder
analysis, whence this uniformity comes. No physicist
would be astonished at the possibility, in dealing with

this question, of managing it fundamentally with the Cavendish-Coulomb law, or alternatively with the Laplace differential equation. For the physicist knows that actually the compounding of the concrete physical fact from the parts, the possibility of which Köhler denies, can be accomplished on the basis of principles; and that, accordingly, the conditionality which holds for the detail naturally suffices also for establishing the nature of the whole.

Köhler therefore, on account of his *gestalt theoretical way of expressing himself*, has lost the eye for the true *import of the physical concatenations of action*. In the so-called quasi-apriori determinateness which Köhler found so remarkable from his standpoint, nothing other is really revealed than *the unitariness of the empirical, elementary law of action lying at the basis of the system*, and the "*summative*" *character of the concatenation of action which ensues*; and this lies at the basis of the whole of physics, *in the shape of the principle of superposition*! [1]

[1] The very manner in which, in the physics of distribution systems, the elaboration of *quite special methods of thinking* eventuated, methods which are appropriate for a most convenient treatment of the problems of such " continuous systems ", can only serve to substantiate this. In particular, the *creation of the concept of potential* points clearly and unequivocally in this direction.

Originally the electrostatic interdependences of action led to the *concept of force*. But as soon as electrostatic systems began to be built up—from the single charges—the extraordinary difficulty of overlooking the effects of the total force emerged; for the principle of superposition, Köhler's principle of the additive that is, now suffered practical complications for the reason that the magnitudes and the forces concerned, that is the vectors, had to be considered both from the point of view of magnitude and of direction. However, after it had been noticed that —to put it in the modern way—these vectors in the electrostatic field permitted of being, immediately and completely, mathematically evaluated as gradients of a scalar, a new possibility was opened up: One could now select statements about new basal magnitudes, the values of potential, instead of statements primarily corresponding to the facts about the forces of the field (," strengths of the field "). Hence it became possible to define the electrostatic field in terms of the fields of its various components *by means of simple superposition*, that is by means of a genuine " additive " procedure.

Thus the introduction of the concept of potential has quite precisely as its object simply the rendering of this very principle of superposition, the principle of additive superposition, applicable here too in the most convenient possible way, just as it is in the remaining provinces of physics.

3.   CONCLUSIONS TOWARDS A CHARACTERIZATION OF THE
PHYSICS OF DISTRIBUTION SYSTEMS FROM THE POINT OF
VIEW OF SCIENTIFIC THEORY

§ 23.   *The distribution systems according to their categorical
import and their intrinsic specificity*

Both our critical appraisement of Köhler's lines of
argument, as well as our positive constructive effort,
lead, after what has been said above, to a very definite
conclusion.

The gestalt concept cannot by any means—as Köhler
imagines—be acknowledged to be a physical category
hitherto ignored, but fundamental, nevertheless, in spite
of that.   A division of physics into two domains of totally
dissimilar categorical structure is out of the question.
On the contrary, we must hold fast to the all-pervading
unity of the whole of physics, as far as its logical constitution is concerned.

To define it positively, the entire body of natural
events accommodates itself to the single, unitary point
of view of the *interdependence of action of the " parts "*—
whether we are concerned with the problems of
"summative" physics, or with the problems of that
physics which Köhler claims to be gestalt-like.   The
elementary category of physics continues to be that of
reciprocal action, or otherwise of causality.   All physical
constructs, in so far as physics investigates them, are—
defined in terms of scientific theory—*units of action.*[1]

And yet the distribution systems do as a matter of fact
present peculiar features which do not occur elsewhere
in physics.   "Distribution," i.e. spatial extension in
"articulation", in "structure", does indeed evince
itself in them.   Furthermore, it is characteristic that this
"articulation", this "structure", reinstates itself and/or
completely reorganizes itself, after being disturbed, always
becomes a "structure" again—in virtue of "inner"
spontaneous "self articulation".

Is it at all possible to do justice to this situation in
any other way than Köhler's ?   Well, it is not necessary
as yet to perceive any "existential" differences in the

---

[1] Cf. the similar position taken up by H. Driesch, in a work which has
in the meanwhile come to my notice, *Ann. d. Phil.*, v, 1925.

matter. It may be possible to comprehend these peculiar properties *materially* by reference to the special physical conditions of the " constructs " involved. And, in fact, we have only to recall that in our discussion in § 21, the singularity of the interdependence of action present in distribution systems was traced back to two principles : (1) To the conditioning topography, and (2) to the multiplication of the number of components up to an " unlimited " number. Here the following observation is pertinent. If, for example, electrostatic fields institute themselves in definite " spontaneous self articulation ", does this depend upon anything other than the periodically fully determined topography ? It is the *topography*, the " boundary conditions " which fix the concrete " complete structuration " of the distribution systems in their " so-being ". *The fact that* " structures ", spatial " distributions ", arise in such and such a "state of articulation ", is due solely to the fact of the *interdependence of the action of all elements with one another*, subject to this regulation by the topography. The occurrence of *spatial* articulation *at all* is simply the consequence of the fact that the *topography* is also *spatially defined*, distributed in space. That the articulation " arises " or else *reinstates itself*, is due to the fact of the *universal* dynamical reciprocal action between all the parts.

The dependence of "what conforms to gestalt ", in the distribution systems, upon the topography is immediately evident, since the question of what the " gestalt " " looks like " in any concrete instance can at all times only be dealt with by reference to the topography.

In this way what conforms to gestalt in the distribution systems is characterized in a perfectly specific manner : something super-geometrical, dynamically-real is in point of fact involved. But, be it noted, this dynamic " being-real " does not by any means signify, as Köhler thinks, that autonomous realities are present here. On the contrary, it is theoretically determinable exclusively " from beneath "—from the elementary law of action, as this is given by the " elementary uniformity " of the physical construct under consideration, which has its roots in " material nature " ; and from the " conditioning topography " which comes to regulate the dynamic course of actions in a binding way.

G

In this sense, then, but only in this sense, may we genuinely speak of a " dynamically real constitution of distribution systems" which gives them their "super-geometrical " character. But the reality which we thus ascribe to the physical " gestalten " is quite different in nature from the reality which Köhler claims for them.

To settle the *signification* in which we speak of *reality* in this connection, it is only necessary to examine in somewhat fuller detail how this reality is tangibly represented in the nomenclature of theoretical physics—to examine such concepts as lines of force, lines of current, field, etc.

When the development of physical theory is impartially considered, it becomes clear that these *at any rate do not represent primary concepts*, which refer directly to the properties and actions of the bodies surrounding us. They are, in truth, *derived concepts*, which are incorporated into theory with a view to the most simple possible comprehension of the facts. We are concerned with *functional concepts*,[1] and *not*, as Köhler thinks, following the expressions used in certain places by Maxwell and others, with *concepts of substance*.

The gestalt category cannot be demonstrated to be a substantive fundamental principle in the *de facto* business of science.

To go further: Not only the gestalt concept, but the concept of the " plus-combination " antithetically co-ordinated with it in Köhler's work, likewise has no meaning from the point of view of scientific theory—at any rate in physics. Physics does not occupy itself with " plus-combinations " either. For a triple division must take the place of Köhler's contrasting of " plus-combinations " and " gestalten ", which proves to be an incomplete disjunction :—(1) Plus-combination ; (2) Interdependences of action ; (3) Gestalten. As for those physical constructs which Köhler himself assigns to the sphere of " plus-combinations ", these, if one seriously applies Köhler's own criterion of " plus-combinations "—the absolute indifference of one part for another—do, in fact, also belong to the sphere of interdependences of action, in so far as there is a physical problem here at all.[1]

[1] Cf. Cassirer, *Substanzbegriff und Funktionsbegriff.*

Thus the scientific-theoretical significance of this distinction vanishes, at any rate for physics. Indeed, we realize that in the distinction developed in reference to psychology between " plus-combination " and " gestalt ", the state of affairs really important in scientific theory, as far as physics is concerned, was entirely obscured. The knowledge of this must have wider consequences, and thus lead to scepticism as regards the adequacy of this distinction to the facts, both in psychology and physics.

One thing is certain. The single, great, far-reaching idea of Köhler's is that it might be possible to assure the position of the new fundamental category of gestalt for psychology by resorting to physics, which has a theoretical apparatus so much better established, by reason of its course of development, than that of psychology. But this idea must be abandoned in its entirety. The gestalt principle does not allow of being conclusively implemented on scientific-theoretical considerations either for physics or for physiology.

There still remains one question for our critical analysis : Whether Köhler's contention does not prove to be *in practice* fertile in the concrete utilization of the physical viewpoint for the physiological explanation of the phenomenal gestalten ; for we have explicitly conceded that the physical constructs considered do, in their factual existence, possess something of " gestalt character ".

CHAPTER II

KÖHLER'S PHYSIOLOGICAL EXPLANATION OF
PHENOMENAL GESTALTEN IN ITS ORIGINAL
PRESENTATION

The gist of Köhler's physiological animadversions is that it seems possible to determine what happens in the neurophysical zone by *hypothetical reconstruction*, starting directly from the stimuli, and this to such a degree that

---

[1] This stands to reason. The " distribution " of articles in a room, prototype of a " plus-combination ", is not a topic of physical research.

the *configuratedness of the phenomenal reality* seems to be made intelligible in terms of this, and in a quite characteristic manner to boot.

I.   KÖHLER'S METHODOLOGICAL PROGRAMME FOR RESOLVING THE PSYCHOPHYSICAL PROBLEM

§ 24.   *Purpose and procedures of Köhler's physiology*

Köhler sets himself the task of determining the physiological happening " from the starting point of physics ". He believes that he can thus arrive quite concretely at a constructional " explanation " of the phenomenally given. He indicates two possible routes by which to attain this object.   In the first place, he believes we could do so forthwith in a way which is conceptually quite clear : " We could set about obtaining *an exact insight into the material nature* of the sort of events which actually take their course in a configured way in the *nervous system*— establish the forces, etc., which are operative in connection with them, and so elaborate a physics of the physiological gestalten."   In the second place, however, he perceives another possible route, which he prefers to the first : " We could make it our object to *get to know* the general properties of phenomenal gestalten *from the basis of the* equally *general properties of physical structures.*"   We can do this " by showing that *physical gestalten* which arise in the nervous system and achieve psychophysical importance, must have " (*in consequence, that is, of the general formal definitions* which may be assigned to them " from the starting point of physics ") " a *constitution* quite analogous and in the widest sense parallel to *that of the gestalten of phenomenal perception* ".[1]

This route may appear somewhat general and indefinite. Yet a well-defined meaning can be attached to it, if one

[1] By explicitly inserting the parenthesis, I believe I have fixed the word " must " of Köhler's formulation, in the sense in which it corresponds to the context of meaning.   Köhler's words by themselves, without the parenthesis, could mislead one to see a logical circle even in this formulation—as if it meant that physical gestalten are supposed from the outset, to adjust themselves in accordance with the phenomenal ones.   But this intepretation, it seems to me, is made impossible by the way Köhler actually proceeds at first.   Cf. Wittmann's (1923) view.

thinks of the methodology of physics in general, and recalls that a similar double route offers itself there. (Cf. the distinction between "pure" thermodynamics and the kinetic theory of heat; for instance, the relation between energetics and mechanism in the narrower sense in Mechanics.)

Methodological scruples cannot validly be urged against either of these approaches. Hence it is incumbent to observe attentively *how* Köhler attempts, in practice, to arrive at something positively new about the neurophysical processes, along these two lines.

Our examination of Köhler's psychophysics will be directed primarily to the core of the theory, to the considerations which lead Köhler to his general *formal* description of the physical process, and to the statements about the possibility of explaining phenomenal gestalten, which were determined by reference to this description.

2. THE GENERAL STATEMENTS TOWARDS A FORMAL DEFINITION OF THE PSYCHOPHYSICAL HAPPENING—THE CORE OF KÖHLER'S LINE OF THOUGHT

§ 25. *The construction of Köhler's line of thought*

The specific points of departure for Köhler's physiological theory only become intelligible in the light of the position he takes up (1924) to the refuted viewpoint. According to this latter, the physiological process of perception builds itself up out of "very many local processes independent of one another", which must be conducted along, each by itself in isolated conduction, from the periphery to the central organ. Thus the process takes its course in the form of a like number of separate physical systems.

Köhler raises two objections to this viewpoint. He makes it clear that it does not correspond to the actual phenomenal effects, on two counts.

Firstly, it goes too far, to a certain extent. It would in effect lead one to expect that these purely anatomically fixed, elementary zones and boundaries of function, which exist quite independently of the constitution of the processes, also become observable on the phenomenal side, as universal constants, in every concrete perception. But such a genuine articulation of elements is not met with in any perception.

Secondly, it does not go far enough. " It omits to take note of a special feature of our phenomenal world, its intrinsic articulation, the fact that we experience things as unitary, and not as a mosaic of sensations."

The fact that the theory could arrive at this view, is explained by Köhler on the ground that one circumstance above all had a dominant influence upon physiological thinking—the circumstance that the field of vision is "not only [organized] in itself" but is so "above all, compatibly with external objects . . . which . . . appear before us as really disparate in optical space" (1924, p. 514). The eye primarily transmits, "purely as a machine," a sufficiently exact point-by-point image of the constituent parts of the environment to the perceiving *sensory surface*. But in order that this correspondence to external reality may be retained in the higher neuro-physical zones, and eventually in the psychophysical sphere itself, the hypothesis of "machine-like" "elementary activities" directed to this end is introduced.

A direct foundation for these hypotheses is not, according to Köhler, possible. At any rate, a direct *histological* substantiation he believes to be "without any force as proof and indeed only an assertion". For "we have no proof of an absolute *functional* separation of any chain of neurones from every other, from beginning to end " ; rather, "there are sufficient facts from which, on the contrary, functionally effective combinations in all grey regions of a nervous sector emerge with certainty " (1920, p. 179).

Therefore Köhler designates this hypothesis of elementary conduction an outright "fabrication", and furthermore, it is the more barren to his mind, since it is just this problem of the "intrinsic articulation " which he thinks should have the central place in psychology.

In order to *solve* this very problem *positively*, he affirms that, "in reality *organization in an extended physical happening* does not require a restriction of local events to unalterably prescribed and isolated paths, but is also possible and realized in coherent physical systems, as *self-organization* or structure of the happening itself."

Köhler's theory accordingly resolves into the new conception that " this articulation could be a *spontaneous self-articulation* of the optical processes, in virtue of their own physico-chemical properties and forces—whereby the mechanistic hypothesis of organization (i.e. the hypothesis which explains the ' organization ' in a ' mechanical ' way, by means of the conduction mechanism) would be discarded " (1924, p. 517).

The possible way of thinking about the matter indicated here does in fact permit of being *positively* realized on directly physical lines, within the framework of Köhler's discussions about physical systems or physical gestalten, by subordinating the neurophysical concatenation of happenings to those discussions.

Thus Köhler comes to characterize the neurophysical happening by the single statement : " The psychophysical areas whose states of excitation represent the physical correlates of phenomenal optic fields, form a *system coherent in itself* " (1920, p. 189).

And this brief statement makes very far-reaching inferences possible; for Köhler simply enquires what he can confidently say, " from the starting point of physics," about the properties of physical systems coherent in themselves.

He summarizes this in the thesis : " *Psychophysical events in the optic sector have the general properties of physical spatial gestalten* " (1920, p. 189). And he specifies what is implied in this by endeavouring to give *a more exact characterization of the psychophysical happening, with this as his point of departure*, as it follows, in his opinion, if gestalt character is ascribed to the psychophysical happening.

From what is generally known about " physical spatial gestalten " on the whole, i.e. pursuing Köhler's second " route ", the following definitions emerge for the psychophysical happening (1920, p. 189 f.) :—

" (1) States independent of the time factor form themselves and persist *for the system as a whole*. The processes in limited regions are carried by what takes place in the rest of the system, and vice versa. They arise and exist, just as they are, not independently as parts, but only in the extended total process as moments of it.[1]

[1] That is, as dependent upon a superordinate whole.

" (2) In every instance of an actual psychophysical happening this is subject to a definite *complex of conditions*. To this belong :—

(*a*) the total retinal stimulus-configuration of the actual instance,

(*b*) relatively constant histological and material properties of the optical-somatic system,

(*c*) relatively variable conditioning factors which must be ascribed primarily to the rest of the nervous system, and secondarily to the vascular system. Just as in physical gestalten, so the psychophysical state periodically arising must be at every point altogether dependent upon these conditions, its local moments must therefore shape themselves in accordance with the *total* " topography ".

" (3) When constant conditions, and a state independent of the time factor are taken for granted, it follows from (1) that the *totality of the extended process represents an objective unity* (not in anyway one that can be assembled arbitrarily, for a particular observer only). For no local moment in the entire territory is completely autonomous or indifferent over against the state of any other region. *The spatial coherence of the psychophysical event which corresponds to a given visual field, has therefore a super-geometrical, that is, dynamically real, constitution.*

" (4) As in the case of physical gestalten, here too the physically real unity of what is configured does not amount to undifferentiated merging or confusion, but is fully compatible with rigorous articulation. The nature of the articulation depends upon the specific nature of the psychophysical event, and the conditions, at the time, of the system. But in every case, for *every actual complex of conditions, the super-geometrical, dynamical articulation of the event is just as much a physically real property of the larger territory as, for instance, the psychophysical colour reactions at one point of the field.*

" (5) In common with all inorganic physical gestalten, the psychophysical ones will have the following *gradations* of inner coherence throughout the system. The moments in the smallest area are indeed in principle dependent upon the conditions of the *whole* system, but according to a scale of a distance function of this kind : They are more powerfully determined by the conditioning forms of an associated area and its vicinity than by the topography of remote areas. In the extreme case (as with physical gestalten) the *detailed* articulation of limited areas is no longer noticeably dependent upon the *formal details* of other areas ; but then it is only that the " total moments " of such areas are determined to a greater extent in their own right. (Distinction between strong and weak gestalt coherence.) As far as spatial articulation or structure is concerned, therefore, such limited and immediately cohering areas can be relatively autonomous—without detriment to the gestalt coherence of the whole system, in accordance with which the total moments are nevertheless still determined, and thus represent, in a very real sense, *more narrowly circumscribed units within the unitary total happening.* No incongruity is to be apprehended here, for as long as the general presupposition is not lost sight of, namely, that the event in the *whole* system manifests gestalt coherence, such units more narrowly circumscribed in themselves may also (as earlier in the inorganic sphere) without ado be designated spatial gestalten.

" (6) However the spatial articulation of psychophysical gestalten may otherwise be constituted, it at any rate certainly also denotes the specific mode of disposition of an *intensity* of a state or happening, and hence of spatial energy densities. Under suitable conditions, the energy densities of the separate subdivisions of the system can be extraordinarily varied. But this, too, is decided by the conditions of the system *as a whole.*" (Cited after Köhler, 1920, p. 189 f.)

Thus far the direct definitions which Köhler lays down for the psychophysical happening.

Now comes the question, what is accomplished by these? To decide this, Köhler enquires to what extent points of agreement exist between these properties of the somatic regions, and the definitions considered to be distinctive of the phenomenal structures.

Once more, in the following paragraphs, Köhler formulates with customary sharpness, in what peculiar characteristics, briefly summarized, the essence of phenomenal gestalten consists. He concludes that (pp. 191–2) :—

" (i) Phenomenal optical fields appear as unities cohering in themselves, and always have super-geometrical properties. Single phenomenal subdivisions never appear completely indifferent, as substantive 'parts'. Thus they correspond to *moments* of the physical gestalt.

" (ii) The phenomenal unity is compatible with organization and structure; and the specific unity of the phenomenal field (correlate of the physical structural state) represents a super-summative property of the field of vision, to which the same experiential reality pertains as e.g. to the colour effects of the field.

" (iii) Without detriment to the unity of the field as a whole, there appear in it phenomenal units of limited areas, which are especially firmly circumscribed in themselves and relatively independent, as opposed to the rest of the field.

" (iv) In particular, vivid, close-knit areas, 'gestalten' in the narrower sense, are wont to segregate themselves clearly from the rest of the optical field which appears as 'mere background', provided that the given stimulus-complex satisfies certain conditions" (pp. 191-2).

A comparison of these with theses (1)-(6) forthwith reveals extensive correspondence between them. Thus the first object Köhler had set himself is attained. In his opinion it proves to be possible to define the neurophysical gestalten "from the starting point of physics" on general grounds; and this to the extent that their "intrinsic similarity" to the phenomenal gestalten seems assured.

Köhler's theory, therefore, seems to be equal to its task in a pre-eminent manner. Through the substitution of the theory of a spontaneous self-articulation of the neurophysical system for that of the conduction mechanism, those very definitions of the neurophysical events emerge, which are required in order to regard the phenomenal gestalten as being physiologically represented in their specific, characteristic properties — i.e. as being "explained".

§ 26. *Köhler's line of argument in the light of the critical conclusions in connection with our characterization of distribution systems*

To be able to appraise Köhler's deductions as to their import, we briefly recapitulate, once more, their conceptual construction. The way they proceed can readily be reviewed.

First of all comes the demonstration that in the neurophysical region we have, in his view, to reckon with a unitary, closed, total system. To this a simple subsumption is attached : If the happening in the neurophysical sector displays itself to be an event in a closed, coherent system, then the properties of physical systems, of physical gestalten, pertain to it as a matter of course. It is immediately evident that, as regards this line of argument, the conclusions reached in our first critical considerations may not be neglected.

It has a definite significance for Köhler when, on the ground of such a subsumption, he makes statements about the properties of the neurophysical happening; for the "physical gestalten" are "realities" to him, realities of the same sort as physical *thing*-concepts in general.

We have had to emphasize, in opposition to this, that what Köhler means by his concept of the physical gestalten, as regards its physical operation, ought throughout to be interpreted only in the sense of a *functional* relationship, in accordance with the character of functional concepts, and this has the effect of rendering the above line of argument questionable as it stands. For, if we take whatsoever may be distinguished as "gestalt-like" in any particular "physical system", its content is, according to this view, not determined in its material form in virtue of the fact that we know that we are dealing with a "physical gestalt". This content becomes tangible only at the moment when we can define more closely, in a *physical way*, and on the basis of its "material nature", that context of action within which the "physical gestalt" "constitutes" itself.

Thus Köhler's contentions lose all their force of proof. On the other hand, our conclusions, too, have only a limited application. We may not by any chance as yet infer that Köhler's physiological affirmations can be rejected *a limine*. We were compelled, it is true, to reject a gestalt physics in Köhler's ontological sense. We could not acknowledge the gestalt concept as a constitutive principle in physics. But this does not amount to a proof that a way cannot perchance lead from physics, along a path through physiology, to phenomenal gestalten. For Köhler was correct on one point: Even if the physical manifestations in distribution systems must always be looked upon as interrelationships of action, they yet retain, in their actual occurrence, a quite specific "gestalt sort" of character, and in a super-geometrical, dynamical sense to boot, as opposed to other physical manifestations. (See above, § 23.)

In consequence, Köhler's theses (1)–(6) (see above, p. 91–3) still remain *possible in respect to their content* even from our point of view, although we cannot in principle acknowledge the concept of a "physical gestalt" as a primary reality. But if these theses are acceptable as materially possible, the proof of their actual *applicability* within the special conditions of the neurophysical sector, *can only be achieved in a quite different way* from that which Köhler essays in the discussions we have mentioned.

If physical "structures"—"physical gestalten" if you will—are scientifically to be interpreted only as functional coherences, based on quite concrete relationships in the interdependence of action of their "moments", they can receive positive definition, as to their material content, only upon a double foundation: Firstly, upon the basis of definite knowledge about the *laws of action of the "material"* which, in its reciprocal action, in its mutual interaction, regulates the building up of that which is gestalt-like; secondly, upon the basis of a definite elucidation of the periodically underlying "conditioning topography" through which, just because of those interdependences of action, the "gestalt-like distribution" ensues, and to which crucial significance for the "so-being" of the consequent distribution must be attributed.

Without a closer consideration of these two factors the conclusions of any discussions of this sort cannot be deemed worthy of examination from a critical point of view.

We turn at once, therefore, to the task thus set, by following out how Köhler attempts to define the neurophysical event directly in the concrete.

3. KÖHLER'S CONCRETE DETAILED PROPOSITIONS IN RESPECT TO THE "MATERIAL NATURE" OF THE NEUROPHYSICAL PROCESSES AND THEIR "CONDITIONING TOPOGRAPHY"

§ 27. *The basic material definitions of the psychophysical processes, as formulated by Köhler, in their theoretical scope*

Köhler's theory of the neurophysical processes on the material side links up, in its basic hypotheses, with G. E. Müller and Nernst, and then develops from that point into a new and individual form of substantiation of the gestalt theory.

Köhler borrows his first argument from theorems which G. E. Müller has introduced as fundamental in psychology, in his theory of colour processes. *Müller's axiom* is that the antagonistic colour processes are to be thought of as being, from the material point of view, the two mutually opposed directions of a reversible *chemical reaction*. The nature of this is such that the state of the somatic field is characterized by defining the momentarily present stationary condition which institutes itself in a state of equilibrium, in such a transformation.

To accomplish his purpose Köhler associates another axiom with that of Müller. This can be described as the *Nernst axiom*. It is the assumption that in the nervous system the medium of solution of the various substances involved is water, and that, therefore, in the neurophysical happening we are concerned with chemical reactions in dilute solutions, in which *ions* participate.

From the teachings of physical chemistry, it is possible fully to envisage what follows from these presuppositions. As soon as one accepts this definition of the state of excitation, it turns out to be "at all times adequately determined by the concentrations of the types of molecules, and also ions, reacting", in accordance with the theory of electrolytic solution systems.

The elucidation of the states in the somatic sector reduces merely to a consideration of the multiplicity of, in the first instance only stationary, ionic reactions thus possible.

It cannot be denied that there is, in fact, a great deal to be said for this view, for it has, of course, been sustained elsewhere in the physiological elucidation of the stimulus processes, in particular since Nernst has advanced analogous opinions in regard to the physiology of stimulation. Indeed, when it is asserted that the neurophysical current must be regarded as electro-chemical in nature, as ionic movement, this view can be accepted, on the basis of electro-physiological experimentation, as more than merely hypothetical.

The essential point, as far as we are concerned, is how Köhler comes from this starting point to discover the configuratedness which is such an urgent problem for him on the phenomenal side, to be concretely represented on the physiological side.

He arrives at this by following up directly and in detail the (photochemical) "control" of the neurophysical electrolytic processes by the stimuli. These processes are discussed as being under the influence of :—

(1) A stimulus action everywhere homogeneous.

(2) A stimulus action inhomogeneous in the various parts of the field.

For the *completely homogeneously excited field*, it is a very simple matter to determine the physical condition. The chemical reaction must have a like course in all parts. The entire somatic field is in itself perfectly homogeneous as regards the concentration of its components, as well as the ionic distribution.

Now for the second case, the *inhomogeneously excited field* :—

" If the sensory surface is stimulated in a spatially inhomogeneous way, but at every point constantly for a time, then dissimilar stationary reactions take place in different parts of the associated nervous field. For the sake of simplicity we shall assume, to begin with, that *only two large areas* on the sensory surface, *of different stimulational nature*, are concerned ; and that these are contiguous along an unspecified but continuous curve. Then two different stationary reactions will take place in the nervous field in two corresponding regions, and the two partial nervous fields likewise meet along a constant curve. Differing stationary reactions are characterized by concentrations of reacting types of molecules which are unequal, at least in part. But the osmotic pressure of each kind of molecule is a simple function of the concentration of this substance itself (in dilute solutions directly proportional to the concentration). Thus there arises a *difference of osmotic pressures along the whole boundary-curve between the two areas.*

If only electrically neutral molecules were present on both sides, there would as a result arise, in brief periods, only a minimal diffusion current of the substances unequally concentrated in different regions. But if, as in the nervous system, reactions in which ions participate are essentially concerned, and if the ionic concentrations are not perfectly equal in the two areas of different reactions, there will at once arise, along the whole boundary-curve, a *difference of electrostatical potential* " (Köhler, 1920, p. 16).

From this, therefore, the *somatic state of affairs* appears to be quite comprehensible as being *dependent in a well-defined way upon the stimulus conditions.* It is characterized by the fact that the areas of different stimulation show themselves to be exactly delimited in the somatic region, and this in a physically real manner, by the occurrence of this sort of potential difference.

Herewith Köhler has apparently achieved a great deal already in regard to the problem of a *theory of phenomenal, or psychophysical gestalten.*

The *inner coalescence* of phenomenal gestalten, their segregation from one another, in brief, the "intrinsic articulation " of the phenomenal field, appears to be physiologically directly represented, in the optical as in all other sensory provinces. For example, " nervous fields which are excited by pressure, pain, and temperature stimuli, manifest electromotive forces when partial areas of the total sensory surface are stimulated, or when the modes of stimulation of mutually contiguous areas differ." Hence :—

" Every contour in the field of touch corresponds to a leap in potential (or a steep fall in potential). And if, for instance, a closed surface or the points of a compass are pressed against the skin, then the area of excitation of an associated nervous field is segregated everywhere from the bounding area, that is, as a circumscribed enclosure, by a difference of electrical potential."

Thus the phenomenal *significance of contours* seems to be happily comprehended within the framework of this electrolytical theory. It is true that from the time of Panum the fact has been known that contours in the optic field are more than simple " curves ", that they " have a special functional significance " which appears clearly in e.g. the phenomena of retinal rivalry (" contour-prevalence "). But now, in addition to this, a direct co-ordinate in the physiological happening seems to have been theoretically obtained, in so far as the corresponding localities are physically distinguished by a very real factor, the potential discontinuity.

It looks, therefore, as if the point has already been reached where a rounded-off picture of the physiological happening, one adequately adapted to the purpose of " explaining " gestalt-articulation, can be constructed quite in detail, built up " from beneath ". But this picture does not remain wholly unclouded, for many of the detailed deductions which Köhler forthwith adds cannot be accepted without objection.

Köhler, in some places, tries to reach " inferences " *somewhat rashly*, as is shown, for example, by the way in which, from this as point of departure, he presently gives a " derivation " for the emergence of " plastic " through " binocularly perceived gestalten ".[1] But apart from such extensions attached to the original propositions, these *propositions themselves still involve important difficulties*, taken in the framework of the whole problem of a physiological theory of gestalt perception. The theorem itself, and Köhler's application of it, are concerned primarily only with the conditions in the *actual sensory surface—* i.e. in optics, with the conditions of the retina.

The crucial question, however, really lies elsewhere. It does not refer to the conditions in the retina or the sensory surface at all, but to the conditions in that zone of the neurophysical sector to which phenomenal facts directly correspond ; that is, to conditions in the actual " psychophysical zone ".

Even if such an internal organization of the happening

---

[1] Observe how he all at once arrives at ascribing a " parallactic displacement " to potential differences (cf. Köhler, p. 27)—and this, too, is supposed to be a concept formed, or a mode of explanation, " from the starting point of physics " !

can be granted for one boundary surface of the neurophysical system on the basis of the hypothesized electrolytical schema, as the purpose of the theory demands, nothing has thus been made out in regard to the *higher neurophysical levels*; for Köhler as a matter of principle rejects the " machine-like " projection of the retinal circumstances by means of isolated conduction mechanisms, and is committed, in place of it, to his principle of a *freely propagated distribution of electrolytical structures throughout the entire extent of the longitudinal section.*

How such a " freely propagated distribution " can be conceived " from beneath ", extracted from the electrolytical theorem in such a way as to give the theory a real finality—this will be the touchstone of the whole of Köhler's physiology.

§ 28. *The supplementary definitions necessary for the comprehension of the higher neurophysical levels, and their empirical physiological admissibility* .

The question now is how the connection between the peripheral and the central " cross-sections " of the neurophysical sector are to be concretely conceived. Köhler makes very exact statements about this. He sees his way to defining quite precisely how the neurophysical happening is constituted, e.g. when a plain white circular disc on a grey background is presented as stimulus.

In this example there is *retinally* present, according to the foregoing discussion, a quite definite, configured " excitation distribution ", which can be designated " symmetrical "—" circle-wise ". On this basis, now, a " gestalt " is *phenomenally* experienced, which likewise exhibits this gestalt feature of " symmetrical-circularity ".

From this Köhler infers that the retinally located symmetry is preserved—on the whole, at all events [1]— right through the entire neurophysical sector up to the phenomenal sphere.

This Köhler regards as a *new* genuine *proof* of the correspondence (" parallelism ") between phenomenal and

[1] That is, irrespective of those " normal " deviations, for example, which arise with vision in markedly extra-foveal stimulus-situations, and also as a result of the normal differences between the vertical and horizontal extensions of the field of vision. (Cf. Köhler, p. 231 ff.)

H

psychophysical gestalten which he upholds—a proof which is above all independent of that previously considered (§§ 26–7). This is what he says, *verbatim*:—

"The psychophysical happening, in the case of a symmetrical gestalt perception, is thus bound to have corresponding super-geometrical properties of symmetry, not, perchance, only for the reason that our fundamental viewpoint shows similarity in general, between optic-phenomenal gestalt and configured happening in the optic-somatic field, to be possible, and presupposes this to be primarily given ; indeed, it is the other way round. Because the super-geometrical, symmetry properties of the gestalt perception are otherwise unintelligible in their co-ordination to the geometrical symmetry of the stimulus-form, we must ascribe corresponding dynamical-functional symmetry to the psychophysical process, which can alone be the mediator of this simple co-ordination. And indeed, in this way, and in this special instance, we *discover once more* that phenomenal and psychophysical gestalten are similar to one another " (p. 234).

We " discover " this result. But in what way ? Clearly, here the methodological relation of the phenomenal and the physiological aspects are fundamentally transposed, by contrast with the original way of posing the question (see above, § 25). Instead of starting directly from what can be physically and physiologically postulated, the phenomenal is now taken as the point of departure, and the physiological pre-ordained to adapt itself accordingly !

At any rate, this is *by no means* still " *building up* " " *from the starting point of physics* " ! This Köhler himself admits. He confesses (p. 231) that a construction such as he originally promised to give, is not possible; for "we are not yet in the position to obtain an extensive knowledge of the relatively constant conditions of conduction, by means of morphological, micro-histological, or physiological research ". He accordingly formulates his own posing of the question for all enquiries, going into details along this line. He poses it in the form of the question: "*How must the conducting system be essentially constituted, in order that the physiological happening should, for any known retinal configuration, take on the structural properties which can be phenomenally observed ?*"

He can reasonably pose this new question, since he now believes it allowable to take it for granted, from his preceding discussions, that it is certainly "a configured happening in the optic sector which is at issue, and which follows the general laws of interrelated physical currents ". And again, the question becomes senseless, involves a vicious circle, if this assumption can no longer be acknowledged as secure.

If the verdict as to whether "gestalten" are or are not involved in the neurophysical happening is still pending, as is our view, then everything that Köhler advances on the basis of this new posing of the question, can lay no claim whatsoever to be of value as knowledge.

Our duty is, rather, to attempt somehow to make it possible actually to trace, directly "from the starting point of physics", whether and how, in spite of the pre-supposed freedom of propagation of the electrolytic processes, a *persistence of the cross-section structure* is possible in *the higher zones as well*. For only so, according to our contentions, can the real accuracy of Köhler's general characterization of the neurophysical happening possibly be retrogressively substantiated (cf. above, § 26, the end).

Definite statements in this connection, adapted to explain *how* such a relationship could allow of being constructed "from beneath", are not to be found in Köhler's discussion.

Our task is, therefore, now to scrutinize Köhler's electrolytical arguments sufficiently to be able to envisage clearly whether, and under what circumstances, an inter-relationship of action of this sort can be so built up, that when free propagation of the happening within the electrolytical system is assumed, the "full configuration" in the central parts of the field institutes itself in the required fashion.

Attempting this leads to a discovery at once : That if it has to be carried through with acceptance of the persistence of the "cross-section structure" (in the sense of a replica of the sensory field upon the neurophysical field) which Köhler tacitly assumes, a further assumption must be immediately added, one *about the "topography"* of the neurophysical longitudinal section.

If we assumed that the whole (say, optic) sector is

homogeneous from the periphery to the centre as far as its conduction conditions are concerned, as perhaps seems more than natural to Köhler, a quite undesired consequence would ensure.

The effect of the stimulus upon the sensory surface, and the electrolytical distribution in the zones superior to it, which must be conceived to arise subsequently through the electrolytical process according to the laws of diffusion, show a quite definite distribution picture (see Fig. 4). The difference in potential rising steeply in the retinal cross-section (concentrated at the " contour "), shows a diminishingly steep drop in the higher zones; the

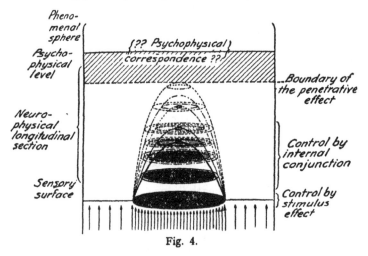

Fig. 4.

prominence, or otherwise demarcation, of the field becomes the less precise the farther one rises towards the central regions; finally, beyond a certain level in the neurophysical longitudinal section, nothing remains detectable of the changes at the receptory surface.

For the peripheral process to have the necessary " penetrating power ", so as to be able at all to become effective right up to the psychophysical cross-section, one has therefore to assume—as actually a *Köhler's axiom*—that the " *conductivity " in the neurophysical longitudinal section is distinctly greater than in the cross-section.*

This, and only this assumption, would enable one to conceive the *required " penetrative effect " as able to prevail beyond the sensory surface*, in connection with Köhler's hypothesis.

But this " Köhler's Axiom ", as it stands, runs counter to the general properties of the neurophysical substance. Direct physiological research has led to the view that, on the contrary, the conductivity is considerably less in the longitudinal section than in the cross-section. Hermann, for instance, concluded that this relationship could be estimated as $1 : 5$.[1] Köhler's presupposition is thus abolished ; for the true conditions are even less propitious for the persistence of the peripheral cross-section in the higher zones as well, than we presumed in our first test proposition (homogeneity in reference to the conduction capacity). (Cf. G. E. Müller.)

Accordingly, " Köhler's Axiom " must now be taken to be refuted. This finding suffices to decide our fundamental position.

4. CONCLUDING ASSESSMENT OF KÖHLER'S GESTALT PHYSIOLOGY

§'29. *The limits of Köhler's electro-physiological theory*

In summing up, one may say that Köhler's theory does not do justice to the requirements it sets before itself. Köhler's final object is to solve the *Wertheimer problem*. The *immediate physiological representation* of " phenomenal gestalten "—in the sense of the proposition " What is within is without "—must be *deduced*. Hence nothing more nor less is intended to be given than a *constructional proof of the correctness of psychophysical parallelism*.

This purpose is by no means attained.

(1) Köhler's actual main proof, which is cast in the form of a deduction of the definitions of psychophysical gestalten in terms of principles (see above, § 26) is not a proof.

It lacks all material content, since it presupposes as a fundamental assumption the acknowledgment of an

---

[1] G. E. Müller (1923) was the first to bring up this fact in opposition to Köhler's theory. But he did so without previously coming to terms with Köhler's physical presuppositions, and this alone really allows one to weigh up the above finding as a decisive point against Köhler, even along the lines of immanent criticism.

ontological significance of the gestalt concept for the physical processes involved; but this assumption cannot be accepted as vindicated.

(2) Köhler's deduction could only acquire material content if one were to reach similar conclusions from a direct consideration of the material nature and topography of physical processes. However, in this respect Köhler's arguments have likewise proved to be unsatisfactory :—

(a) Köhler's discussions in definition of *topography* on the contrary make it particularly clear how it is impossible to determiné physiological-psychophysical "gestalten" "from the starting point of physics", conclusively. They eventually lead to a position where that which has to be proved, viz. the correspondence of "phenomenal and physiological", is taken outright for granted in defining the topography.

This confounding of assumption and proof may not, for Köhler himself—just in so far as the deduction of this correspondence in terms of principles is accepted as already accomplished—appear so dangerous. But if the deduction in terms of principles depends upon the elucidations of material nature and topography for its yitality, then all the force of proof of Köhler's deliberations becomes illusory.

(b) What Köhler says in regard to the *material nature* of the psychophysical happening, in so far as it concerns the adoption of the Müller-Nernst axiom, proves to be physiologically possible and also to a large extent fertile, as a point of view. But it is not sufficient to provide a conclusive foundation for Wertheimer's thesis. The Müller-Nernst axioms as applied by Köhler, do not reach beyond the peripheral sphere, since the structure properties, which Köhler thus hypothesizes to be characteristic, are directly dependent upon the effects of the stimulus as "conditioning topography" of the retinal event. A persistence of retinal structure in the higher cross-sections too, as this should be made conceivable if the problem is to pass for solved, cannot be deduced. It would only be possible, under acknowledgment of Köhler's principle of the free self-articulation of all events in the neurophysical sector, if the conditions of conduction in the neurophysical substance were different from what they really are. The central problem, the persistence of the point-by-point arrangement from the retina up to the phenomenal sphere, can at all events not be solved along Köhler's line of thought.

On the whole, Köhler's attempt to " deduce " the phenomenal gestalten physiologically from the spontaneous self-articulation of the neurophysical process, must be deemed a failure,[1] as far as those methods of establishing principles and concrete facts are concerned, which were developed in connection with Köhler's discussion of " physical gestalten at rest and in a stationary state ".

But we have not yet reached the end of our consideration of this side of the gestalt theory. For it requires amplification, in view of the fact that Köhler has recently again dealt with the matter, and in a new form.

CHAPTER III

THE PROBLEM OF GESTALT PHYSIOLOGY IN KÖHLER'S *GESTALT PSYCHOLOGY* OF 1929, AND ITS APPRAISEMENT IN THE LIGHT OF A RECENT FUNDAMENTAL EXPERIMENT IN BIOLOGY

Köhler's extensive review of the gestalt theory, published in 1929 (*Gestalt Psychology*, Horace Liveright, New York); on the one hand, and, on the other, certain findings of experimental biology, have carried the appraisal of gestalt physiology to a new stage, beyond our preceding considerations.

---

[1] So also Becher, in his " popular " account, devoted to Köhler's theory (1921), has essentially weakened Köhler's treatment. By reducing the concept of gestalt to his own concept of " causal coherence " he has abolished the primary significance of the former. By further declaring insulated visual conduction paths for retina and central sphere to be indispensable for the connection, he has flatly rejected Köhler's notion of the free propagation of " lines of current " in the total field of the optic sector. At bottom he retains only that part of Köhler's contentions which follows directly from the Müller and Nernst axiom—everything that is " gestalt-theoretical " in the specific sense, is at bottom omitted by him.

An elucidation of the situation thus created, permits one to clarify the points of departure, and the tendencies of Köhler's ideas consonantly with the present position of research, far more comprehensively by immanent analysis than was possible before.[1] It permits one also to assess their significance and to confront them with empirical findings in regard to the specific facts of central nervous functioning.

I. GESTALT PHYSIOLOGY ACCORDING TO KÖHLER'S RECENT EXPOSITION. ITS PREMISSES AND PRINCIPLES

§ 30. *The general position of gestalt physiology in Köhler's* Gestalt Psychology *of* 1929

A comparison of Köhler's statements upon gestalt physiology in his previous publications with his train of thought in this latest book, clearly reveals a characteristic shift in outlook. The change here encountered may be briefly described as an emancipation from dogmatic deductivism.

The characteristic feature in the position of gestalt physiology in relation to the total endeavour of gestalt psychology, has hitherto been the following idea : It is possible to achieve a positive foundation for the reorientation that is being striven for in psychology, in distinctive fashion, by starting from beyond the field of psychology. A special " gestalt theoretical " province could be indicated in physics and the altogether unique doctrinal possibilities arising therefrom could be evaluated as to their bearing upon a new interpretation of nervous events.

Thus gestalt-physiology rested upon a special sanctioning of the gestalt concept as a basic category for the analysis of reality, derived from physics. Gestalt physiology provided directly "from beneath", from physics as starting point, in deductive form, free from any pre-judgment from the psychological side, exactly those definitions of the central nervous happening which were necessary if the gestalt-theoretical view were to be secure in its ultimate basis. Moreover, through this concurrence it lent a weight to the gestalt view, which was held to be the more valuable inasmuch as here the

[1] At the time the German edition of this book was published (1929).

peculiar intellectual dignity of the exact natural sciences could be advanced as a measure of comparative worth.

All of this is altered in the new exposition. The effort on behalf of gestalt physics appears to be altogether more subsidiary, occupies a less dominant position in the whole body of theoretical considerations. The idea that it is possible to establish the significance of the gestalt category by recourse to physics is no longer put forward, nor is any attempt made to build up a concrete physiology in a positive, deductive way from that starting point— one to which a gestalt character could be attributed as distinctive of its processes.

This attenuation of the claims as to the potentialities of gestalt-physiological views is too important to allow of being construed as fortuitous, or as a concession to extraneous circumstances. On the contrary, it obviously marks a process of transformation in the gestalt theory. To be sure, this process concerns only the manner of establishing a foundation for the theory. It is momentous enough, however, to necessitate an examination of the new situation thus produced. Let us review this new kind of foundation in more detail.

§ 31. *The gestalt physiology of* 1929, *and the principle of psychological isomorphism*

It is a point of considerable interest to realize how *the approach to gestalt physiology* is now sought. A general methodological discussion, intended to define the boundaries between the gestalt theory's position and behaviourism, breaks the ground. This, in reference to Köhler's positive purpose, is mainly preliminary and presents a negative orientation. Two crucial chapters follow, which may be looked upon as the theoretical nucleus of the whole book. The first, under the somewhat colourless and formal title " Psychology as a Young Science " (pp. 35–70), arising out of a critique of the behaviourists' scientific creed, with its two articles— limitation of the basis of enquiry to "objective" experi- mentation, and of the means of explanation to the associated concepts of " reflex " and " conditioned reflex " —presents the need for a fertile working hypothesis. " It is not probable that an observer looking upon human and animal behaviour without prejudices, would find reflexes and conditioned reflexes as the most natural, or as the only, types of function by which his observations might be explained."

The pivotal question emerges : " But how shall we find more productive concepts, if the gap between the observable stimulating environment and observable overt responses is as huge as we find it in the present stage of physiology ? . . . even the more recent discoveries about the all or none law and the metabolism in nervous activity do not give us just that basis which we need for our purposes."

This basis is then established in a very characteristic manner, that is, in an axiomatic, wittingly hypothetical, manner.

At the outset of his positive considerations, Köhler sets his course expressly in the direction of physiology (p. 60).

The ultimate point of departure for every scientific apprehension of " reality " he considers to be what he calls " direct experience ". This is the " raw material of both physics and psychology " ; and in his opinion, therefore, psychological theory is concerned with making the transition from the given characteristics of " direct experience " to corresponding characteristics of " concomitant physiological processes ".

In order to be able to accomplish this transition, however, he commences with a *general leading principle*, that of *psychophysical isomorphism*. This is the assumption that a co-ordination exists between the domain of the experiences and that of the physiological processes, each regarded as a systematic order, and that it is a co-ordination in the sense of congruence or isomorphism in regard to their systematic properties.

The introduction of this conception is based directly on Hering and on G. E. Müller's " psychophysical axioms ". He thereupon proceeds to apply the conception immediately in specific examples. His first example is the problem of the intensity of sound.

" A sound of given qualitative properties is produced in various degrees of experienced intensity or loudness. The systematic order of all these different experienced intensities may be represented by a straight line, which means that following that order, we have the impression of moving continually in the same direction. What may correspond to loudness in the underlying processes ? The principle decides that whatever the concrete nature of those processes, the physiological fundaments of all the experienced degrees of loudness must show the same order as these show themselves, i.e. that of a straight line. More especially : If a definite loudness is situated between two other loudnesses in the systematic order of experiences, the process corresponding to the first shall be between the processes corresponding to the two others in the order of underlying physiological events. That gives the congruence or isomorphism between the two systems " (p. 62).

Köhler believes it possible directly to utilize the argument here applied, still more comprehensively, " in a much more general, and at the same time much more concrete, form than either Hering or Müller would have done." He correctly insists that Hering and Müller referred the principle merely " to the *logical* order in which we arrange certain experiences after abstracting them from their context, and judging about their similarities ". It merely requires the assumption of a multitude of possibilities of variation within the psychophysical happening, which is not less in its dimensions than the empirically demonstrable multitude of variations within the sphere of experience.

Köhler, however, wishes to apply the principle in a new way, to the " real concrete order of experiences which is itself experienced ". As a first application, he sets down how, from such a viewpoint, he conceives a verdict should be reached on the *space problem.*

" At this moment I have before me three white points on a black surface, one in the middle of the field and the others in symmetrical positions on both sides of the centre one. This, is an order again ; not an abstract, logical order, but a concrete, experienced order. As experienced it depends upon physiological processes in my organism, so that some feature of a physiological function must correspond to it. And applied to this concrete order our principle says that correlated with the visually experienced symmetry there is an homologous symmetry of dynamic context in the underlying processes. Or in the same example : One point is seen *between* the others, this relation being experienced exactly as the white of the point is. Again in the underlying processes there must be something functional which corresponds to that 'between'. Applied to the *concrete* order our principle claims that the experienced 'between' is accompanied by a functional 'between' in the concrete dynamic context of concurrent physiological events. If the principle is applied strictly to *all* cases of spatial order in experience, it will lead to the general statement that *all experienced order in space is a true representation of a corresponding order in the underlying dynamical context of physiological processes*" (p. 64).

Thus, to begin with, the space problem is for the time being in principle settled.

Five pages follow in which the outlines of an analogous physiological theory are similarly developed for temporal order, for the experiences of order in the "belonging together" or closure of objective units, and for the articulation and orderliness of language processes.

He writes : "The temporal position of one experience as 'between' two others is frequently experienced in the same way that spatial 'betweenness' is. Now as far as it is experienced, time must have a functional correlate in underlying physiological processes no less than experienced space. . . . And . . . we will arrive at the proposition that *experienced order in time is a true representation of the corresponding concrete order in the underlying dynamical context*" (p. 65). This is simply a straightforward application of the basic principle.

Furthermore, "more order is experienced than that of space and time. Certain experiences 'belong together' in a concrete manner, whereas others do not, or at least, belong together less intimately. And again this 'belonging together' may be experienced itself. . . . In this case our principle applied formulates the proposition that *to a context, experienced as 'one thing' belonging together, there corresponds a dynamical unit or whole in the underlying physiological processes*" (p. 66).

Reviewing all that is here laid down, we reach the following conclusion. We are, in the first place, here confronted with a procedure which leads to nothing but purely formal pronouncements about the physiological happening. Moreover, it proves to be a procedure which can in fact lead to nothing but "propositions". All these considerations "*prove*" *nothing* in principle. The actual nucleus of what Köhler calls his theory—or else, obviously moderating the word intentionally, his "working hypothesis"—that is, the tenet of fundamental psychophysical isomorphism, consists *in no way in "considerations"*, but merely in a *variety of formulations of a petitio principii.*

The only thing that seems to give these enunciations any sort of real content, is the word "dynamical context", which represents the physiological happening itself. But even this does not, on the face of it, offer anything more than a word. What connotation the word has is, from the outset, vague and undefined. And the manner in which Köhler has made positive use of this word in another connection (cf. below, § 54 ff., § 58 ff.) is not calculated to arouse any special confidence, from the outset.

It is necessary to enquire more fully, in what sense a closer definition of what we have just expounded may ensue, in the further course of the argument, at the point occupying us here.

§ 32. *The gestalt physiology of* 1929, *and the principle of dynamical self-distribution*

When we turn to the relevant concrete utterances of Köhler upon what he subsumes under the general caption of "dynamical", we discover, once again, the long familiar formulas which previously appeared in connection with the corresponding examination of the domain of physical facts. But these formulas now also stand in new—and indeed more carefully weighed—relationships.

They appear here exclusively in the framework of the antithesis between "machine theory" and "dynamical theory". Köhler finally develops his physiological views from the starting point of this antithesis, and he illustrates it by examples from physics itself.

The total aspect is thus essentially altered. There are no longer, as Köhler originally would have it, two kinds of physics, a "usual" one of the atomistic-elementary operations of forces, and another one of different categorical structure, viz. a physics of gestalten. This conception, formerly made the avowed basis of his entire point of view by Köhler (cf. *supra*) is now simply passed over in silence.

Only one feature which had been basic to this former distinction is substantially retained, but in a new form Köhler frames all his considerations upon the basic thesis that it is possible to characterize every physical fact according as it is determined, in greater or less degree, on the one hand by " limiting topographical conditions ", and on the other by " the play of actual forces ".

In detail, he develops this as follows (cf. p. III ff.) : " In physical processes we find two sorts of factors determining events at every moment. In the first class belong the actual forces of the process itself ; they represent the *dynamical* side of it. In the second class we have those properties of the system which may be regarded as *constant conditions* of its events." (Where these constant conditions may be either material properties like the charge of an electron, or the conditions of the conductor, i.e. topographical conditions ; and where either the one or the other of these two kinds of constant conditions of the system can *de facto* determine the total state more or less predominantly. An example of the preponderant influence of the topography is the " piston's motion strictly confined between the walls of the cylinder ", a case where " nothing but the motion as such is determined dynamically . . . whereas its direction is strictly enforced by topographical arrangement ".)

Such propositions, in Köhler's opinion, lead to the following inference, which is entirely sound :—

" This leads to a *classification of physical systems* which is decisive for our problem. In all of them the process is to be regarded as necessarily determined, but among the various cases we find enormous differences in the relative influence which *limiting topographical conditions*, on the one hand, and the play of *actual forces* on the other, exert upon the course of events."

This observation is a matter of essential consequence to Köhler. For it permits him to demonstrate how those specific " one way processes " which are in current nerve physiology reckoned as the sole issue, merely represent a very small section of the entire range of possibilities which must actually be taken into account, physically speaking.

His observations become particularly impressive, in

that he reminds us how such a state of affairs in nerve physiology can be directly compared with very primitive, long vanquished forms of explanation in physics. He refers to Aristotle and Descartes. " It is the same idea which occurs to Aristotle when he views the remarkable order of celestial movement. His spheres are topographical conditions enforcing that order. And since Descartes neurologists have worked with the same concepts wherever they have dealt with orderly organic function in higher animals and in man." [1]

He is anxious to prove one particular idea by means of these considerations. This is the idea that an orderly physical event can be attained not only through parallel and serial circuits of " one-way-processes " of the stated sort ; but that on the other hand, physical systems are equally possible which have, to put it briefly, various and infinitely numerous degrees of freedom; and that rigorous determination of the details, and hence orderliness and organization, obtain in such systems too, in " free " self-articulation of a " dynamic " nature.

All of this, however, as we immediately perceive, proves nothing more than the *possibility* that such a solution of the problem could, in certain eventualities, be taken into account.

Köhler now quite lucidly proceeds *a step further* showing anew that the pure machine theory of central and peripheral nervous co-ordination is by no means so clear and so well-rounded, as is commonly assumed.

Taking his stand on the viewpoint thus developed, he describes the rejected theory as follows. Like the Aristotelian sphere theory of the movement of the heavens, this theory traces all effects to anatomical arrangements functioning *ad hoc.* These are, firstly, primarily inborn, " pre-established machine arrangements " ; and secondly —taking into account the phenomena of learning, habit formation, etc.—secondarily acquired arrangements, where these very arrangements are assumed to be directly adapted for the appropriate point-by-point retention of organization in the successive neurophysical levels.

---

[1] Lewin has elaborated this observation in a fairly full historico-systematic study, where he describes and evaluates the contrast between the Aristotelian and the Galilean point of view from this standpoint. (Cf. *Erkentniss*, vol. ii, 1931.)

Köhler advances four arguments against the utility of such a theory, two general and to some extent formal ones, and two empirical ones, of concrete import.

The first deals with what would follow on the assumption that the schema of the absolute one-way-aggregate be actually conceived as perfectly satisfied. "How empty and dead does the organism appear in this theory . . . an indifferent stage for actors indifferent to the stage, as well as to each other." Such would be the state of affairs, on this assumption. Merely to envisage it is tantamount to revealing its inherent improbability. According to it, a soap bubble would be a more complicated unit than the entire nervous happening.

The second argument refers to the fact that in the concrete elaboration of the theory the absolute isolation of the single, to begin with atomistically substituted, "one-way-processes", is not really preserved. "Mutual influences" are introduced, which are, on the whole, always conceived in accordance with the schema of the concept of irradiation. But this is essentially dangerous. For the object of the theory, viz., the explanation of the retention of organization throughout all the levels of the psychophysical happening, is thus seriously called in question, since mutual influences of such a kind must inevitably result in more or less far-reaching disturbances being sustained by the ordered distribution—in "interfusion", that is.

The third argument concerns the facts known about special self-regulation, which ostensibly transcend purely elementary regulation. The *constancy* in the phenomena of brightness and size with *varying retinal situations*, and conversely, the fact of the dependence of what is experienced upon attitude, when the stimulus constellation remains fixed, similarly prove, according to Köhler, that pure elementary automata do not suffice, once the difficulties in the "meaning theory" of the cited phenomena have been perceived (see above, § 5).

The fourth argument embraces all the facts which show, in any way whatever, that "local processes depend upon sets of stimuli in a bigger field of our visual sector". As far as observation goes the properties of local stimulation do not simply determine the size, the form, the localization and the brightness of local experience. So also all the " well-known illusions " can be adduced—such as the familiar phenomena of colour-contrast and the numerous experimental devices which have become known through the researches of the gestalt theoretical school.

The situation, in the train of reasoning we are discussing, reached by all these considerations—in parentheses we may note, none of them worked out in much detail even by Köhler himself—is now as follows : It has been shown how little adequacy the atomistic theory of the " one-way-aggregate " really has, how little satisfied one can actually be with the theoretical apparatus hitherto current, the apparatus of "inherited machine arrangements " and "secondarily acquired arrangements " to which the rejected theory resorts.

But—what positive achievement does this represent ?

The question as to whether there is really a *third positive alternative* or not has not yet been adumbrated at all. It is only the more emphatically implied, presented as a task, the more Köhler has succeeded in demonstrating that the current ways of looking at the matter are problematical.

His proceeding in this manner gives a great advantage to Köhler's exposition. He himself puts forward quite clearly the question : " If we are not satisfied by the alternative between order enforced by pre-established arrangements and order determined by acquired arrange-ments, what else can produce order ? " (p. 133). And then, with lucidly marshalled precision in the further development of his conceptions, he produces the answer to this question—within the framework of the statements of the particular facts already known to us in their content.

The formulation of this answer is based on physics ; on the previously developed ascertainment that in physics besides the " one-way-systems " characteristic of the " little world of man-made machines ", " there exists an immense world of other physical systems in which the direction of processes is not completely determined by topographical arrangements."

Indeed, there can be no doubt that in millions of instances of natural physical systems " not only movement or process as such (as in the one-way machines, e.g. steam engines) but also the direction and distribution of process is determined by interaction " through the internal control of the forces between the separate particles (cf. above our examples, §§ 9–11 ; § 18 ff.).

The special point in Köhler's line of thought is the emphasis he lays upon the possibility of order explicitly emerging here in a clear-cut way. He shows that this is possible by reference to numerous examples, e.g. the order in astronomical movement, the order in the configuration of the atom, the order in the alignment of electrical currents through mutual dynamical interaction, the order in the structural formation of a drop of oil, freely floating in a liquid with which it does mix, which conglobates into a sphere under the influence of the forces of surface tension.

From these examples he deduces his basic thesis : " Dynamical interaction, undisturbed by accidental impacts from without, leads to orderly distribution, though there are no special pre-established arrangements " (p. 139).

To prove this thesis he resorts to an observation by Mach, who has emphasized apropos of this that, " In orderly and regular distributions the totality of internal stresses will be more balanced than in a state of disorder." For indeed every change in the system ensues on the basis of the internal forces, either in the direction towards equilibrium, or in that of a stationary state. And if Mach's general formulation has any justification, then an orderly distribution must emerge as a result.

Köhler thus arrives at the *general result* : " Dynamical self-distribution is the third kind of functional concept which I propose to add to psychological theory, in addition to distribution enforced by inherited arrangements and order determined by acquired arrangements " (p. 140).

Thus the framework for his own theory of nervous processes has been achieved. Though, to be sure, it appears rather as a general possibility than as a concrete theory. But this, of course, is from one point of view decidedly a source of strength. Methodically, too, the procedure characteristic of it is at any rate essentially more satisfactory than the seemingly more concrete and definite one which we entered into in connection with Köhler's book on *Die physischen Gestalten in Ruhe und im stationären Zustand.*

One point is certainly significant, for critical reflection ; and this must now be brought to the fore. The thesis of Mach cited above will have to be very clearly envisaged, as to its intrinsic import, and as to the manner in which it attains importance in Köhler's disquisition, if one wishes to assess the line of argument justly in accordance with its import. For this thesis is actually the major premise upon which Köhler's entire discussion depends, in spite of its being disguised by many examples.

If we take the observation as it stands, as it has been developed up to this point, no one will be able to make any objection to it. That " order " emerges with the inner equalization of the forces of the system by means of self-regulation, must indeed be admitted.

The essential point for the application Köhler forthwith makes of this, is the question as to what is understood by the term " order ".

To be able to grasp this pivotal point of the set of problems, we must go farther and trace out what the concrete aim of the whole thing is ; we must see how Köhler advances towards the *direct application* of his considerations to the *nervous happening*.

Here again the whole thing seems to proceed quite simply and without difficulties. Only a simple transference of what has previously been developed, for example, to the events in the visual sector, seems necessary.

Thus there immediately emerges the proposition : " From this viewpoint the processes underlying the visual field in a state of *rest* represent the *equilibrated distribution of sensory dynamics* under actually given conditions." And, he continues : " When *not at rest*, sensory dynamics will be in a state of *developing dynamical distribution* " [1] (p. 140).

He continues the consideration of this proposition suggestively rather than otherwise. So that the electro-physiological theory, which we have previously been led to distinguish as the nucleus of Köhler's doctrine, now merely appears as one of the " particular assumptions

---

[1] Here it remains an open question whether this self-distribution arises in peripheral nerves already, or only beyond the area striata, which then functions to some extent as a sort of "central retina", forming the starting point for the establishment of the self-distribution, whereas the transmission may be " a matter of isolated pathways " up to that point (p. 141).

concerning process, force, and interaction, to be made for the course of the theory ", in order that a more detailed mode of explanation may be possible. This theory is thus very distinctly curtailed in its claims. Köhler himself says that these particular assumptions are not regarded by him as specially important, that he is concerned rather with the basic thesis alone, the thesis of self-regulation through dynamical interaction, in general. It is thus actually entirely barred from criticisms—by means of the explicit warning " that all the perplexities we may find in our way and all the mistakes we may make in its course are not to be referred to the fundamental concept of self-distribution by interaction ", and the tacitly implied idea that all such difficulties would consequently have a merely subsidiary significance, and could not be used to test the theory in its essence.

Nevertheless, we cannot ignore the details, when we reflect upon the matter critically. For only in this connection does it become manifest whether the theory can be brought into function concretely, or whether it offers merely a new general formula, the application of which is still at issue.

Here two questions arise, relevant to the preservation of organization through the distinguishable levels of the central nervous system, in the sense in which the concept of organization is of importance to Köhler in this connection. There is, firstly, the question of the circumscription of the separate areas of the field, typified e.g. in the phenomenal delimitation of figure from ground ; and there is the second question as to how the properties—i.e. the totality of differentiating characteristics—of such a figure, such as its symmetry, etc., can be preserved throughout the conductor.

In regard to the first question, a consideration arises which we have not hitherto encountered, seeing that the question has not hitherto been posed in the physiological discussion. Here it is explicitly raised with reference to physiological dynamics : " How can one set of processes remain detached from the rest in dynamical theory ? "

We immediately observe that this question directly touches upon our previous consideration in § 28, where we were led to conclude that, on Köhler's assumptions, and having regard to the constitution of nervous substance, the delimitations are not transmitted beyond a certain critical boundary stratum. Let us look at what Köhler has to say to this.

We are given an astonishing answer. We discover that nothing in the way of definitive presuppositions as to processes, forces, dynamical uniformities, etc., is made the basis of his considerations. On the contrary, the solution ensues simply by way of an *ad hoc* assumption, resting upon a mere superficially adduced analogy.

Köhler's actual words are the following : " Generally processes corresponding to a definitely colored area will have definite properties as a class of processes, different from the properties of a class of surrounding processes which corresponds to another color. They will remain segregated in the nervous network if we suppose that in the ganglionic fields where they ' touch ' each other, their differenial properties provide *separating forces of contact*, so that they mutually exclude each other." And in support of this observation, he continues : " Take as an example the contact of oil and water. Here interaction is so strong that the form of the surface is determined by it ; but this surface as such remains a sharp boundary and the drop of oil remains detached from the water by those same molecular forces. . . . I shall assume, then, that, in optical processes, contours are preserved by *similar* forces of antagonistic contact, depending upon differences in the properties on the two sides of the contour " (pp. 143–4).

Such a solution of the problem must of course be most emphatically rejected. It is not enough that the corresponding "separating forces of contact" are simply assumed without more ado ; in addition, by referring to the oil and water example he makes it appear as if the phenomenon in question were something quite simple and self evident. This, of course, can in nowise be entertained until a justification for the analogy is truly provided, on the ground of the material nature, and the laws of action, which one proposes as the substructure of the nervous event.

Thus critical reflection makes it clear how Köhler is here already transgressing the bounds of scientific responsibility.

The same holds good for his observations on the second

of the above-mentioned special questions, that of the preservation of gestalt differentia in nervous organization. It is treated in a manner familiar to us. The example of Köhler's colour disc, which we shall discuss more fully hereafter (§ 42) is brought up once again, with the object of showing that there is nothing to be astonished at, if e.g. the property of symmetry of the circle is indeed preserved, in this dynamical self-distribution, on the way from the retina to the cerebral centre.

This reasoning is of the very same kind as that which we have already met and criticized in reference to the closure of figural units. And as before, we can only once more conclude that in the present case, too, we are dealing solely with *ad hoc* assumptions ; indeed, that the whole argument presents itself as a vicious circle. Any positively satisfactory, or in itself valid, new general interpretation is nowhere to be found here, in so far as concrete application in the field of problems of nervous physiology is the issue (cf. §§ 42-3, below, for more detailed discussion).

If we turn back to the general features of his theory, those which Köhler would primarily bring forward as the only essential—and hence secure—parts, according to his present formulations, we shall before all have to pose anew the question of the nature of the " order ", as we have previously met with it.

We have already indicated that pivotal significance was attached to a proposition of Mach in Köhler's general remarks upon the possibility of dynamical self-regulation, and upon the possibility of orderly distribution emerging thus. Compare now what Mach himself means by " order ", in his thesis, and, on the other hand, the goal ahead of the deductions in Köhler's discussion. One cannot but conclude that these do not coincide ; that at bottom there is no direct bridge leading from Mach's concept of order to Köhler's.

For Köhler the whole point of the matter, when all is said and done, is that we are enabled to perceive how the peripheral order imposed by retinal regulation can *maintain* itself as far as the higher strata of the neurophysical sector.

But Mach's main point is that in general, in a system left to itself " order ", i.e. distribution according to relatively simple and geometrically discernible laws, *arises* as a result of the balance of internal forces of the system.

These two principles are at bottom incompatible, apart from the fact that Mach's concept of order still requires further clarification, which we shall have to take up hereafter (p. 236).

Hence from this point of view, too, we cannot unconditionally admit the validity of Köhler's considerations. And this holds, even though we are bound explicitly to recognize that these *general considerations*—these conclusions about the *formal* possibilities of propounding theoretical concepts in this sphere, which are expressed in the principle of " dynamical self-distribution "—are, as far as they go, essentially more lucid than they were before.

We can make this concession without any hesitation, the more so since Köhler himself now remarks : " At the present time only the first steps have been made . . . and it will take a long time before we feel firm ground under our feet." One can even go further and declare explicitly that the general enunciations, in the cautious mode of elaboration in which Köhler has presented them here, actually amount to a positive advance. That is, in so far as they have elucidated the scientific case for a dynamic way of regarding the neurophysical happening, a viewpoint directed towards the play of internal forces, and have established this viewpoint as a problem of the future.

However, in talking of Köhler's theory, we are concerned not only with these generalizations relative to the formal definitions of his point of view, but, in addition, with their concrete working out as actually offered in regard to the neurophysical processes. As to whether this concrete theory does indeed represent the facts, in the form in which Köhler attempted to develop and substantiate it in 1920 and 1929—this, from the results of our total examination of it, must still be considered very questionable.

To be sure, we must, for the time being, leave open the question of whether these difficulties, which have been revealed by our immanent *criticism*, actually suffice to dispose of the concrete application of the dynamic doctrine, as this presents itself to Köhler's mind, *a limine*. It is perhaps impossible fully to justify any such rejection of the theory on the basis of purely immanent criticism, in view of Köhler's recent more cautiously balanced exposition of it.

However, even if we are perhaps not prepared to decide upon so apodictic an " impossible " on the basis of immanent criticism, criteria are still available, *which show more cogently than any of the considerations hitherto advanced that Köhler's doctrine cannot fit the facts.* We can adduce findings from recent research in experimental biology, which though primarily concerned with totally different purposes and tasks, yet in their implications have direct relevance to our field of problems, and are not compatible with Köhler's doctrines.

In order to reach a really valid conclusion in this network of problems, we must now turn our attention to these findings and their evaluation along these lines.

2. KÖHLER'S GESTALT PHYSIOLOGY IN THE LIGHT OF WEISS' EXPERIMENTS ON CENTRO-PERIPHERAL CO-ORDINATION IN THE NERVOUS HAPPENING

To Paul Weiss is due the credit for experiments which may well be of immeasurable positive significance in connection with the appraisal of the general problem of centro-peripheral co-ordination in the nervous happening. They provide a direct empirical foundation for the problem, distinct from all the merely speculative enquiries —as they are, when all is said and done—such as Köhler's ; and at the present juncture it becomes necessary to determine accurately what are their implications.

To begin with, we shall give an account of Weiss' fundamental experiment ; we shall then proceed to his own general inferences relative to reaching some conclusion on the problem of nervous " conduction " ; and finally, we shall consider the consequences which emerge, after weighing up the facts, with reference to concrete statements about nervous physiology, such as those of Köhler.[1]

[1] Cf. Weiss, *Sitz. Ber. Wiener Akad. Anz.*, Nos. 22–3, 1922 ; No. 10, 1923, *Arch. f. mikr. Anat. u. Entw. mech.* 102, 1924, pp. 635–72. His " Erregungsresonanz und Erregungsspezifität ", *Erg. d. Biologie*, vol. iii, 1928, pp. 1–151, gives the most detailed account, and his " Neue Theorie der Nervenfunktionen ", *Nat. Wiss.*, 16, 1928, a conspectus of

The fundamental experiment is of a purely biological nature. The inferences emerge by way of a *functional analysis* of the events concerned, as a concrete natural happening in the living organism.

§ 33. *The general results of Weiss' experiments*

Weiss experimented with the possibility of transplanting entire, fully developed extremities in Amphibia (Salamander larvæ, with success in seventy cases). He amputated entire limbs and transplanted them in such a way that a transplanted limb was always placed beside a normal limb. (The cases in which the transplanted limb took the place of the normal limb are not of interest to us here.) The result was that perfect healing ensued, the transplanted limb being wholly retained in its particular new position.

To begin with, thus, the " local " limb and the " transplanted " limb hang side by side from the body, the latter at first, in consequence of the total disruption of all its nervous connections, as a mere " appendage " of the body.

After a few weeks, however, something entirely unexpected occurs. The transplanted limb commences to give signs of movement, at first weakly, and then more distinctly, until finally, it is in no way inferior to the intact limb functioning normally, being well co-ordinated in itself, and moreover not defective in its degree of strength.

Furthermore, a remarkable, uniform relationship between the co-ordination of the movements in the normal extremity and in the adjacent transplanted limb, is revealed. The transplanted extremity (provided it is at all capable of functioning) and the normal, local extremity *always and without exception* function *simultaneously and homologously.* At every instant of time each limb itself makes the very same movements as the other, so that we may speak of an absolutely " homologous function " of the two ; and this, by the way, occurs wholly independently of the anatomical relation of the transplanted limb to the organism.

the facts. For confirmation of the facts, see Detwiller, " Co-ordinated movements in supernumerary transplanted limbs," *Jnl. Comp. Neurol.*, 38, 1925, and G. Hertwig, " Funktions- und Regenerationsfähigkeit artgleicher und artfremder Extremitätentransplantate," *Sitz. Ber. u. Abh. d. nat. forsch. Ges. Rostock*, iii, Ser. 1, 1926.

What does this phenomenon signify ? In the first place it makes it evident that in the meantime a connection with the central nervous apparatus must have been resuscitated for the transplanted limb.

Upon closer investigation of the peculiar features of this nervous reunion, we further discover that quite unique problems are here involved. In connection with these problems, it is necessary to follow out more closely the processes of nervous regeneration, as they are actually to be met with in a concrete form in this case.

From general experience of degeneration and regeneration of the nerve supply in operations of the above-mentioned kind,[1] we know that, to begin with, at any rate, nerve fibre no longer connected with its cell of origin undergoes involution, and degenerates, in its course towards the periphery. And we also know that any subsequent regeneration can only occur commencing from an injured nerve stump that has been cut. Normal and uninjured nerve fibres do not participate in any process of regeneration. But nerve fibres which have been .severed, while degenerating on the. distal side of the section, at the same time commence to sprout again from the proximal stump sending offshoots to the periphery, which rapidly divide dichotomously. " The newly formed branches proceed to grow through the connective tissue of the scar and sometimes cease there. Their tracks, the determination of the paths which they take through the scar, depend entirely upon the chance topography of the surroundings they reach. . . . Thus, at first the branches of the fibres grow wildly and untrammelled into their surroundings " (*Erg. Biol.*, pp. 13–14). . . . " One bifurcation follows upon another, and long before the periphery is reached, the single original fibre stump can have become ramified into sixty or more branches. The multitude of branches, however, does not remain neatly together, but each follows its own path . . . criss-crossing through the connective tissue ; many a one comes to a stop *en route*, and many another becomes attached to a nearby organ " (*Nat. Wiss.*, p. 628).

" But when a fibre in the course of its advance meets an old, degenerated, peripheral stump, the picture is

[1] Cf. Boeke, *Nervenregeneration und verwandte Innervations-probleme. Ergebn. d. Physiol.*, issued by Asher Spiro, 19, 1921.

changed. For if it has once entered through the proximally directed open end of a Buengner bundle, it cannot again escape from the neurilemma. Indeed, it seems as if it finds this an incomparable conducting tissue, for now it shoots ahead with . . . greatly enhanced speed, and thus soon reaches the end organ (which has in the meantime also degenerated) to which the Buengner bundle leads. Since it is a matter of chance whether the branch of a central fibre stump encounters any Buengner bundle, and which it does encounter, in its outward growth, it is also *a matter of chance which terminal point it is conducted towards.*

"But no matter which end organ the fibre eventually reaches, it is capable of forming a new end apparatus there . . . even though this terminal belongs to a functionally quite different organ to that which it originally supplied." This end plate corresponds not to the origin of the nerve fibre, but solely to its functional value at the point in question. Thus, to cite a crude instance (after Boeke) "even the afferent fibres of the nerve, when they are conducted into the degenerated peripheral hypoglossus and thus to the tongue musculature, form motor end plates there . . ." (cf. Weiss, *Erg. Biol.*, pp. 13–15).

These general results of various investigations of nervous regeneration, taken in connection with Weiss' observations, are now subjected to further tests, and at the same time become the source of most important complications of the problems of centro-peripheral parallelism of excitation.

To begin with, the concrete checking of the anatomical relationships in regard to the nerve supply of the transplanted limb, arises for consideration. As to this, Weiss' report is very definite. He writes: "As could subsequently be incontrovertibly gathered from the microscopical investigation and reconstruction of the course of the nerves in the original limb and in the transplanted limb, this is what took place. The severed nerve fibres in that spot had vigorously *split* up in the scar at the place of grafting. The branches had pressed forward, and had eventually in part met the degenerated nerve paths of the transplanted limb. *As fortuitously as they were located and distributed*, they had penetrated into these and so had reached the muscles . . . the most extraordinary and indiscriminate tangle. . . . Moreover, the few paths belonging to the local extremity which had also to be interrupted previously (as a general means of obtaining an injured nerve stump capable of regeneration in the vicinity of the transplanted limb), these, too, were filled with fresh nerves. In the end, therefore, the relatively small number of ganglion cells, which originally led to a diminutive, limited section of muscle of the local extremity were now connected not only with this very section of muscle again, but, in addition, with the entire musculature of the superfluous limb T " (p. 629, *Nat. Wiss.*).

It is necessary to be quite clear as to how this new anatomical co-ordination presents itself in comparison with the original one. " It is not only that now the ganglion cells involved have to serve a terminal area several times as large as before ; and it is not only that muscles altogether different from the previous ones now belong to them," above all, this must be borne in mind : " The previous rule, that one ganglion cell had connections with only one muscle, now becomes the exception. Instead, the rule now is a *boundless confusion of conduction paths.*

One functional significance of this can be very clearly stated with the help of a diagram given by Weiss as summarizing the anatomical findings. The diagram

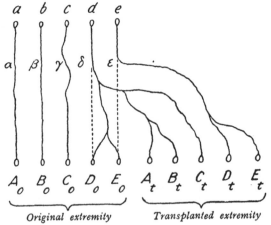

Fig. 4a.—Connection between the C.N.S. and the muscle system, according to Weiss' grafting experiment. Index o = belonging to the original extremity; t = belonging to the transplanted extremity. (Weiss' diagram.)

shows the connecting conduction paths to be found between the central cells (a, b, c, d . . .) and the peripheral nerve end-organs of, firstly, the original limb [$A_o B_o C_o$ . . .] and, secondly, the transplanted limb [$A_t B_t C_t$ . . .]. Normally we have the co-ordination $a-A_o$, $b-B_o$, $c-C_o$, etc. After the operation more complicated connections are developed. (See Fig. 4a.)

The diagram shows clearly the following : " If we accept the current geometrical point of view, then every co-ordinated movement in O would have to be accompanied either by an unco-ordinated spasm in T, or else, if the centre with which T is united is not involved in the particular movement, T would simply have to remain motionless.

" Actually, however, something altogether different happens. All transplanted extremities function without exception, showing complete co-ordination in themselves. And not only does this occur, but there is perfect identity between it and the neighbouring original extremity " (p. 630, *Nat. Wiss.*). " The co-ordinated function of the periphery continues to correspond perfectly to the central determination of co-ordination, even when the connections cease to be orderly and take an entirely fortuitous course " (p. 631).

This means that the *structural, part-by-part co-ordination between musculature and nervous system*, upon which theories have hitherto been based, must now be regarded as " having no leg left to stand upon ". After what has been said above, it should no longer be utilized as the foundation of the orderly functioning of centro-peripheral nervous co-ordination. On the contrary, a different construction must be put upon the matter.

" If . . . it is no less satisfactory without orderly connections, then, surely, one cannot in the normal case attribute to the manifest order of the connections the rôle currently ascribed to it, in regard to the mediation of co-ordination " (p. 631).

To put it in other words : " The means by which the C.N.S. maintains concord with each muscle individually, does *not* consist in *separate paths* of concatenation. The law of peripheral discharge must be more complicated. The principle hitherto made use of, that of the " *inexorable subjection of the end-organ* to every nervous impulse arriving there ", must be looked upon as an *unwarranted* " *prejudice* ", and a different kind of principle must be substituted for it. We must now endeavour to outline this principle.

§ 34. *Weiss' experiments evaluated in terms of principles, with reference to the uniformity of the centro-peripheral co-ordinations in the nervous happening*

How then, may we well ask, is the co-ordination between centre and periphery to be understood under these circumstances ? Weiss' answer is an altogether unequivocal one. He says : " If one and the same nerve cell has to supply excitation to several organs simultaneously ; but if under these circumstances, only one single route common to all these end-organs is at its disposal, be it even for a short distance ; and if, furthermore, the individual end-organs are capable, separately and independently of one another, of draining excitation wherever they require it ; . . . then it is logical to assume that the periphery is so constituted that a control of its functioning in a co-ordinated manner inheres in itself " (p. 39, *Ergeb. d. Biol.*).

" We require . . . a mechanism of *positive selectivity in the end-organ*, which must be able to enlighten us as to why, when two muscles in the same state are given, one of them enters into function and the other does not, although both, being connected with the very same nerve cell, receive excitation equally " (p. 40).

Purely formally, as a direct consequence of the facts, the position may be described as follows. In the nervous motor event " we must postulate some sort of *specific*, individual excitation-constitution for each end-organ, distinguishing one from another ; and we must assume a corresponding multiplicity of forms of excitation for the nervous happening, so constituted, that *any drainage takes place only selectively*, in accordance with a pre-established mutuality." To state it in other words : " The nature of every muscle is such that—given natural excitation—it does not react to every excitation, but only to excitation of a quite definite form, characteristic for it " ; and it only succeeds in obtaining excitation when excitation of the form specific for it arrives from the C.N.S., but not when any other sort of excitation arrives.

These two assumptions—that there are present excitations of various and distinctive specificity, and that there is a corresponding multiplicity of distinct, and for the time being adequate, excitation-constitutions for the various end-organs of the periphery—emerge directly, without any accessory considerations, as the only appropriate inference from the facts.

To establish this specificity of discharge in a corresponding "mechanism", one naturally turns to the concept of *resonance*. Taking this concept in its widest sense, we can say that the facts cited lead to an interpretation of centro-peripheral co-ordination which may be defined by the two terms *specificity of excitation* and *resonance of excitation*. These two concepts are, as the facts demand, the central concepts of the new theory of nerve function proposed by Weiss.

Indeed the interpretation of the facts offers no difficulties in such a framework. It must be worked out on the analogy of the resonator analysis of a complex clang in an accoustic resonator system, which proceeds in accordance with the fact of the specific response of each particular resonator to the peculiar tone characteristic of it.

Weiss accordingly assumes that "the total impulse flowing towards a particular peripheral region from the C.N.S. can, figuratively, forthwith be designated an ' excitation clang '. The ' excitation clang ' consists of the ' excitation tones ' for the muscles which are to be activated at a given moment, and hence it is constantly fluctuating in its composition ".

" The process, now, is as follows : At the very same time, the same ' excitation clang ' flows through *all* the motor root fibres (at least those within a considerable territory) towards the periphery. It flows *equally* through *all* the fibres as if it had been indiscriminately poured into a canal system and were flooding all the channels. Thus it arrives at all the muscles which are in any way whatever connected with the centre. But when it gets to this point it is *analyzed*. Every muscle, in accordance with its constitution, selects the components appropriate to it, from those eventually arriving, and acts as if these components alone had arrived. And thus, although the very same impulse streams to all the muscles and across every available route, only that combination of muscles comes into action—as is now intelligible—which the C.N.S. has provided for " (p. 632, *Nat. Wiss.*).

The particular results of Weiss' experiments are fully covered by this theory. It is superfluous to remark that Weiss has, naturally, checked all previously known findings of nerve physiology, as to whether they do not conflict with his new theory. In this connection he came upon something of direct positive import for the new theory, in so far as our experience of the naturally " adequate " nerve-impulse is taken into primary consideration. At first blush, the results of the electro-physiology of the nerve which are based upon artificial stimulation, contradict the new doctrine. However, they allow of being reconciled with it, when we reason that we are not here dealing with the naturally adequate impulse. " If we wish to picture to ourselves the contrast between the naturally and the artificially elicited impulse, we can compare the naturally ' organized ' impulse . . . to a clang, and the artificially evoked ' unorganized ' impulse . . . to a noise or, better, to a blast. Just as, both with the clang and with the noise, the substratum carrying the movement always is the same, viz. the air, so, obviously, the medium in which both the organized and the unorganized nerve impulse run their course, is always the same, viz. the conductive substance of the nerve fibre. But, just as the clang sets a definite selection of resonators vibrating, whereas a noise or a blast causes them to resound all at once and without an exception ; so also, only the organized impulse, built up of specific impulse-tones, is capable of bringing a co-ordinated selection of muscles into activity, while the artificially induced, *unorganized* impulse, by contrast, forces *every muscle whatsoever* which it reaches into function. On these grounds, findings about the consequences of naturally adequate impulses, and those about the consequences of inadequate, artificially evoked impulses, must be kept strictly apart " (p. 645, *Nat. Wiss.*).

At all events, only the assumption of the new point of view leads to a comprehensive and unitary picture of all the phenomena, whereas, according to the old theory of conduction, the findings of Weiss at least, remain fundamentally inexplicable, and, furthermore, many other results seem to be explicable only by artifices.

When we consider carefully all the concrete facts known to us to-day, from the functional analysis of nervous activity, we are, in my estimation, compelled to acknowledge the more complicated explanations of Weiss' theory as inevitably following from the body of facts. And we must, it seems to me, base future discussions in the field of nerve physiology upon it, or else reinterpret all the available material on the basis of it, as Weiss has already in part done. (Cf. his writings upon fundamental data of nerve physiology such as the " all-or-none law ", etc., as well as his accounts of confirmatory experiences in the provinces of embryology and surgery in his paper in *Erg. d. Biol.*, pp. 129–44.)

Here one other point must be expressly stressed. Weiss never extends his considerations so far as to attempt constructionally to propose a mechanism for the " specificity " of reaction in the nervous system postulated by him, or for the definitive correspondences in the end-organ.

He discusses in detail, but purely hypothetically, the various possibilities which come into question at all. These include the possibilities of a *purely materially determined specificity* (like the specific local dependence, analogous to the present case, of the processes in the hormonal or, speaking generally, endocrine system) ; and, secondly, the possibilities arising out of the assumption of *specific temporally formed processes, " vibrations,"* the specific *induction* of which can be established by the principle of *vibration resonance*, no matter what the processes concerned are like, as to their material nature. He refuses, however, to go farther and reach any conclusion. He is content to have indicated the general possibility of corresponding processes of *specific induction* in the organism.[1]

But even though lacking any conclusion, the results of this theoretical evaluation of the experiment are

---

[1] Here he is thus explicitly propounding a *functional-analytical interpretation* of the facts, free from more far-reaching hypothetical subconstructions, in the same sense in which we, too, at the end of our enquiry demand this, as a matter of principle, for psychology. (Cf. § 67.)

K

sufficiently far-reaching. In particular, it permits us, in a negative sense, to adopt more decisively than before, a standpoint towards hypotheses elsewhere propounded for the constructional interpretation of the centro-peripheral nervous happening ; that is, above all, in the present connection towards Köhler's statements about the psychophysical happening.

§ 35. *Köhler's contentions, in the light of Weiss' results*

When we set out to utilize Weiss' results for the purpose of appraising Köhler's theory, we must note, at the outset, that Weiss' investigations and inferences primarily refer only to processes in the motor sector of the neurophysical happening.

But, in the first place, Köhler himself claims to embrace the motor happening as well, in his theories. And secondly, it must be admitted that no reason could be found for restricting Weiss' statements solely to the motor sphere. There seems no reason why we should not, logically, have a basis of corresponding doctrines in regard to the perceptual sectors, subject to further direct clarification hereafter.

We may, therefore, draw upon these new findings in their full import, in order to appraise Köhler's ideas. And when we do this, definite consequences bearing upon the tenability of these ideas emerge.

In arriving at our position, it is essential to bear in mind particularly clearly the distinction elaborated above, between the formal delineation of Köhler's leading conceptions, and the concrete, material theory. *Köhler's purely formal leading ideas* are, to a certain extent, in agreement with Weiss' views. And Weiss himself has referred to them in this sense. More exactly, Köhler's first line of orientation, the *leitmotif* " *abandon the purely geometrical excitation represented in elementary conductors* ", receives decisive and impressive affirmation in Weiss' results.

Furthermore, Köhler's second line of orientation of a formal kind, the *proclamation of a " dynamic " interpretation of the nervous happening*, receives immediate justification in Weiss' manner of statement. Indeed, it is formulated in its general sense as the nuclear import of the new theory by Weiss himself, in his exposition—directly in connection with the concrete considerations.

But if we go further and ask how Köhler's general ideas fare as to their concrete embodiment, in the light of Weiss' contentions, we arrive at entirely opposed results.

The reason for this is that the formulas of the two investigators, ostensibly referable to a common basic position, really have a totally different significance in their actual import. When all is said and done, the kinship remains a purely formal one, while the connotations of the two formulas are completely different.

To substantiate our contention, we need only investigate that one among the common formulas which seems to have a positive import. This is the second formula, that of the " dynamic " interpretation of the neurophysical happening. What does " dynamics " signify for Köhler, and what does it signify for Weiss ?

To both it stands for something more or less indefinite ; namely, a mode of explanation which expounds relationships by postulating some sort of mutual influence of partial processes in the total nervous happening. Here, conformably with the meaning of the word " dynamics " they have in mind some sort of " forces ", though extraordinarily indefinitely, in both cases. The significance of " dynamics " in the two senses, so far as it can be more concretely established at all, can only be grasped by taking into consideration the particular form of the " explanation " adopted by each of the writers. It then becomes immediately evident where the distinction lies.

Weiss has in mind a pattern of nervous events, in itself not further definable in detail, but proceeding in accordance with quite definite laws, those of a characteristic resonance specificity. These laws are furnished solely as the end result of a very careful and close analysis of the facts.

Köhler, on the other hand, in his dynamics, deals with a state of affairs which is incorporated into the discussion of the nervous happening by a very vague transduction. He is primarily concerned with a concept—one, moreover, devoid of any clarifying elucidation—borrowed from physics. Its concrete significance in the discussion of nerve physiology, however, receives absolutely no closer definition, apart from the very vague analogical statements given in the consideration of electro-physiological fields, where the fact that the word " field " seems applicable in both spheres provides the chief foundation for the erection of the correspondences sought or, possibly, desired.

When we place Köhler's observations in this connection side by side with those of Weiss, they must be regarded as very unconvincing, as far as their inner clarity and validity are concerned.

Weiss' enquiries can serve as more than a merely methodological standard. Since they present direct factual findings they can also serve as a standard with immediate reference to content.

In this regard we can at once resort to them by asking : Are Köhler's premises and lines of thought sufficiently wide and complete in themselves to be able to accommodate Weiss' results, which refer solely to the pure facts ?

Merely to pose this question is to answer it in the negative. For indeed, Köhler's considerations nowhere embrace anything which permits the radical possibilities directly demanded by Weiss' findings.

We may say that Köhler's theory has indeed got rid of the point-to-point co-ordination between periphery and centre. In one respect, however, it still remains " geometrical ". It accepts the total conduction process, as a whole, with its anatomical-geometrical arrangement, as foundation. But in this total conduction process, in. accordance with the dependence of the physical " distribution processes " solely taken into account by Köhler upon the topography of the material system carrying it, it is obviously by no means irrelevant for the general issue of the distribution of excitations whether and how the separate partial conductions are aligned and integrated. It is by no means possible for the same result to be achieved irrespectively of whether these partial conductions are integrated in one way or another, as can immediately be perceived from the example of the system of tubes of current adduced by Köhler.

Weiss' facts, however, inevitably demand the complete discarding of any constantly recognizable influence of the geometrical-anatomical connections—not only in regard to the elementary constituents, but also in regard to the general nature of the integration of the partial conductions. The conflict of Köhler's theory with these facts, which is thus revealed, conclusively proves that we are not dealing with a formulation which is indeed intrinsically adequate.

In Weiss' observations we see the *experimentum crucis* which quite clearly controverts the possibility of a doctrine of nervous physiology after the style of Köhler's proposals and considerations. And in them we at once discover the critical material, looked at from the purely physiological and biological side, which decides our question as to the validity of Köhler's contentions in the negative.

Taken as a whole, Köhler's theory strikes us as a first bold attempt—but one not sufficiently buttressed by biological and physiological facts—to transcend the atomism of excitation geometry in nerve physiology. It must be valued as a pioneer attempt which will remain so for the reason that a goal of that sort was for the first time pursued on a large scale in it ; an attempt, however, that only stimulates, but leads no farther, since it does not achieve the direction which must really be definitive for the solution of the problem. This direction must be sought in a conscious and adequate consideration of the specificity of drainage, which appears to be equally fundamental for the detailed happenings in the nervous system, and, in a larger way, for what is given in our experience (cf. the final chapters in my book *Das Gestalt-problem in der Psychologie im Lichte analytischer Besinnung,* 1931).

PART TWO

TOWARDS AN APPRAISEMENT OF THE CONCRETE EMPIRICAL FOUNDATION OF THE GESTALT THEORY

If we wished to attempt to form some judgment as to the empirical basis of proof of the gestalt theory, the discussion would have to take on truly large proportions. For the researches of the adherents of the gestalt theory have, during recent years, brought together factual data from the most varied fields of psychology, intended to furnish a basis for the substantiation of the theoretical enunciations at issue. The undertaking is made still more difficult by the fact that up till now a comprehensive and systematic incorporation of the facts in question, according to their status and their value as evidence, into the system as a whole, has hardly been accomplished in those works which are intended to serve as a general foundation for the new theory as a whole. For, actually, all the basic enquiries of Koffka, Köhler, and Wertheimer, have a conceptual point of departure—the polemic against the elementalist standpoint—and not an empirical one.

For our enquiry, it is only pertinent to elucidate to what extent the various conceptual tenets of the gestalt theory allow of being developed by *starting directly from the experimental findings*, to what extent these tenets can be empirically reached by a *direct route* from experimentation as the starting point. We must therefore endeavour to accomplish, by ourselves and in our own way, a suitable *ordering of the facts within the body of the system*, of such a nature as to make it clear what status can be assigned to them within the whole. And we shall then have to develop our criticism within the framework of this classification, bearing clearly in mind what weight is to be attached to the conclusions emerging from it.

In thus traversing the various fields of experimentation relevant for us, the standpoint of internal organization, which is all we can still consider essential in the building up of psychology in accordance with the systematic principles of the theory, as a matter of course serves as our guiding line. We mean the distinction between *static gestalten at rest in themselves* and those *gestalt processes* which run a temporal course with *dynamic development*.

SECTION ONE

ON THE STATICS OF GESTALTEN

CHAPTER I

FIGURAL STRUCTURES AS THE FUNDAMENTAL PHENOMENON OF THE GESTALT THEORY

I. THE PHENOMENON OF FIGURAL STRUCTURE IN ITS GESTALT-THEORETICAL APPLICATION

The first question that arises within the purview of an examination of the empirical material offered in support of the gestalt theory, naturally relates to the phenomena which we are accustomed to denote by the word " gestalt " even in everyday speech. These are the " gestalten " in the narrowest sense of the word, apparent e.g. in optical perception, " figural structures " as, to lend more precision to the terminology of the gestalt-theoretical school, we propose to call them in contrast to the other " structures " to be treated of hereafter.

§ 36. *The phenomenal basis of the problem of figural structure*

We need not explain what is meant by such a " figural structure ". One immediately knows what sort of presentations are here had in mind. One knows that something of this kind is present, e.g. when a solid object confronts one in space ; when any cut-out colour patch upon some sort of background is before one ; when a " figure " is outlined upon a homogeneous white surface by means of drawing a contour, and so on.

But the very fact that everybody is familiar with the phenomenon is the reason why it was not made an object of scientific enquiry until relatively late, and why the analysis of it had indeed at first to be approached in a roundabout way before its significance could be fully comprehended.

The merit of having accomplished the first step in this connection belongs to Schumann. He entered upon the analysis of this phenomenon for the first time (1900), in the course of investigations upon the psychology of space, when he analyzed more exactly what was phenomenally present when looking at simple line drawings.

We shall consider his results in connection with the observations he published upon an example in which a series of equidistant parallel lines were presented (Schumann's Figure).

Upon looking at this figure, one does not simply get the impression of a juxtaposition, a row of straight lines; on the contrary, a specific articulation within the field of .vision presents itself. " Any two lines *combine into a group* with striking ease; and this in such a manner that every white patch lying between the two lines of a group forms a *unitary whole with these lines*, and *stands out in consciousness*, while the white patches between the groups recede and appear quite otherwise. One has the impression of *seeing* something like a ' fence ' ".

This analysis of the parallel-line figure by Schumann, already includes, in a characteristic manner, all the special points which are in any way essential from the descriptive side for the consideration of figural structure. It has, moreover, been in no way superseded by more recent analyses.[1]

It is important in more ways than one as a point of departure for our discussion.

In the first place, viewed from the gestalt-theoretical standpoint, the essential feature of this stimulus situation is that *it is not simply an* " *additive* ", " *plus-summated* ", " *there* " *and* " *there* " *and* " *there* " of single lines which appears, not simply a " juxtaposition " given in a " piece-meal " way. We have here a paradigm of a *specific* " *collocation* " into characteristic " unities ", a " collocation " in which the single lines, the single constituent

[1] Cf. Wittmann, 1921 (cf. below, § 40), Rubin, 1915 (German edn., 1922)

parts, appear *no longer* as *unrelated* "*elements*", but *rather* as "*participants*" *in something* "*whole*"—as belonging, for the time being, to the white area of the patch with which they appear, for the time being, to be coalesced in pairs.

In the second place, as regards the *total field*, this too shows itself to be not simply "compounded", as it were, of juxtaposed plane stripes ; on the contrary, an *articulation* is involved, which pertains to the field as a whole. The receding "areas" do not appear isolated, but coalesce on their part, as more exact analysis shows, into a whole, into a more diffuse background cohering in itself, within which the lines actually possess no significance, but which stretches out "invisibly", that is, "concealed," behind the protruding stripes. The prominence of the "fence", on the other hand, the "collocation" of every pair of lines, is not a phenomenon pertaining only to two of these lines, for the time being ; this coalescence ensues "automatically" to a certain extent, over the total visual field. The *visual field as a whole* here undergoes an *articulation*.

In the third place, the *peculiar qualitative mode of manifestation of the parts of the field* is especially distinctly characterized in these findings. They lead to the phenomenal *distinction* between the "figure" character and the "ground" character of the differentiable areas in the field, i.e. the divisions of the visual field which appear as "object" and as background respectively. "The figure is more strongly configured than the ground, it is bounded by the contour, and the ground not so ; it is more insistent, firmer, more thing-like. The ground is more simply configured or more chaotic than the figure" (Rubin, Danish edn., 1915 ; German, 1922).

All this was available when the gestalt theory had developed to the point where it was seeking to link up with empirical findings. Thus the observations upon Schumann's figure (generally, it is true, without mention of Schumann), and Rubin's formulations on the basis of his observations with plane figures, were fitted into all the more empirically biassed discussions (e.g. Koffka, 1922).

But this merely indicates the beginning of what it is believed can be accomplished for the theory with the aid of these findings. Apart from the endeavour to achieve a direct physiological explanation for these phenomena on the basis of gestalt physiology (Köhler, 1920), effort is also devoted to the exact empirical investigation of them, directed towards resolving the functional moments which can be traced in them. This, firstly, raises the question (in reference to those stimulus conditions which—analogously to Schumann's figure—consist of a configuration of single 'lines, points, etc.), of how "states of collocation" arise here at all, what conditions the kind of collocation depends upon, and whether there are any principles for the collocation of such "discontinuous stimulus groupings" (Wertheimer, 1924).

Secondly, the question is taken up as to whether the, internal closure, the unitariness, occurring with plane figures, cannot be made more precisely intelligible. It is found possible to place these "continuous stimulus groupings" in a definite general context (Köhler, 1925).

We shall, to begin with, turn immediately to this second question, that concerning the closure of homogeneous areas of the field, since the answer to it in part covers the first question as well, and we can in this way gain a general idea of the problem at issue in its implications and treatment.

§ 37. The phenomenon of closure in homogeneous areas of the field and the problem of mosaic

Köhler, in 1925, attempted, in a very characteristic fashion, to make the "intrinsic articulation" of the visual field, as this appears e.g. upon presentation of a homogeneously coloured plane figure against a ground of different colour, intelligible as regards its "real foundedness". He is naturally closely concerned with this problem, for in the formula of the articulation of what is given according to "natural units" he has plainly succeeded in grasping the problem involved in its most precise form.

The treatment of the problem proceeds in a very noteworthy manner, which advances more deeply into the specific gestalt-theoretical interpretation of the "figure-ground" phenomena. Köhler begins with simple drawings, modelled on the Schumann figure, and aims at approaching closer and closer, in a uniformly progressive series, to the conditions present in apprehending a surface appearing homogeneously black or grey.

Three "principles" are, to begin with, derived—in reliance upon the work of Wertheimer (1925) to be discussed hereafter—from the consideration of the drawings (Fig. 5) ; and these are held to be the "*decisive factors*" *for the modes of* appearance of the figures (p. 696).

(*a*) The fact that in No. 1 the more closely adjacent parallels come together into unitary groups, appear in units, leads to the first factor : The factor of " distance ".

(*b*) No. 2, where the supplementary small horizontal pieces which are added " bring about " a directly contrary impression, leads to a second possibility. " Perhaps we

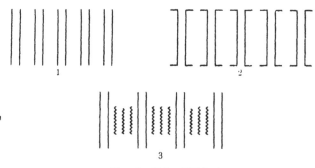

Fig. 5. (After Köhler.)

have two different principles, that of distance and *that of enclosing* " (p. 696).

(*c*) No. 3 illustrates a third principle : " Members of the *same* " *quality* ", whatever it may be, form groups " (pp. 697-8). " Neighbours of equal properties given, group units are formed " (p. 699).

These three principles, that of " nearness ", that of " enclosing ", and that of " likeness ", are thus looked upon as the " decisive factors ", the " effective causes " [1] for the coalescence observed in connection with combinations of lines.

These provide the starting point for Köhler's main quest. A simple line of thought leads to the goal : " The groups formed in the series of parallels included

---

[1] They " are seen working (!) " Cf. p. 699.

pairs of them. We add third parallels in the midst of each group and find, as one may have expected beforehand, that the three lines so close together still form groups and that the grouping is even much more striking now than before. We may add two more parallels in each group between the three already drawn. Not much of white is left now in the group and the stability of group formation is still increased (Fig. 6). Some steps more and

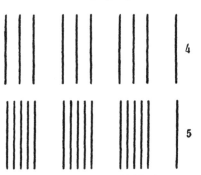

Fig. 6. (After Köhler.)

the areas of our groups are uniform black rectangles. There would be three of them ; everybody looking upon the page would see these ' three dark forms '. And our gradual procedure has taught us that *to see the black content of each of those areas as ' one thing '* united in itself, outstanding as one from the ground, *is only a very extreme case of the formation of group units* which we were observing first."

The problem of " natural units " is completely settled herewith.

" It is *an extreme example* of the fact *that, with neighbours of equal properties given, group units are formed.* This principle was seen working with increased effect the denser we filled the area of the group."

Thus we see here how that " primitive experience in vision "—" that continuous, uniformly coloured areas or spots in differently coloured homogeneous surroundings appear as wholes, as units," that fundamental fact of the " being one " of a homogeneous colour field, appears to be conclusively traced back to those three principles, in particular to that of " likeness ".

The very same consideration leads also to the "explanation" of another peculiarity in the mode of appearance of such a colour field, the explanation of the "thing character".

Köhler harks back to the same figures and evaluates them in another respect. After what has been established for Nos. 1–3 in regard to the three principles, Köhler concludes that "the description of our observations is not yet complete. If we look upon the series of parallels we see that the formation of a group is not an affair of those parallels only. The whole area *in* a group, half enclosed between the parallels nearer to each other, and white like the surrounding paper, still looks different from it and also different from the area between two consecutive groups".

It is thus the distinction between "figure" and "ground" which is here explicitly invoked, the special "'figure' character* as something solid, outstanding from the empty ground" (p. 700)—in contrast to, or rather in supplementation of the fact hitherto alone considered, that of the impression of coherence between the "elements" of the groups, the parallels.

This "figure-character", too, is carried over from the "discontinuous groups" to the "continuous groups" so that "wherever a thing is visible as 'one' and as something *solid* the same principles are concerned which we first became acquainted with in the formation of groups" (p. 700). Thus is deduced, up to a certain point, the reasons for which continuous groups too, that is, homogeneously coloured areas, show figure-character; and a substructure for a further characteristic aspect of the problem of natural units is thus provided.

At all events, it is evident here how the problems of the "being configured" of homogeneous parts of a field appear to be transferred to a very wide context. The question, now, is to what extent these considerations actually lead, in a precise way, to conclusions in accord with the gestalt-theoretical orientation of principles.

We are put on our guard when we observe that G. E. Müller in 1923, thus before Köhler, contrived to deduce the "being configured" of homogeneous areas of a field by an exactly similar trend of thought—but from quite different theoretical premisses, within the framework of his theory of "Coherence", which is avowedly synthetically orientated.[1]

The suspicions thus aroused prove, upon closer conceptual analysis, to be in fact concretely confirmed by Köhler's explication. Two objections might present themselves at once. Firstly, it seems questionable how far the whole treatment of the matter can be accepted as secure *in its foundations*, how far it is at all cogent in itself. When Köhler perceives a logical sequence from discontinuous to continuous stimulus conditions, does he not commit a methodological error which he had already, with the greatest emphasis, branded as impermissible in 1913, in connection with his denunciation of psychological atomism? Does he not tacitly make a "constancy hypothesis" reaching beyond the sphere for which it is justified? With the discontinuous stimulus conditions definite "parts" can still plainly be indicated as the foundations of the state of collocation, as "elements", "constituents", directly and perceptively. In the homogeneous stimulus field, in which such foundations of the state of collocation are not perceptively given as such, a correspondence is simply imputed to "be present", in spite of Köhler's own earlier polemics against transferences of this kind.

Secondly, even if we concede this constancy hypothesis to Köhler, the *bearing of this view* does not appear to be correctly assessed. For Köhler's actual aim is undoubtedly to lead up pointedly to the gestalt-theoretical thesis that "these units cannot be deduced from an aggregate of independent local states", by means of his discussion.

But it is not difficult to perceive that Köhler's stepwise procedure is in truth exceptionally adapted to defend just such an "aggregate" standpoint. If mosaic structures are given in the stimulus—however subtle the merging may be—the case is exactly the same as with the "collocation" of pairs of parallels, etc. If now one imagines a "mosaic" structure to be active physiologically, owing somehow to histological conditions of the receptor apparatus, etc., also in the case of "objectively" homogeneous stimulus fields as well—where would be the

---

[1] After he had already given—in a different connection, it is true— an enumeration and exact description of the "Coherence factors" here brought forward, in his *Analyse der Gedächtnisstaetigkeit*, 1911.

grounds upon which one could adjudge it impossible to derive the " being configured " from the mosaic hypothesis ? [1]

Köhler's sequential treatment can contribute nothing to the endeavour after a foundation for the gestalt theory that would not be already included in the " figure and ground " phenomenon. In fact, taken in conjunction with the " Köhler constancy hypothesis " at the back of it, it has the effect of actually reinforcing the " bundle thesis " of the " old psychology " ! Thus the whole discussion leads back to the distinction between " figure and ground " in discontinuous stimulus constellations. It rests upon the decision as to whence the state of collocation comes with " macro-conditions ". But nothing conclusive has been made out in this regard in what we have referred to above. When Köhler posits his " decisive factors " of " distance ", " enclosing " and " equality " for that state of collocation, this does not offer any conceptual clarification of what is really the main problem. It is necessary, therefore, to determine the significance of these statements about the " decisive factors " more exactly. To this end, we must test the foundations of these factors ; and do so by reverting to their actual source, the studies published by Wertheimer on this matter in 1923, from which Köhler's enunciations derive.

§ 38. *The conditions for the building-up of the figural unity, according to Wertheimer, and the concept of figural structure*

In his " Untersuchungen " of 1923, Wertheimer explicitly poses the question, in regard to the phenomenal inter-articulations of discontinuous stimulus constellations : " Are there principles that account for the manner in which ' states of collocation ' and ' states of disparateness ' thus result ? If so, what are they ? " (p. 302).

---

[1] This is not called into question by the fact that in the " macro-conditions " of the homogeneous stimulus situation the " independent parts " are not given as such perceptively. Even in the presentation of e.g. two parallel lines, these are, in the " collocation ", not there merely as such " lines ", but in their specific function in the whole of the discriminated unity, as limiting " inwardly ", etc. In both cases they appear in the form in which they seem to be incorporated into the total context—on the ground of their " state of collocation ".

He bases his answers to this question upon a series of illustrative experiments on "discontinuous stimulus constellations" (isolated dots, lines) in the most different arrangements, varied according to a plan. This series is so selected, that by means of a "series of simple characteristic instances" the "effective factors" of that "state of collocation" should be exhibited, in a systematically progressive sequence.

To begin with, Wertheimer gives the factors utilized by Köhler :—

(1) *The Factor of Nearness* : "The collocation (in rows of dots, and of lines) ensues in terms of the least distance."

(2) *The Factor of Likeness* : "If rows of stimuli with constituents of different sorts are given, there is a tendency towards the form in which the like ones appear grouped together."

Then follows a new factor of a very remarkable sort.

(3) If, for instance, the following constellation is presented, obvious in its form as determined by the factor of nearness :

$$\overset{\cdot\ \ \cdot\ \ \cdot}{a\ \ b\ \ c}\quad\overset{\cdot\ \ \cdot\ \ \cdot}{d\ \ e\ \ f}\quad\overset{\cdot\ \ \cdot\ \ \cdot}{g\ \ h\ \ i}\quad\overset{\cdot\ \ \cdot\ \ \cdot}{k\ \ l\ \ m}$$

Fig. 7.   (Wertheimer.)

and if now, without the cognizance of the observer, a common alteration in the constituents is produced before his eyes, e.g. a sudden, small, equal shifting of several dots vertically upwards, two kinds of measures stand in marked contrast in respect to their effects :—

(*a*) "Structure-befitting" alterations such as involve the groups objectively intended here ; e.g. *d, e, f*, are moved slightly upwards (or *d, e, f*, and *k, l, m*).

(*b*) "Structure-violating" alterations, in which the common destiny of the change does *not* involve groups in accordance with the ostensible grouping, e.g. *c, d, e* are simultaneously moved slightly upwards (or *c, d, e*, and *i, k, l*, or *h, i, k*).

Those of the second sort typically occur "by far not so smoothly" as those of the first sort. While the first are often easily and simply "cognized" (obviously, therefore, nothing exceptional is evinced by them), a characteristic process, on the other hand, is usually manifested in the case of the second sort. It is as if a special (much stronger) " resistance " to changes of this sort were present. A suspense ensues, and eventually perplexity, a confusion of the rows, frequently an over-balancing. " *The components affected by a common destiny result* (acting in opposition to the law of nearness) *in a state of collocation.* Upon shifting c, d, e, i, k, l, m, the row does not remain in the form a, b, c/d, e, f, but now has the form a, b/c, d, e/f, g, h/i, k, l/m " (pp. 315–16).

What is evinced in these last instances ? What " principle " lies at the basis of the new " state of collocation " which arises ?

Wertheimer offers a very simple reply. He says :—

" We propose provisionally to designate the *factor* displayed as that of the ' common destiny '." Constituents which have a common destiny of this sort, result in a collocation of such a nature, that in it the factor of " nearness ", as well as that of " likeness ", is deprived of its influence. In this factor of the common destiny we have therefore a new, autonomous, primary principle for the state of collocation.

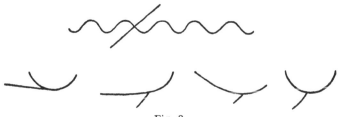

Fig. 8.

(4) Furthermore : If the position of a component is systematically varied in a configuration, by equal stages, there does not ensue, phenomenally, a corresponding, regularly changing—i.e. by analogous stages—number of individually characterized impressions, but on the contrary, definite *stages of precision* occur. For example, a series of dots is presented in a circular arrangement ; if now the position of one of these dots is so changed, in successive exposures, as to be gradually progressively displaced from the periphery towards the centre, this dot in

the first instance still appears to be decidedly a part of the continuity of the curved line, in no way extraneous to it ; but then—with a sudden change—it immediately appears as quite decidedly projected into the plane surface, more so than would directly correspond to the stimulus situation.   Here a new factor is evinced : A *tendency towards precise form* determines the nature of the state of collocation.

(5) In patterns of continuous points—continuous lines or curves—a principle related to the preceding one manifests itself, the *principle of the good, whole gestalt.* A state of collocation results in conformity with a good, a " curvitally proper " continuation.   It takes place in such a way that, for example, when two curves are drawn to cross one another, the way the constituents belong together is unequivocally fixed : " Supplementary " or " cross lines " do not disturb the state of collocation of the main curve (Fig. 8).

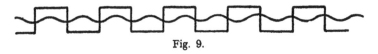

Fig. 9.

When two curves intersect, it results in the separation of one from the other (Fig. 9) ; that is, a state of collocation of constituent gestalten in conformity with the " inner belonging-together " (Fig. 10), or in conformity with a " ' closure ' of the run of the curve "—in brief, in conformity with a " good curve ", a " good gestalt ".

Rivalry may arise between these " principles " or

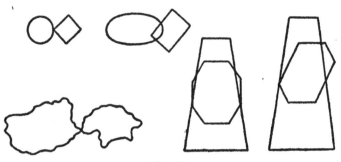

Fig. 10.

"tendencies", e.g. "nearness" and "likeness" can oppose each other in a figure. In such a case a "compromise of forces" to a certain extent ensues; the "stronger" tendency "triumphs", the other is "weakened".

The state of collocation can also have a *temporal after-effect*, depending upon its constitution: "*A factor of objective attitude*" exists. If a row of pairs of dots, like this . . . ., is presented, so that the factor of nearness is obviously critical; and if a series of other figures is then successively presented, in which from time to time the right hand dot, say, of each pair is shifted somewhat further to the right, in successive stages, then when the stimulus situation has passed the stage of an equidistant distribution of dots, a new grouping together does not arise—in accordance with the altered effects of the factor of nearness. Instead, the previous state of collocation still continues to assert itself, even when the distances are relatively large. Because of the preceding figural processes, so Wertheimer interprets the matter, a control upon the later instances is "objectively" set up, a "state of being set" of the receptor apparatus (see above, § 15) which now determines the event. The explanation thus resorts to a figural after-effect, a notion which had already, by the way, been introduced into the explanation of gestalt phenomena by Rubin, 1915 (with reference to his general observations in regard to figure and ground).

Figural after-effect, in exactly the same sense, is also invoked—and, in this case, as active over even greater stretches of time—when we speak of a *factor of experience* being critical for many states of collocation.

. The collocations which arise in connection with these principles, according to Wertheimer appear as *effects of an entirely primary sort*; as effects which are established directly as a *result of the specific properties of the stimulus situation*—without the intermediation of any sort of synthetic function, purely as a result of the general conformity to law of the happening which leads from stimulus to impression. In these states of collocation, an event is concerned which falls under the heading of *spontaneous self-articulation*.

Furthermore: These primary forms of collocation prove to be *unequivocally bound to the stimulus conditions*,

objectively controlled by them—either straightforwardly
in accordance with the so-being of the stimulus constellation at this moment, and/or by the detour through figural
after-effect in the co-operation of the present stimulus
constellation with corresponding temporally precedent
stimulus effects.   They are *absolutely* " *objectively* "
founded.

From these singular features of the matter—not yet,
it is true, formulated explicitly in this way by Wertheimer—as a starting point, the investigation thus seems
virtually to lead up to the theoretical framework which
the gestalt theory would gladly wish to establish empirically—the more impressively, as Wertheimer emphatically
points out, since in the entire building up of it only
questions of fact seem to be involved.

But do the " facts " really purport so much ?   We
must, so it seems, forthwith settle some points in this
connection.   To begin with, if we review the concrete
results which Wertheimer has put forward in regard to
the gestalt-forces, gestalt-tendencies, gestalt-principles
revealing themselves in these states of collocation, we
cannot avoid noting, that a peculiar *lack of homogeneity*
inheres in them.   The first factors, those of likeness, of
nearness, and of the common destiny, are patently of
quite a different sort from the others, the " tendency
towards precise form ", " towards a good curve ",
" towards a good whole gestalt ".   The latter, in fact,
relate to specifications which can obviously be employed
only in respect to the totality, the whole of the
" constituents ", in so far as they can be rationally applied
at all.   The former, on the other hand, relate to specifications about the single points, specifications which can at
all times be rationally applied " in a piecemeal fashion ".
In principle, they can be so interpreted as to allow one
to state that whether or to what extent a " tendency
towards a state of collocation " exists " between " (!)
two dots, in accordance with the principle of nearness,
depends, to go by this canon, solely upon these two dots,
and in no way upon anything else.   In the total configuration such tendencies at bottom arise between all the dots,
and the kind of state of collocation which appears as
the end result can thus pass for a pure resultant effect.
The factor of " nearness ", and likewise that of " likeness "

and that of the "common destiny", on this interpretation thus have a palpably synthetic character, as regards the conceptual structure of their underlying premises. They are actually, therefore, thoroughly incompatible with the basic tendency of the gestalt theory. One does not under these circumstances rightly understand how those principles can, on the contrary, be put forward as standards for a verdict consistent with the gestalt theory.[1]

Furthermore, when Wertheimer advances the claim that nothing but a "*straightforward problem of fact*" is involved in the enumeration of these factors (p. 302), this can by no means be assented to. Much more enters into his work. It embraces *not purely* facts, but *in addition the interpretation of facts*. And this interpretation is not introduced for the first time with the elaboration of the general specifications of the facts of the matter, as we have explicitly presented it above, but is already introduced in the concrete findings communicated by Wertheimer himself, which lie at the basis of this elaboration.

What is implied when Wertheimer introduces " factors " of " nearness ", " likeness " and so on ? It is not that a concrete finding is simply being formulated ; this finding is also at the same time traced back to an " effective principle ", a " tendency " underlying it and coming to expression in it. And the true import of what *Wertheimer* puts forward lies only in this reduction to such a " principle ".

Hence the *manner* in which Wertheimer believes the task to have been thus accomplished, is bound forthwith to elicit the sharpest criticism from one who takes up the standpoint of scientific theory. Even the categories selected for the purpose are bound to stir suspicion.

What, for instance, does it signify, psychologically, when Wertheimer talks of " common destiny " ? Is it legitimate to speak of " destiny " purely with reference to what exists in the stimulus objectively ? Perhaps yes,

---

[1] One further point appears of importance as characteristic of these principles. Starting from them, Wertheimer is led to a methodological conception which is especially characteristic of the system of the particular psychological orientation which he most strongly combats. He attempts a quantitative comparison of " tendencies " which are operative side by side ; and this in a way which is identical with Ach's procedure for determining the " associative equivalent " ; that is by means of a specifically synthetically orientated procedure.

for something obviously "happens to" this objective thing in the experiment. But how does it present itself, if we try to imagine, along the lines of Köhler's theory, the gestalt processes which are supposed to correspond to the phenomenal gestalten physiologically? What sort of appreciable reality can there be assigned to the "common destiny"? And also, is anything really definite to be understood by "good" curve, and "good" gestalt? What "material" criteria have we for deciding which of two continuations of a curve is the "curvitally proper" one?

Such concepts make all exactitude of thinking illusory, and throw open the doors to arbitrary interpretations. They cannot claim any explanatory value, in the genuine sense.

Their explanatory value becomes even more questionable, when we examine more closely in what relation fact and explanatory principle actually stand, from the point of view of scientific theory. When Wertheimer believes that he has made the fact of like constituents appearing grouped into a unit theoretically intelligible by means of his explanatory principle, the "factor of likeness", this is a procedure identical with the one which explains the soporific action of opium by means of the *virtus dormitiva*.

Surely we must demand somewhat more than such a scholastically hypostasizing treatment in psychology too. Physics itself is not satisfied when, for instance, the fact that hydrogen spontaneously ignites upon contact with a platinum sponge, is "explained" by a "catalytic action" of the platinum sponge.

In physics the residue of Aristotelean ways of thinking inhering in this terminology has long been eliminated. It retreats before keener analysis of the conditions. Ought we not perhaps to take this path in psychology too? It seems as if the real problem only commences with Wertheimer's results—and, as a matter of fact, as a genuine "problem of fact", in the sense of a most searching exploration of the conditions.

Thus our discussion is bound to lead us to refer the quest for gestalt factors *de novo* to the forum of experimental research.

2. THE GESTALT-THEORETICAL INTERPRETATION OF THE FIGURAL PHENOMENA IN THE LIGHT OF A COMPREHENSIVE ANALYSIS OF FACTS

In virtue of our last-mentioned considerations, it is our duty to enquire once more into the conditions of the " collocation " ; and this with keener analysis, in order thus to settle the question whether or not Wertheimer has really said the last word about these facts. The experimental material for this task does not even need to be gathered together ; it is already at our disposal, at least as far as the first group of gestalt factors is concerned ; and we shall discuss only these to begin with.

§ 39. *The Wertheimer " gestalt factors " and my findings on spatial collocations*

In an experimental research carried out in the summer of 1919 (published 1923), I was able to elicit observations which must be brought into direct relation with Wertheimer's submissions of 1923. I also investigated— to use Wertheimer's expression—" articulations " which arose upon presentation of " discontinuous groups of stimuli ". Complexes of discs (circular, white and grey-toned surfaces, background as homogeneously dark as possible, merging into the frame of the diaphragm without noticeable contour) in varying spatial distributions in indifferent space (depth 16,00 m., field of regard ca. 60°) were exposed to my observers for monocular regard. The " articulations " with which I thus dealt, however, covered not only juxtaposition, as in Wertheimer's line and dot figurations, but also the sequential position of visual objects in visual space. I was concerned with " collocations " in respect to spatial depth, that is, with " collocations " the experimental explication of which has not yet been undertaken by Wertheimer and his colleagues.

The results stand in a special relation to the discoveries of Wertheimer which we have considered. They can be so represented that exactly the same " factors " should appear to be critical as those Wertheimer put forward in 1923. Here, too, a " factor of nearness " proves to be apparently operative.

This showed itself when one of the discs objectively within a given constellation of discs, differentiated in some way according to visual depth, was objectively moved in a direction parallel-frontal to the observer :—

E.g. Obs. Fe. regards six discs of equal depth and brightness. The *objective* conditions are given in the table below, the distribution in apparent juxtaposition in Fig. 11 :—

Disc no.	1	2	3	4	5	6
Diameter cm. . .	14	18	6	7	8	14
Distance cm. . .			750			

The following distribution of the visual objects was *seen*, to begin with :—

Discs 1 and 2 at one level, about 4 m. away.

Discs 3, 4, and 5, again almost at one level (about 7 m. distant).

Disc 7 perhaps a little nearer.

Disc 6 approximately in the centre between these.

The illuminated curtain above hanging at a depth of about 9 m. If disc 6 is moved (Fig. 11) depth displacement appears. " The disc retreats slowly towards the second level of discs (3, 4, 5). Now (at about M) it suddenly turns about, and is at the level of 1, 2. It remains there. Hallo ! now all at once it quite suddenly jumps backward ; it is now twice as far distant." The startling jump occurs at the moment when the disc approaches nearer to the illuminated cloth above and touches it. " Now it is at the level of the curtain." (Petermann, Arch. 46, p. 371).

Thus in fact : " The disc which is moved, from time to time shifts, more or less distinctly, to a depth position which is determined by the seen distance of those discs

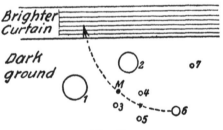

Fig. 11.

in the *proximity* of which it successively appears while being observed. When it comes into the proximity of the *coulisse*, it is seen either advancing or retreating, gradually or more saltatorily, drawing near to it in depth too " (p. 371)—quite conformably to Wertheimer's " factor of nearness ".

Similarly, a " factor of likeness " is apparently revealed. If we consider the original distribution of the seen depth of the discs in the cited protocol, we notice at once that the discs which are " equal " in respect of size, that is, numbers 1 and 2, on the one hand, and 3, 4, and 5 on the other, appear to be assembled in a uniform depth stratum : *Likeness of size determines collocation.* And furthermore, if a combination of discs of equal size but of different brightness (grey toning), is objectively exposed, a corresponding coalescence shows itself. " Bright discs lie far to the front, dark discs far to the back, *equally toned* discs appear arranged *for the time being in one depth stratum*, as a uniform group, screenlike, with large distances in depth between the groups."

Finally, there seems to be a *factor of common destiny.* For example, in the case of a combination of discs, arranged according to brightness, as follows (see the distribution of stimuli) :—

Obs. He.   Distribution of stimuli.

Diameter .		14	cm.			20	cm.		25 cm.
Brightness	5	3	2	1	5	3	2	1	1
Distance .	420	425	425	435	570	575	570	585	800
Designation									
of discs .	i	h	g	f	e	d	c	b	a

Scale of brightness : No. 1 = pure white ; No. 5 = dark grey.

When a group of discs placed objectively at one level of depth (e.g. the 20 cm. group) is suddenly transformed as a whole, by interposing illumination from a projector, the following occurs : Previously the discs of brightness 1 (pure white) appeared conjointly, right in front, palpably in one uniform stratum of visual space, and the two darkest discs (brightness 5), for example, also formed a unit, a screen-like stratum, right at the back ; but now this state of collocation is suddenly upset. Wertheimer's description fits exactly : " A suspense ensues, and eventually perplexity, confusion . . . frequently an over-balancing. The components affected by a common destiny result in a state of collocation." Now the group of (objectively belonging together) discs e, d, c, b can stand out as a new and stable spatial distribution, a stratum of visual objects, demarcated as such.

Thus far Wertheimer's statements receive confirmation ; his "factors" indeed seem in some way to give an accurate account of the matter.

But to *indicate* these "factors" by no means brings the analysis to an end. My researches inevitably led me to the *establishment of further facts* and consequently to a *quite different viewpoint for appraising the results*. It became clear to me, forthwith, that these very findings only link up to give a completed picture when the stated "objective depth motifs", "nearness", "likeness", and "common destiny", are considered in relation to the subjective conditions, the conditions of apprehension —" when the proposed factors are regarded not so much as 'depth motifs', but much rather as at bottom 'cognizance motifs', which only become secondary to 'depth motifs'. The true condition for the monocularly seen depth distribution lies in the direction of cognizance, in the mode of apprehension, in these cases too."

In my work, I was able to take the movement experiments, and thus the "factor of nearness", as point of departure in order to explain this all-inclusive orientation. Moreover, in giving a unified account of all my findings, I was able to base it upon this orientation, as the mainspring of the whole ; and I could with justice in the title state the topic of the research to be " The significance of the conditions of apprehension ".

" Unless these primary conditions of cognizance are taken into account, a conclusive analysis of the monocular seeing of depth is wholly impossible " (Petermann, pp. 397–8).

Wertheimer himself—and indeed all the gestalt theorists —is not aware of this aspect of the question at issue. But for this reason the way to a true psychological analysis of the facts of the matter is blocked to them. Their proposals do not do justice to the range of the actual relationships among the conditions. When the analysis of the facts is carried through to the finer details, it necessitates transcending Wertheimer's formulas, if these phenomena are to be thoroughly understood.

§ 40. *The fundamental dependence of the gestalt phenomena upon the mode of apprehension, as the main difficulty of the gestalt theory*

However, the foregoing considerations not only lead to our having to go beyond Wertheimer in a purely factual respect ; they also bring us to a crucial point in regard to the verdict *in the matter of principles.* They call for a clarification of the *question as to what significance the fact of the primary dependence of the quoted " collocations " upon the regulation of apprehension, has for the fundamental position to be taken up towards the gestalt theory.*

Here we must, to begin with, consider whether the facts thus established may at all be directly brought to bear upon the gestalt problem. For they were developed, first of all, only in reference to a perhaps quite different problem, the problem of the spatial distribution of visual objects ; and, moreover, under special circumstances perhaps particularly favourable in the approach at issue, that is, for monocular vision.

On the other hand, observations like those of Benussi and Rubin upon " gestalt-ambiguous figures ", or those of Wittmann upon " apparent solids ", show that as a matter of fact a general conditionality, critical especially in the simplest of all " articulations " of " figure " and " ground ", is here present, one which has significance for all gestalt phenomena (figural structures). Wittmann has, as it happens, fundamentally emphasized the significance, from the point of view of principles, of these observations, for the appraisal of the gestalt theory. He quotes a very simple and impressive experiment in illustration, in which this conditionality emerges particularly clearly. (Cf. Wittmann, 1921.)

In this experiment circular discs with variously coloured sectors (e.g. Disc I, white 180°, black 180° ; Disc II, white 240°, black 120° ; Disc III, black, red, and blue each 120°) were exposed while rotating (period of rotation varying from 1·3 sec. to 0·08 sec.). The experiment is noteworthy, in the first place, for the fact that it shows the " intra-configuration " of what is given, in the sense of the separation of a "figure" from a "ground", with exceptional distinctness ; and it has a particular interest for us, because in it this separation can at the same time be comprehended as conditioned by the mode of cognizance. Wittmann states : " The Observers have, to begin with, only the indeterminately sustained task of fixating the midpoint of the rotating disc, while, however, uniformly regarding the whole disc. This uniform, receptive manner of regarding the discs was experienced as unpleasant by all Observers ; they pass on, of their own accord, to pay special regard to one (and even two) of the rotating sectors. The more successfully this sector is apprehended in its configuratedness and, simultaneously, its movement in isolation, the more does the other sector lose its particular configurational—as well as movement—character. The single, successive, appearances of this sector seem to be more or less at rest, and in the course of one or more revolutions coalesce, in a way that can be clearly followed, into the startling total appearance of a resting, even, full disc, before which the isolated sector seen in movement rotates independently at a second level." This impression is remarkably precise. " The temporarily complete disc is seen so perceptually that it seems quite impossible to apprehend the sector constituting it as such. If for instance, in the case of Disc I a full white disc with a black semi-circle (sector) rotating in front of it is seen, then the perception of a rotating white semi-circle is found to have completely vanished " (p. 31). Furthermore, " If the impression of the full disc has once arisen, the gaze can wander over it at will. Henceforth it is also immaterial whether the sector here seen in movement continues to be attended to or not in its often very distorted form. Very frequently, with brief periods of rotation, the latter is not even seen at all for the duration of a number of revolutions. The surfaces of the full discs are markedly perceptual before the eye, to an extent which an ' objective full disc ' of the same colour could hardly surpass. This perceptuality is reinforced by the high degree of saturation with which the in itself at the time less saturated sector-colour appears, with the impression of the full disc " (p. 33).

From this it is clear how " a separation of the contents of perception into complexes of visual objects which have the character of objectivity in varying degrees, comes to pass; one part of the contents is seen as objective things, the other as ground, formless, level, or even possessing a certain depth, as visual field or else as visual space " (p. 33) only in specific temporal extension.

But above all this analysis shows that this process of separation is patently subject to the influence of cognizance. How the phenomenon will eventuate is an ambiguous matter, depending upon whether cognizance is directed predominantly to the white or predominantly to the black sector. In fact it is possible by means of appropriate voluntary direction of the mode of cognizance, to conduct the process in an arbitrarily predetermined direction in an outright " intentioned " way. The process of separation is therefore not by any means determined " in itself ", that is from the stimulus as starting point.

Moreover, even if it has once ensued in one way, the mode of appearance is by no means thus finally settled. The existing separation can be broken down and another separation produced. It is possible to experience an inversion of the phenomenon, that is, to see a rotating white sector in front of a black full disc, and also intentionally to induce this inversion to take place. This transformation process is characteristically and quite regularly determined by the mode of cognizance.

To begin with, according to Wittmann's observations this process cannot arise at pleasure. For—to repeat once again—in the meantime, in experience " the perception of a white rotating semi-circle has completely vanished. To regain this, one has in the first place wholly to ignore the black sector ; but this is not, as a rule, always easy, since the white sector happens throughout not to be given as such in the percept, but is seen as a full disc internally no further differentiated. One very often does not know how one could elicit a moving white sector out of the resting white full disc. With practice this transition can soon be more rapidly accomplished " (pp. 31-2).

Thus the mode of cognizance operates simultaneously to decompose and to assemble together—in brief, in an articulating way, for the mode of manifestation of the visual objects.

That the articulation of visual reality in circumscribed

wholes of visual objects, fully formed in themselves, is essentially bound up with a function of cognizance, a function of the mode of apprehension, can accordingly be subject to no doubt.

This conclusion has consequences for the foundations of the gestalt theory. For originally it has no place for such findings. At bottom—ever since Wertheimer's work of 1912—the main orientation of the theory is selected with reference to the stimulus. From this starting point it is proposed to deduce the whole of neurophysical and psychophysical reality, e.g. when Köhler strives to deduce his views about the configuration of "lines of current" in the neurophysical sector. (See above, § 28, below, §§ 42-3.)

A *primary* influence of subjective factors, such as we have had to draw attention to here, is nowhere positively acknowledged in principle. Either the facts in question are not mentioned at all, or else they are slightly touched upon by the way ; but they are thus expressly introduced as if it were *merely secondary*, at bottom incidental, and *as far as the theory is concerned unimportant, accessory conditions* which were at issue—conditions which to a certain extent accrue as disturbing moments to the genuine, pure, stimulus-controlled "gestalt processes", and deflect it.

Hence the facts quoted above seem to embrace findings which are essentially opposed to the general presuppositions of the gestalt theory. How weighty these findings are, can be judged by the extent to which the gestalt theory has been capable of coping with the facts in question in the manner we have indicated.

§ 41.   *The position of the gestalt theory in regard to the inversion phenomena, and to the dependency upon the subject of figural structures in general*

A position in regard to the inversion phenomena is directly taken up, in gestalt literature, for the first time by Koffka, 1922. Koffka starts from a definite interpretation which derives from Titchener. The latter gave a characteristic figure (Fig. 12) as a clear-cut example of the interchange of " figure " and " ground ".

This figure reveals very impressively how at one time one can see a row of black T's, and how thereafter, with a sudden reversal, a row of white leaves on a black background, can appear. Titchener's " explanation " of this phenomenon makes use of the *differentiation of various degrees of consciousness, which is related to the old-fashioned concept of Attention.* In his opinion the emergence of the T's has a very simple cause: "The black T's are on the upper level of consciousness, while the rest is at a lower level"; and so, also, he imagines the reversal to be easily explained ; all that has occurred is merely a change in that " level ".

In agreement with Koffka, serious objections can be developed against Titchener's interpretation of the inversion phenomena. Wittmann, Rubin, and Zahn have already indicated with due emphasis, that even from the purely descriptive side the case is essentially otherwise.

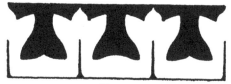

Fig. 12.

When the T's disappear and we see in their stead a bare background, they have no degree of clearness whatsoever in consciousness—as T's they are simply not there any more (cf. above, p. 161, Wittmann's analysis of analogous phenomena). The formulations upon which Titchener bases his interpretations are therefore not plain description, but already theory. But this theory is undoubtedly burdened with a quite dangerous presupposition. In so far as existence in consciousness is ascribed to the black T's—be it even " at a lower level "—when they are not apprehended as the figure, an assumption underlies the whole train of reasoning, the dangerousness of which Köhler discussed thoroughly in 1913, viz. the constancy hypothesis (see above, § 15). But we cannot reject the line of argument about the danger inherent in the constancy hypothesis, which derives substantially from the principle of " fundamental determinability " hitherto invoked by us as a decisive standard ; on the contrary we must agree with Koffka's remarks about Titchener's way of interpreting the inversion.

But when Koffka believes that he has thus shown the concept of Attention to be of no use at all as a principle for the theory, this claim must by no means be left unchallenged. For Koffka's submissions are relevant only to the quite definite theory of attention upon which Titchener takes his stand. This, in the last resort, derives from the body of conceptions of the Herbartian ideational mechanism, and is, accordingly, to a certain extent a relic of an attitude in all respects unempirical. But objections to it can of course not be directly transferred to what has in the meantime—subject to far less confined presuppositions—been achieved by means of empirical analysis of the facts.

From such analyses of the facts, it is well established that the modes of appearance of the figural structures depend upon the conditions of cognizance, of apprehension, of attentional attitude, in general upon subjective factors ; and we need only be concerned with the question of whether and to what extent the gestalt theory is capable of accounting for these in a positive way. These results do not permit of being facilely explained away. in any perfunctory manner.

The obligations thus imposed on the gestalt theory are, as we have seen, foreign to its original basic point of view. Nevertheless attempts to cope with them have in the interim been made. The general framework for these is already provided by Köhler's disquisitions on gestalt physiology, 1920. For in his hypothetical construction of the structures in the neurophysical sphere, he in principle concedes a co-determining influence to " other moments as well ", besides the retinal configuration (see above, p. 92). These are, firstly, the " relatively constant histological and material properties of the optical-somatic system " ; and secondly, " certain *relatively variable* conditioning factors which are to be ascribed primarily to the rest of the nervous system, and secondarily, to the vascular system." The introduction of such " variable factors " does indeed provide the *possibility* of " explaining " e.g. " gestalt ambiguousness ". Nevertheless, this " explanation " is abundantly vague. If one

adheres to the viewpoints developed within the framework of the gestalt theory in connection with the scrutiny
of other points of view (Köhler, 1913), one will needs
require more than this. One will demand that the
concrete configuredness of the contents of experience
should be reduced to an equally concrete account of the
conditions. For unless this is accomplished, the criterion
of fundamental determinability remains unsatisfied in
this case too ; and this is regarded as the scientific-
theoretical touchstone of the value of any theory
propounded.   However, Köhler's amplification fails in
this. He does not give a concrete theory of the phenomena
in question, but merely guarantees their general possibility
within the bounds of the fundamental orientation. On
the other hand, an apparently concrete treatment of
the phenomena occurs in another connection, in the
form of a special functional interpretation of them.

We shall review this interpretation, to begin with, in
connection with a somewhat different example, viz. the
question of how it happens that in observations upon sense
discrimination, within a definite critical region and with
the same pair of stimuli a, b, the three judgments $a>b$,
$a=b$, $a<b$ are all equally possible ; so that in one observation the first judgment and in another the last can occur,
although the stimulus conditions are not altered.

Koffka offers a quite definite functional interpretation
of this problem. " These facts, they show that the
organism's structural reaction to a pair of stimuli depends
upon its *attitude*. If we generalize from all the data, the
attitude may be such as to favour either a stepwise or an
assimilative structure (each to the detriment of the other),
or it may be indifferently advantageous to either one."
And from this he draws the "conclusion ": "Before the
subject is confronted with the stimulus, the structure that
will eventually ensue must be prepared for by a mental
attitude, and this attitude consists mainly in a readiness
to carry out a certain structural process."

This "readiness to carry' out a certain structural
process " is supposed to represent what really underlies
the ostensible influence of attention. Hereby is functionally
settled what Köhler vaguely intended by his "relatively
variable factors " in the neurophysical sphere. And
indeed, it is at the same time conceived as very concretely

M

defined. The appearance of e.g. the black parts of the T-illustration as figure here receives an explanation. "In attending to the black parts we adopt a '*figure attitude*' *toward them* by making them the centre of our interest." (Koffka 1922. Cf. also Rubin, 1916 already, or 1922.)

The "figure attitude" is thus the grounds of explanation and the grounds of existence of the mode of manifestation of the example. And in general, an appropriate "gestalt disposition" is correspondingly co-determinative of the phenomenally experienced gestalt in any sort of gestalt perception, under certain circumstances. It operates in such a way that a "gestalt phenomenon corresponding to it" also ensues "even if the stimulus situation would evoke another phenomenon in the indifferent individual."

Moreover, be it noted, each of these gestalt dispositions, these gestalt "attitudes", is characteristically defined as a "readiness to carry out a *certain* structural process"; each one is individually differentiated from every other, and this in accordance with exactly the same features which characterize the corresponding realized gestalten. Thus the specificity of the end product seems, on the face of it, to be functionally established in a very concrete way.

However, this manner of conceiving the "relatively variable factors" as functionally determined in the individual gestalt perception in a concrete way, is still no more than a mere apparent explanation. Koffka's "figure attitude", his "readiness to carry out a *certain* structural process" cannot fulfill the requirements one has to make of a scientific concept. For how is one to know in any concrete instance that a "figure attitude" of this sort, a figural *disposition constituted in this or that particular way*, is present? Surely only from the fact that a corresponding "figural *experience*" *subsequently* arises. By interposing a gestalt disposition corresponding to this "end product" as a condition, the problem has of course not been solved, but only obscured. Directly, we know just as little about such dispositions as about Köhler's variable physiological factors. They can, that is to say, never furnish positive means of explanation, provided that Köhler's scientific-theoretical principles should not simply be surrendered in this connection.

The concept of gestalt disposition and all its "derivatives", such as e.g. Wertheimer's explanation, as far back as 1912, of certain movement phenomena in terms of a specific "attitude"—physiologically conceived as a dispositional reality—must fundamentally be rejected as *not proven from the viewpoint of scientific theory*. Moreover, they do not satisfy the criterion of determinability, but are on the contrary of exactly the same character as Titchener's concept of attention which Koffka rightly rejects.

Furthermore, these concepts also fail to hold their ground *when set against the facts*. For the point of the matter is not only that an "explanation" must merely be found for *the fact that* a given arrangement of stimuli can at all be variously experienced on the phenomenal side; it must also be made intelligible in what way a change in the transmission of what is given can be directly *intentionally* induced. In regard to this question, the gestalt-theoretical conception is an utter failure. Only direct and exact analysis leads beyond this. This shows (cf. Wittmann) that such re-articulations are initiated by quite definite, voluntarily attainable or accomplished alterations in the mode of cognizance, and that they can therefore only be understood from the starting point of the concrete conditions of cognizance.

Thus we see that the means by which the gestalt theory seeks to adapt itself to the facts of subjective variability of phenomenal figural structures, are by no means satisfactory. The endeavour to fill the gaps met with in the theory at this point ends in a purely verbal solution.

As against this, we must emphasize that every positive discovery emerging in empirical research, however unpretentious, patently has more value as knowledge than this conception. And if such discovery suggests a relationship between the gestalt phenomenon and distinct, *specifiable*, "attentional" conditions, one will certainly —despite the efforts of Koffka and Köhler to bring discredit upon the concept of attention in scientific theory —by straightforward acceptance of this relationship, contribute more, and in a more positive way, to the clarification of the true circumstances of the genesis of the separation of "figure" and "ground", than if one believes the situation to have been cleared up in virtue of conjecturing "explanatory concepts" of the other type. It is true, one would not be able to take the concept of "attention" in the narrow sense in which the gestalt theory discusses and rejects it. It would not be possible at all to retain it as an explanatory concept of a theoretically constructive kind. "Attention" should not be regarded as a mysterious x, a force in itself unknown, which—in itself throughout detachable from the contents —exercises influences on these contents, forms, controls, regulates them in their mode of appearance "from without". For then everything can in truth be explained by it. *This* concept of attention psychology must indeed disown ; it is a relic from the days of faculty psychology ; in this we are entirely at one with e.g. Rubin in his polemic at a recent congress. But it is at all times necessary to take into account as a psychological problem, and to do justice to, the data which lie at the back of that concept. They are *empirically detectable* in every analysis of *concrete* conditions of *cognizance*, can be characterized in a psycho-logically wholly genuine manner ; and also, they are of decisive importance for the functional consideration of psychological coherences. To do justice to this importance it is necessary, in giving an account of the gestalt facts, to acknowledge—purely as a result of actual analysis of what is experienced—the *regulation of apprehension*, the *mode of cognizance, as a condition of the acquisition of form by what is given.* It must, at the same time, be borne in mind that the problem of attention should not, in this way, be conceived as allowing of isolation, but that, on the contrary, it is just from such findings that new viewpoints for the approach to the problem of attention itself, may emerge.[1] In regard to the gestalt problem, however, it follows from this that it is necessary to repudiate a purely physiological, image-like genesis of the structuration of what is perceptually given. The theory of Wertheimer, Koffka, and Köhler cannot do justice to the facts of the matter.

[1] Cf. in connection with the above, Wittmann, 1921, *Scheinbewegungen und Scheinkörper*, as well as Petermann, 1923, "Bechterews Theorie der Konzentrierung, ein Beitrag zur Analyse des Aufmerksamkeits-problems." We return to this question in another book, *Gestaltproblem*, 1931, Joh. Ambr. Barth, Leipzig.

3. KÖHLER'S ATTEMPT AT A POSITIVE CONSTRUCTIONAL THEORY OF THE "FIGURE" CHARACTER

The dissenting position we have taken towards the gestalt theory on the grounds hitherto advanced, is even strengthened when we investigate one of the latest forms in which the gestalt theory has been elaborated, with reference to the problem of "figure" and "ground". This is Köhler's attempt at a constructional foundation for this fundamental differentiation, by resorting to physiology.

§ 42. *Köhler's physiological proposals*

In his book of 1920, Köhler gives a derivation for the figure-character, through a very simple example. He takes

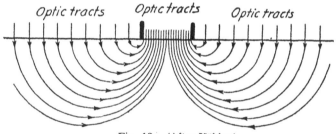

Fig. 13. (After Köhler.)

the case where a white circle against, say, a homogeneous grey-coloured ground, is regarded.

He develops (p. 206) the appropriate theorem for the retinal processes. " The retinal image yields *one* kind of reaction on a similarly circular area, and a second kind of reaction extensively around that." Herewith electromotive forces arise along the course of the contour, which bring about electrostatic displacements in the optic sector after the fashion shown in the diagram.

And " now this is what it comes to : *The same total electrostatical displacement must ensue* through the homogeneous surrounding of the circle, as through the retinal circle-field itself ; and since by assumption the figure has a moderate retinal extension, compared with the differently coloured surroundings, the average density of current through the circle-field is throughout very much greater than through the surrounding field. . . ."

Thus " in the *configured happening*, as far as it is of an electrostatical nature, a *much more lively state corresponds to the figure area than to the ' extended ground ' "*. Hereby a physiological definition of the peculiarity of the figure-area is achieved, which seems the more illuminating, to begin with, since to a certain extent the " phenomenal forcefulness " of the figure area is seen to be " directly " represented in a correspondingly enhanced liveliness of the physiological event.

§ 43. *The scientific import of Köhler's proposals*

It cannot be denied that this possibility does at first sight have a persuasive effect. But the greatest anomalies are, nevertheless, very soon revealed in its further elaboration. Thus, if we consider the fact of the ever possible reversibility of figure and ground in a stimulus constellation of the kind in point,[1] very great difficulties appear.

Köhler does not discuss these cases, but merely erects the general principle for them, that the already developed explanation " gestalt area of high psychophysical energy density " must be universally taken as their basis. But if we do not acquiesce in this, and on the contrary apply, in this matter too, those principles which are supposed to enable us to arrive at a deduction of the physiological singularity of the figural areas directly " from the starting point of physics ", we very soon come upon the sharpest contradictions and obscurities.

" From the starting point of physics "—that is in so far as one does not, from the outset, keep in view what " ought to supervene "—it would follow that this time the region physiologically parallel to the phenomenal " figure " area would be the one in which the amount of energy is spread out in the least density. For the distribution of the flux of current, and its density, are regulated, according to the whole theorem, simply and solely by the cross-section of the areas of excitation concerned which are compared with one another. A modification through the " relatively variable conditioning factors which are

---

[1] We know that this white circular disc is equally well and insistently capable of appearing as "ground" for instance, and the grey of the surrounding as a very firmly configured "figure". In this case one experiences an orifice in a fixed grey frame which permits a free view into a brightly illuminated space.

to be ascribed . . . to the rest of the nervous system ",
which Köhler grants in addition to the main conditions
of formation of psychological gestalten, cannot be
adequately incorporated into this treatment. For it is
inconceivable how such a "controlling action" of these
other factors should be fitted into Köhler's scheme, seeing
that the factors in question are wholly indeterminate.

And if, on the supposition of such accessory conditions,
we could perhaps come to the conclusion, that we are
indeed dealing with a different case from that which was
first considered, this in no way renders it intelligible how a
straight transposition of the circumstances in the two
cases could occur.

But this is not the end of the matter. This consideration affects the original hypothesis retroactively, and must
dispose us to be critical towards the possibility of adopting
this theorem in this form at all. For if, in the second
instance, "other factors" ostensibly have such great
influence upon the circumstances in question, have we the
right to ignore "other factors" altogether in elucidating
the first instance? We are certainly not justified *a
priori* in this, but simply lull ourselves in silent security,
"because it fits so beautifully," when we show ourselves
inclined to accept Köhler's line of argument as sound.
Hence, as actual support for Köhler's assumption, there
evidently remains only the analogy between "phenomenal
forcefulness" and "enhanced psychophysical energy
content "—an anology which can indeed have a persuasive
effect, but nevertheless possesses no significance for a
scientific train of argument.

Thus, in respect to the physiological side, too, the
gestalt-theoretical treatment of the problem of figural
character leaves as great gaps as it does in respect to the
descriptive-functional side. On the whole, the problem
"what *is* figural character, descriptively, and *what is its
genesis*, functionally or else physiologically ", is by no
means cleared up in this way, nor even so comprehensively
prosecuted in the analysis of the conditions as one would
expect from the claims of the gestalt theory.

This, however, does not exhaust the factual material
on the "figure-ground" problem, in reference to its
vindication of the gestalt theory. The singularity of the
figure areas is supposed to be evinced above all in the fact

that certain effects appear in connection with such presentations, which seem to be quite conspicuously traceable
to the figural unit as a whole—that is, which seem to be
attributable to the independent functional significance
of the figural unit.

CHAPTER II

THE FIGURAL STRUCTURES AND THEIR FUNCTIONAL EFFECTS PROPER TO THE STRUCTURE

According to the results of experimental research,
effects seem to be demonstrable with figural structures,
which deserve to be described as inherent in the structure,
as transcending the " elements ". Hence these have been
regarded as supporting the gestalt theory. We proceed
to consider certain findings upon the influence of gestalten
on the qualitative determination of the single points of
the field. In these findings it is shown how the single
points of the field are determined in their colour quality,
not by the single, specific action of the stimulus at the
particular place concerned (cf. the constancy hypothesis),
but by some sort of " gestalt moments " which transcend it.

I. SIMPLEST COLOUR PHENOMENA AS EVIDENCE OF THE FUNCTIONAL UNITARINESS OF " GESTALTEN "

In the question as to a direct influencing of colour
phenomena by the figural structure of the field, a series of
findings can be adduced, which have emerged partly
before the advent of the gestalt theory, and partly in
direct consequence of problems posed under the influence
of the theory. They include problems of contrast effects,
of " colour assimilation ", and of " colour thresholds ".

§ 44. *Gestalt context and colour contrast*

The theory of colour contrast, which has since the
time of Hering followed certain very definite conceptions

—the notion of an induction effect of the single points of the retina upon one another—is shifted into entirely new domains on the basis of experiments by investigators with the gestalt-theoretical point of view.

Hering's theory is throughout "atomistically" and "additively" aligned in its approach : The induction effects are effects which pertain to the retinal points as such, in their isolation. The induction consequent at a

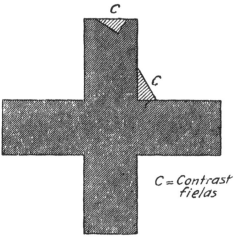

Fig. 14.

particular place, which comes to expression in the qualitatively given hue, is conceived as a total effect, resulting from the superposition of the single induction values which enter the contrast-field from the various points of the surrounding parts.

As against this, Benary in 1924, stimulated by Wertheimer, communicated specific findings which contradict such an atomistic-additive view. Using a black cross upon a white ground he introduced small, grey-coloured, right-angled triangles of equal dimensions, as contrast-fields, firstly in one angle of the cross, and secondly upon one of its arms (see fig. 14).

The result was that the grey field lying in the angle of the cross appeared dark in comparison with the field introduced upon the arm of the cross ; although the extent of the black area contiguous with the triangle in the corner is substantially greater than the black area adjoining the other triangle.

Wertheimer and Benary conclude : Obviously the contrast effect cannot therefore be regarded as compounded of elementary induction effects in the manner indicated at the outset. On the contrary, the effect proves to be dependent upon the gestalt-context in which the contrast-field belongs.

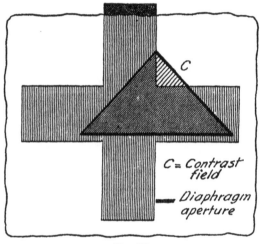

C = Contrast field

Diaphragm aperture

Fig. 15.

Benary shows this perhaps even more distinctly in a slightly modified experiment. A black cross upon a white ground is presented to the regard, with a grey contrast field in a corner between the arms. This is now suddenly covered over with a white screen which leaves the contrast field and a homogeneous black triangle visible, say, through a triangular aperture (see fig. 15), but otherwise covers a considerable part of the original black area out of sight. In this second situation the grey field in turn appears brighter than in the first situation, in spite of the fact that in comparison with the first distribution of colour, black is subtracted and white added in the "inducing" colour areas. Exactly analogous phenomena appear with coloured areas.

Accordingly, a new condition seems to be important for

the genesis of the contrast effect. In addition to the amounts of the effective colours, " the configured whole as a part of which the portion of the field presents itself " is also critical (p. 141). The effect depends upon how the surface " belongs together " (p. 142).

These facts are irrefutable. But what do they prove ? Do they needs implicate acknowledgment of the gestalt theory ? To begin with, they are obviously evidence of nothing more than the fact that the characteristic unitariness which phenomenally marks gestalt areas also possesses some sort of significance in functional respects. But more far-reaching inferences could not be drawn from them. Benary himself emphasizes, that one would have " to have more exact knowledge than is the case at present about the quantitative conditions of contrast . . . far too little is known about how the contrast effect for various distances should be statistically treated ".

Indeed the import of these observations of Wertheimer and Benary will have to be even further limited. That the colour is influenced in relation to the configurational organization must be admitted ; but in doing so the *gestalt-theoretical* interpretation of these facts has not really been touched at all. The question is, *how* the operation of the gestalt moments is to be construed.

That this " how " need not be interpreted in the sense of a physiology of gestalt processes, is specifically vouched for. I shall only refer to one of Wertheimer's experiments,[1] quoted by Koffka in 1915. In this, a grey circular disc was introduced upon a half green and half red ground, so that it was exactly symmetrical about the dividing line between the two fields. This experiment clearly reveals how here too the *influence of apprehension* plays a rôle. " If the complex is apprehended in such a way that two contiguous semicircles, each upon a different ground, are seen, these two semicircles display strong contrast. If the apprehension is changed so that a full circle is seen instead of the two semicircles, then this is only very weakly, or not at all contrastively coloured, that is, corresponding to the unitary figure, it also has a wholly or almost wholly unitary colour " (p. 40).

[1] For that matter Wundt made use of a quite analogous experiment in his lectures—for the purpose of demonstrating the *central* conditioning of the contrast phenomenon (cf. Sander, *Bericht X. Kongress*, 1928, p. 38).

This comes out even more clearly in a variant of the experiment by Benussi. In this, about 20 grey discs arranged in a circular form were exposed upon an equally apportioned green and red field. Here too, with appropriate cognizance of the circle gestalt the contrast effect entirely disappears [1] (*Arch.* 36, p. 61).

Thus it is only possible to say that a quite *specific internal*, if one wishes, " dynamic " *closure* pertains to the gestalt coherence, and that this closure makes itself apparent along with the qualitative mode of appearance of the colours—assuming *that* a coherence of such a kind *is* present. And it might also be emphasized, that the question *whether* such a coherence is *present or not* must be elucidated essentially in terms of the problem of the influence of apprehension.

Thus no essential reinforcement for the actual theoretical position accrues from these facts.

§ 45. *Colour assimilation under the influence of gestalten*

The connections between colour and gestalt have been more systematically followed out by Fuchs (1923—1, 2). His attention was first drawn to such connections in his work on " the simultaneous seeing of things behind one another in the same line of vision ". In this work it appeared—in experiments utilizing Hering's reflection method—that a simultaneous post-position of two colours in the same line of vision does occur ; i.e. that " transparency " may be spoken of in a precise sense, and this only under quite definite circumstances.

" The condition for this is that the *transparent object* and *the object seen through it* be apprehended as *two gestalten* ! " " It is possible to achieve a colour transparency in which one colour can even be seen through its complementary colour. In a successful experiment, a closed and uniformly coloured gestalt is seen through a

---

[1] Similarly, Johann Köhler had already established in 1904 (*Arch.* 2), " With a not too small neutral field, exposed on one side to a colour induction, it is possible to bring about the following—where the contrast effect has to be compensated by an inserted colour sector. The half adjacent to the inducing field appears contrastively coloured, while the other half appears of the colour of the inserted sector, when a thread is held before it, dividing the field in the middle like a dark line. When the thread is removed, the field appears unitarily coloured."

similarly closed and uniformly coloured gestalt. When the experiment is less successful the colour of the anterior surface often appears flaky, in such a way that colourless, glassy patches between the flakes make the surface a gestalt which is nowhere disrupted, and which simultaneously appears before a likewise fully closed, and for the most part uniformly coloured gestalt, in the rear. Furthermore, another case is possible where 'nothing' is seen between the coloured flakes. Hereupon the closure character of the anterior surface is, as a rule, lost, in such a way that a series of transition stages can be observed between this and the preceding stage. Finally, still keeping to the same stimulus conditions, the anterior surface can appear to be interrupted at the (critical) place correct for the line of vision, so that only one gestalt, and with it only *one* colour is visible there " (Summary of 1923—2, p. 250).

Thus a significant result seems to have been obtained, one which points to the gestalt theory. Only when the " separation conforming to gestalt " asserts itself, does that differentiation of spatial localization which Fuchs made the object of his investigations, arise. Similarly, it' always lapses—" compulsory conjunction " of " unity of colour " and " unity of line of vision " (in the sense of Hering's researches on colour-mixture) sets in—when through the deficiency of dominant parts the possibility of such configurational isolations is in any case eliminated.

The way in which gestalten, under the circumstances here in question, coalesce for a time being, or are demarcated from one another, the way in which gestalten are " picked out ", is therefore of decisive importance for the impression. It determines the impression of the colour—and this not only in reference to the mode of appearance of the transparency, but also purely in respect to the quality. " The dominant parts make possible not only the configurational separation as such, but soon after the commencement of the research it appeared that they also have some sort of influence on the colour of the critical part. If e.g., a yellow line is exposed behind a transparent blue line crossing it, and if the critical part has a whitish-grey colour when regarded through a perforated screen, or when picked out in isolation, this is reversed, as soon as the whole blue or the whole yellow gestalt, or both gestalten at the same time, are picked out. The critical part then takes on more or less strongly the colour of the gestalt to which it is attached. It thus becomes either yellow or blue ; whereupon it can, in the extreme case, fully take on the colour and mode of appearance of the dominating parts of the gestalt concerned. Or it splits, as it were, into one portion belonging to the anterior and one portion belonging to the posterior gestalt, in which case each portion more or less takes on the colour nuance of the gestalt to which it belongs " (p. 251).

Hence there arise, in correspondence with the inter-articulation of the field of vision according to whole gestalten, "reciprocal colour assimilations in the (objectively) differently coloured parts, which in the extreme case give rise to an entirely unitary colour of the gestalt which is picked out " (p. 208).[1] And moreover, " the colour of the dominant parts [influences] to a far-reaching extent the colour of the critical part, inasmuch as the latter, through assimilation, partakes, as it were, to some extent in the colour of the dominant parts " (p. 264). Alongside of this, however, it is shown (p. 286) " that the colour of the prominent part, that is the apparently true colour, is influenced also by the colour of the covered part, and this the more so as the covered part increases— even if the covered part is appreciably smaller than the prominent part " (p. 286).

" The assimilation is a consequence of the gestalt apprehension " (p. 264). For on the one hand the reciprocal assimilation is " proportionately stronger, the better the precise apprehension of the total gestalt of each surface succeeds ". On the other hand, this assimilation disappears completely if the prominent part is picked out by itself as an independent gestalt. The colour is then independent of the rest of the field, it does not change when the size of the covered area is made to increase or diminish.

Here too is impressively shown, once more, how the *configurational* " *being-at-one* " manifests itself *as a crucial condition for the qualitative determination of the colours* of the parts, exactly as with the Wertheimer-Benary findings on contrast. The question is whether

---

[1] Cf. also a brief communication by Koffka about analogous colour assimilations with objectively typical inhomogeneous colour disc surfaces, in so-called " pseudo-Masson discs " (1925).

the theoretical evaluation goes further in this case than in that.

Without a doubt, these findings furnish significant material for the *substantiation of the thesis that it is not possible to build up the whole from the parts in a synthetic manner*. We almost think that Fuchs, who in principle grounded himself upon the gestalt theory even in his first work, does not stress this consequence enough, nor with conceptual clearness and definiteness. Throughout, his phraseology is that of an additive mode of thinking (1923). He speaks of " super-position " of colours, or of the " subduing of memory colour ", of " compensating " and " overcompensating ", quite as if Köhler had never uttered polemics against the constancy hypothesis.

But even if the antisynthetic orientation finds further support in this work, still it establishes nothing in regard to the *gestalt theory in the specific sense*. For, as with the contrast results, it is again evident, that the *really central question*, the question of *how* gestalt coherences constitute themselves, cannot be more exactly settled from the starting point of the facts here under review.

Fuchs himself does not pose this question. From the outset he employs the gestalt concept as understood by Wertheimer and Köhler, as a means of explanation. He assumes, that is, that the gestalt theory is already sufficiently well founded. And if, conversely, one seeks among his results for findings calculated to furnish material towards the solution of that problem, one cannot reckon upon great profit ; since for this purpose the analysis should from the outset have been carried through in greater detail in this direction. Nevertheless one finds enough that is noteworthy, as it is.

It appears that Fuchs' observations lead to the very same question which we encountered in connection with the contrast findings—that of the " relationship between attention and gestalt apprehension ".

Many of Fuchs' more exact conclusions point towards this question. Thus Fuchs' result, according to which a mixed colour is essentially determined by the size of the partial field involved, proves to have exceptions. " The dependence of the mixed colour upon the size can undergo a change, by reason of the colours' having different intensities and insistence " (p. 259). This is so far-reaching, that e.g., on occasion the less extensive but more insistent colour tone can even entirely " prevail " over the extensive colour, in determining the mixed colour.   Furthermore, the same result can ensue because of the smaller field's being conspicuous in reference to the configurational coherence, in an appropriately clear way ; that is to say, when it comprises the "centre of gravity of the gestalt ". The smaller part can also be reinforced in its influence relatively to its proportion by reason of its being " the more important part of the gestalt " (p. 259).

Since we are already aware, in a general way, of the significance of the conditions of apprehension, it becomes difficult not to bring these observations into relation with them.   Fuchs has very well perceived that there are moot questions in this connection.   He himself grants that the gestalt apprehension has something to do with attention.   But he unfortunately dismisses the question with the brief remark that the relationship between attention and gestalt apprehension " which enters into these matters, still requires clarification ".   He has not yet come as far as methodically investigating this relationship, obviously because, in his bondage to the gestalt theory, he misjudges its significance (see § 48).

Thus Fuchs' investigation, too, comes to nothing conclusive. It leads up to the same problem as the Wertheimer and Benary contrast experiments—and leaves them equally open.   The findings quoted in the foregoing paragraphs in regard to the effects of gestalten upon the quality of colours, can therefore not be deemed evidence of the correctness of the *gestalt theory*, even if they quite palpably demonstrate the *positive significance of the antisynthetic orientation in general*.

§ 46. *Figural structure and colour thresholds*

Gelb and Granit have given an account (1923) of the other experiments which are taken to be evidence of the influence of specific gestalt processes on colour, in the sense of the gestalt theory.   They are concerned with the question " whether colour *thresholds* do not behave differently, according as the grey field (to which the colour is added in just noticeable strength) has more the properties of a figure, or those of a ground ".

Pictures were presented which showed a brighter or else a darker figure like a Maltese cross upon a homogeneous grey ground. The pictures were so constructed, that for every fixed brightness-constellation of figure and ground (e.g. figure 340°S, ground 36°S—" positive picture ") there was always available a corresponding one in which the brightness relationships were interchanged (e.g. figure 36°S ; ground 340°S—" negative picture "). Thus paired grey fields of equal brightness were always available for the supplementary colour stimuli ; the fields being differentiated only in that they appeared once as figure and the second time as ground. The supplementary colour was introduced—by means of reflectors—once on the figure field of a positive picture, and the next time on the ground field of the associated (and therefore objectively equally bright at the place in question) negative picture, each time covering a small circular patch within these fields.

In the determination of the colour threshold—i.e. that particular stimulus intensity at which a *true colour impression*, not, perchance, the appearance of a colourless patch or of one not exactly definable as to its quality, was observed—the *main result* that emerged was : " The colour threshold for a field of given brightness which remains objectively constant varies in magnitude according as the field concerned appears as figure or as ground." And *always* moreover, " the *figure threshold is greater than the threshold for the ground field* (p. 93) in such a way that the *difference between the threshold for the figure field and that for the ground field*, for a field of fixed objective brightness, *is the greater the more lively the effect of the difference between figure and ground* " (p. 95).[1]

In order to give a positive *explanation* of this fact, Gelb and Granit resort to the gestalt theory, and this in a noteworthy manner, *along two lines*.

Firstly, they make use of Köhler's theory of the *neuro-*

---

[1] An essential point here is that, for the observed difference, the objective variation, as stimulus, of the white content of the fields does not alone suffice for the explanation of the effect. It was possible to produce conditions which show how " the influence of the figure-ground factor compensates directly for the influence of the objective brightness of the fields " (p. 96), a circumstance which is particularly stressed by Gelb and Granit, as an instance in opposition to the theory advocated by Revesz.

N

physical character of figural structure, his notion that the phenomenal singularity of the " figure " areas can be neurophysically represented by " ascribing to the ' figure event ' a higher physiological energy density than that ascribed to the, as it were, feebler happening which forms the correlate of the ground impression " (p. 104), Gelb and Granit readily accommodate their results to this : When the colour patch becomes noticeable this signifies the arousal of a new " figure ". What happens is that " the new figure-formation [must] in the one case be engendered upon a field which already has figure character ; in the second case, upon a field which has the psychophysical properties of the ground. The physiological process which corresponds to the new figure-formation must in the one case assert itself against a psychophysical event which is in itself already more lively, i.e. denser ; whereas in the contrasted case it has only to overcome a feebler happening " (pp. 104–5).

Thus the varying degree of resistance of the already present psychophysical state to the new figure-formation, would, according to this line of reasoning, be the reason why the threshold for the figure field is higher than that for the ground field.

This first interpretation is, however, forthwith abandoned by Gelb and Granit themselves—in favour of a second, more general one. To obtain a uniform explanation not only for their own results, but also for those of Fuchs on colour assimilation, they take up general gestalt-theoretical viewpoints. They want to " reduce all of it to a general conformity ", " namely, the *tendency towards precision* of the gestalt."

Hereupon an entirely *new* " *explanation* " arises. It is very simple, to begin with : " Since an inhomogeneity in colouring detracts from the precision of the figure fields used by us, the *tendency to appear as homogeneously as possible* asserts itself, and for that reason the field-threshold for the figure fields is, in our experiments, higher than for the equally bright ground fields " (p. 105). Here the previous interpretation seems at first sight merely to be characteristically transformed and extended. " From this point of view, the ' resistance ' of which we previously spoke is only a resistance against a change in the psychophysical event of a sort which threatens to prejudice the precision of the figure " (pp. 105–6). Thus the neuro-physical theory seems to be still retained.

But a little later (pp. 109), in the course of coming to terms with Revesz' suggestions for explaining similar findings on the ground of an inhibitory effect of the white content of the critical surface,[1] they declare : " According to the law of precision of the gestalt, a figure has the *tendency to appear in as precise a colour as possible,* that is either truly free of tone or properly coloured. For that reason it offers ' resistance ' against a change of its (already present) tone-free colour, until the amount of the supplementary colour is large enough for it to be able to appear in a new, approximately precise, colouring " (p. 109). Thus a formulation is given which has nothing more to do with the preceding one. The precision-tendency, which according to these last reflections determines the raising of the figure-threshold, is undoubtedly quite different in nature to the tendency towards precision previously under consideration. Here—in the antithesis " truly free of tone " and " properly coloured "—*precision in respect of the mode of appearance of the colours* is meant, whereas previously it was *precision* patently *referring to the configurational aspect of the fields* in the narrower sense of the word, the character of being a figure.

We have, therefore, to come to a decision about *two entirely different conceptions.*

If, in the phenomena described above, *precision in respect to the coloration* of the fields is the issue, then other findings may be adduced which totally refute Gelb's analysis, the observations of Ackermann (1924) which, it deserves to be noted, likewise emanate from the gestalt-theoretical school.

Ackermann, stimulated by Koffka, and independently of Gelb and Granit, carried out analogous experiments in con-tinuation of some made by Stumpf in 1917. By means of the colour top, he presented upon a homogeneous grey " surrounding field U ", a ring-shaped grey " test-field J ", where he continued to add colour to grey until the moment coloration was observed. In their general outcome his observations agree with those of Gelb and Granit. " Besides the properties of the test-field itself, the structure

---

[1] Cf. the foot-note on p. 181.

of the total phenomenal field exercises a decisive influence upon the colour threshold." But in addition a phenomenon occurred which Gelb and Granit had not observed. Ackermann states that the J, even when it has the most precise figure character, as when J is white and U a deep black, *by no means* behaves quite indifferently towards small increments of colour, and appears suddenly in an *approximately precise coloration* only with larger ones. The *exact opposite is the case* : the white becomes blurred, then somehow drops out of the black-white series, then acquires a " weak, still wholly uncertain coloration ", until at length it shows " the clear colour character " (p. 78).[1]

It is clear, therefore, that we cannot by any means speak of an " effort after precision of coloration " in Gelb's sense. The facts which more exact analysis brings to light stand in opposition to the theoretical tenets basic to Gelb's second explanation.

The first interpretation given by Gelb and Granit, which hinges on Köhler's work, is equally unsatisfactory. Köhler's pronouncements can, according to our previous contentions, by no means be accepted as already secure in themselves. When, therefore, Gelb and Granit set out to bring their observations into relation with them, this is naturally a highly uncertain " explanation ". But, conversely, it can as little be said that Köhler's proposals are necessarily implied by these observations. These observations contain nothing more than the general confirmation of the phenomenal finding that the threshold has a different altitude in the gestalt context than in the ground. If one simply chooses to hypostasize appropriate *ad hoc* " tendencies ", " resistances ", etc., one naturally does not arrive at a genuine explanation. The situation is then no different from that of the previously considered facts of colour psychology.

The findings in regard to colour psychology, and their connection with gestalt phenomena, must so far still rank as intrinsically not at all satisfactorily explained. Here lie urgent tasks for further detailed, experimental analysis.

---

[1] For that matter, these facts have already been observed by Katona (1922, *Ztschr. f. Sinnesphysiol.*, 53, pp. 145–6).

2. THE PHENOMENA OF GESTALT DISPLACEMENT

The functional singularity of the figural structures in the gestalt-theoretical sense, is supposed to be detectable in still another connection. The gestalt processes were observable, in the cases considered, in the gestalt interior, in an influence upon the quality of the separate field localities. They are held to be operative *also " outwardly "*, in respect to the relation of a gestalt to other gestalten of spatial nature. They are held to determine the position of these in the total phenomenally given spatial arrangement. Just as gestalt processes, as opposed to stimulus conditions, are held to evince themselves in the *conversion of the quality evoked by the stimulus*, so they are held to be able to display themselves in a *displacement counter to the spatial situation required by the stimulus*.

Fuchs (1920) was the first [1] to evaluate such spatial displacements under the influence of gestalten, in terms of the gestalt theory. He bases himself on the material which he obtained—in the institute of Gelb and Goldstein [2]— in investigating the vision of hemianopic and hemiamblyopic subjects with brain injuries. Indeed, Fuch's assessment of the pathological findings throughout creates the impression that the gestalt theory gets to the heart of the matter, and that it stands the test in an unexpected and extraordinarily impressive manner.

---

[1] Although Wertheimer in 1912, in his " Exkurs " had already hit upon something similar, and even provides Fuchs with many concepts which play a rôle in the latter's " explanation ", no connection with " gestalt theory " can as yet be perceived in 1912 ; so that Wertheimer can only rank as a pioneer, and not as a precursor, from this point of view.

[2] The works of Gelb and Goldstein themselves hardly come into question in the discussion of the gestalt theory. They do indeed contain personal confessions in which the authors decide in favour of the gestalt theory ; but nowhere do they lead to positions from which anything conclusive in support of the theory materially follows. Even though Gelb and Goldstein in their first work formulate the " fundamental theoretical conception " of their researches along the line " that we are dealing with the possibility of a singular pathological change, a disturbance of what the normal person encounters as *firmly configured impressions* in his optical perception " ; and even if this conception is directly traced to Wertheimer ; yet a true inner relationship with the gestalt theory in the specific sense, is nowhere to be found. This, in fact, is evinced only in the works of Fuchs.

§ 47.   *Fuch's findings and their gestalt-theoretical interpretation*

Fuchs' enquiries are concerned with very simple experiments. He dealt with the straightforward question of how people with brain injuries of this sort see when certain simple stimulus-complexes are presented to them tachistoscopically. These included both closed, coherent gestalten (rectangular or radial figures), and point-constellations of definite gestalt organization (linear series of points, rectangular and triangular arrangements, etc.). The exposure was so arranged that when the regard was fixed upon a fixation mark, the figures fell either totally, or partially, or not at all within the area of relative impotence of the retina (amblyopia).

In the case of an almost exactly hemiplegic amblyopic disturbance for example, which had persisted after almost complete homonymous hemianopsia, the following discovery emerged, which is sufficient to characterize facts of the matter.

If the stimuli were selected so as to fall entirely within the functionally competent part of the retina, the perception was normal.

If the stimuli were exposed so as to fall fully within the area of amblyopia (left half of the visual field), they were seen, but were localized not in their true position in space but displaced towards the right—into the sound half of the visual field.

And finally: If the objects are so chosen, that both the amblyopic and the normal sections of the retina are involved, the result—at all events as given at that time, in the first publications of the tables in question—is that " the displacement extends to the parts of the figure falling in the functionally competent halves of the fields as well, which parts were not displaced upon being exposed alone. In other words, a rightward displacement of the *total gestalt* takes place " (p. 263).

This last result is, for Fuchs, the most important one. With this as starting point, he develops a very pregnant train of reasoning, which aims at proving the gestalt-theoretical interpretation to be the only adequate one. He says: " If we were to explain these results in terms of the traditional anatomical-physiological views, it would not be intelligible why the displacement here extends to both halves of the visual field. For according to the first results, . . . a stimulus is displaced by our patients only when it falls in the damaged half of the field, whereas it is correctly localized in the sound half. If now, in our experiments, a stimulus falling simultaneously in the two halves of the field is also displaced as to the part of it lying in the sound half of the field, this result can only be the effect of a total process. This total process consists in the gestalt process " (p. 263).

The line of reasoning which is believed thus to lead to the acknowledgment of the gestalt theory, is again very simple. Its basis is the datum that like retinal points at different times have very different "space values", according as they are stimulated by themselves, or in connection with other points falling in the impotent half of the retina. From this the conclusion is drawn, that : 1, the traditional anatomical-physiological view, this very theory of " space values ", is inadequate ; 2, instead of it, only an explanation in terms of " gestalt processes " deserves positive consideration.

At any rate, to Fuchs it seems satisfactory to assume that the localization is determined on the basis of such total processes as these of Wertheimer. " If the impression of a unitary gestalt which corresponds to such a total process is localized, an alteration of localization affecting one *part must* (!) be critical for the total gestalt ". He proceeds to the interpretation, " In these manifestations, the way the processes run their course in the cortex is not such that the damaged and the sound visual spheres function by themselves, a purely summational effect thus being present ; but characteristic total processes, super-ordinated to the single excitations (which occur only in abstraction) exist " (p. 263). And with this he arrives at formulations, according to which an illustration for Köhler's thesis of the free propagation of lines of current appears directly in these findings—in so far as they can be cited as warranting the affirmation that a strict point-by-point transmission, fixed in isolated conduction, from the retina to the psychophysical level, does not exist.

Thus Fuchs' factual results appear to lead directly to an inductive proof for the gestalt theory, both in regard to the general, somewhat vague idea of " total processes ", as Wertheimer enunciated them, and in regard to the concrete, constructionally erected theory of Köhler.

It cannot be denied that these pointed statements which we have thus far considered, do indeed appear to betoken something of the sort. However, if we go beyond these, and bring Fuchs' material in its entirety under consideration, and test the suggested consequences by it, the state of affairs does not seem to be so wholly clarified.

With Fuchs himself, it is true, all of it seems to be capable of being uniformly comprehended under the gestalt-theoretical viewpoint ; but we should not allow ourselves to be lulled into security by this. The plan of Fuchs' work is a quite specific one. It starts avowedly from a precise, particular instance (see our account), and arranges all further findings that follow within the theoretical framework which, in the exposition based on that precise, particular instance, seems already established in § 2. Through this plan Fuchs' results as a matter of course acquire far more the character of corroborative ascertainments than that of experimental and empirical findings. An inductive procedure, mounting gradually from the facts to the theoretical issues, is in nowise striven for, let alone attempted. The consequence of this is, that it is almost impossible to obtain a clear picture of the relation of fact to theory, from Fuchs' disquisitions—unless one takes the trouble specially to separate the two, in studying Fuchs' writings. For in spite of the empirical character of the investigations, the theory permeates the whole of it from the outset. The danger of this manner of exposition is that, in virtue of the theory, many of the facts can appear to be already coloured in a definite way, although in and by themselves, in their true factual import, they could certainly not be regarded in that light.

If, therefore, we wish to evaluate Fuchs' work in a sound way, it seems unavoidable to follow up further, in more detail, his particular findings, while deliberately adhering to the viewpoint we have indicated. It amounts to testing Fuchs' results in their entire bearing, while keeping facts and theory apart as clearly as possible, so as to see whether the facts really lead to the theory as cogently as Fuchs would have it ; and also to see whether, in the whole compass of the empirical material assembled by Fuchs, the consonance of facts and theory asserted by him proves to be intrinsically accurate.

A scrutiny of Fuchs' statements on these lines, has indeed very surprising results.

§ 48. *The tenability of Fuchs' interpretation*

A critically discriminating assessment shows the gestalt-theoretical position to be essentially less surely founded in Fuchs' work, than one should at first sight believe it to be from Fuchs' own account. We shall limit ourselves to the more detailed discussion of only one central question, the question as to the possible significance of subjective conditions. That such conditions play a rôle is evident again and again at every step from Fuchs' statements ; and that they are in some way connected with the core of the displacement phenomena as a whole, is even implied in Fuchs' own elucidations, which finally culminate in an attention theory of hemianopsia.

Even the first communications about the more exact details which Fuchs established in regard to the localization conditions in the hemiamblyopic visual field, those referring to the displacements with constellations of dots, point in this direction. Fuchs, it is true, manages to classify these facts entirely in a gestalt-theoretical concatenation, when he reports the various possibilities which arise in the matter. He distinguishes (besides the insignificant case where, with tachistoscopic presentation, nothing at all is seen of the elements falling in the amblyopic zone, and consequently none of the seen parts of the dot-figure are displaced) two main cases, which he forthwith finds it possible to set out explicitly as results of the activity of the total process. He reports :—

(*a*) " If anything was seen of the elements (presented to the left of the fixation point) falling in the amblyopic zone, then *the whole point-gestalt* was often displaced to the right. The displacement then also affected the elements situated in the sound half of the field, which were never displaced when given alone. The localization of the whole was in these cases determined *by the elements falling in the damaged zone.*"

(*b*) " The displacement could, finally, not take place at

all, even though something was perceived of the elements situated in the amblyopic half of the field. Under the *influence of the total gestalt*, for the localization of which the *elements situated to the right* were now *critical*, the elements situated to the left were then also correctly localized."

Here everything thus accommodates itself to the " total processes ", and apparently, therefore, substantiates the gestalt doctrine.

And yet this ranging of the facts with the gestalt theory is actually not so very satisfactory. For, *firstly*, let us assume that, in the displacements, the phenomenon can be understood in terms of the " physical gestalten " or alternatively, their direct physiological effect. Hereupon it becomes unintelligible why no change of localization occurs in the case cited as insignificant and incidental, in the results. Physiologically the " total gestalt " is of course operative in this case too, since the amblyopic zone is at all times sensitive enough, in the cases in point, to receive stimuli. *Secondly*, one cannot rightly perceive how it happens that, in the two cases, the localization ensues once in one way, and the second time in a quite different way. Here one requires a more exact record of the concrete conditions—a requirement which certainly does not seem to exist for Fuchs, since he believes himself to have " explained " everything with his records.[1]

Fuchs' belief in the complete competence of the explanation goes so far, that in a report on cases of a displacement of *parts* of the dot-gestalt, he still adheres to it, and sees in them nothing other than " characteristic evidence of the correctness of these statements ". And yet, in spite of using gestalt-theoretical terms, intrinsically and in his own formulations too, he already fundamentally abandons the ground of the gestalt theory. Thus the following sort of case came under his observation, e.g., upon presentation of a group of four dots, arranged to form the apices and the midpoint of the base of a right-angled triangle (without connecting lines), which was so set up, that—in a case of exact hemiplegic amblyopia—only the left hand dot fell into the amblyopic area. Hereupon, in addition to the types of effects mentioned above, there occurred the new

---

[1] Cf. below, p. 193, where this question arises again, though in a different context, in connection with the influence of the " anchoring moments "

possibility "that only the lower row of dots appeared displaced to the right, so that its left hand dot came to lie vertically beneath the upper one ". Obviously, therefore, it is not in every instance that the localization of the total gestalt is determined according as this is present in the *stimulus* conditions.

Fuchs, nevertheless, disregarding this difficulty, maintains that these cases, too, are at least evidence in favour of the gestalt theory, in so far as they do not readily permit " of being understood . . . [from an] atomistic mode of approach in psychology, which builds up perceptions from single sensations only, and does not look upon them as characteristic total events " (p. 269). Yet he tacitly introduces a certain modification in the theory. He says " that dots in the sound half of the field become displaced *only when they form a characteristic unitary whole* with the dots falling in the amblyopic zone " ; that contrariwise, " co-exposed dots, otherwise still in the undamaged zone, which in the presentation in question for some reason or other do not belong to a distinguished or obtrusive gestalt, do also not become displaced " (p. 268). For the rest, however, all is still the effect of the " total process ".

It is just this modification, however, which conceals an essential point. What lies behind it becomes clearer from what is expressly stated elsewhere—that the temporary localization or displacement phenomenon ensues " just according to the mode of apprehension which is effective ". When Fuchs thereupon actually traces the effect to the fact "that the *apprehended gestalt* (!) is different, from time to time, and this for the reason that the upper point in the first presentation does not *subjectively* (!) belong to the displacement gestalt, but in the second is incorporated in the group " (p. 265), he thus himself abandons the sphere of genuine gestalt-theoretical explanation. With a remarkable lack of clearness and distinctness in thinking he completely overlooks the implications of his earlier theoretical standpoint.

It is worthy of note how with Fuchs this difficulty is at once concealed in the terminology. Fuchs finds a way of very simply introducing into the gestalt-theoretical phraseology a factor calculated to cover these special circumstances. To a certain extent, he interpolates *a new*, *supplementary, explanatory concept* into the theory, *that of the " unit character "* of the particular gestalt impression. According to this the relationship ultimately appears to be of such a sort, that to begin with the elements are indeed singly present in the stimulus process, and that the " unit character " then accrues to them ; and this can, for the time being, be involved in such or such a way, and even arises as an independent condition, if it is a question of localization or displacement.

From the standpoint of the gestalt theory, one cannot help being amazed to find the unit character, which is appended to the original theory as an auxiliary " moment ", here treated as something special, described as something quite new.   For the unitariness, the closure, was surely the first and most clear-cut characteristic demonstrable in the gestalt or the total process.   It is true that Fuchs too at first (p. 270) speaks generally of the " togetherness of the stimuli " as the foundation of the phenomenon, and he directly identifies this togetherness of the stimuli with the " gestalt impression ".   In addition, however, he himself actually distinguishes the " unit character " as something quite special, in some way separable.   He establishes that this " unit character " can be absent in the " apprehended (!) gestalt ", or can arise in varying manner, unaffected by fact that the very same " togetherness of the stimuli " is always present.   Thus the " unit character " is completely dissociated from the real basis of the theory.   It is substantiated in a remarkable manner, and to such degree that Fuchs appears to regard it as a new, necessary condition for the occurrence and nature of displacements.

In this way a quite extraordinary situation is created. For this unit character of the gestalt is supposed to be deduced immediately from the Wertheimer-Koffka-Köhler theory, as a result.   But here it comes to the fore in a wholly different fashion, not as the objective of the explanations, but as a new, independent condition, specifically contrasted with the action of the stimulus.

Fuchs is able to extricate himself in a similar way in other instances, where in the face of the diversity of the modes of localization, the means of explanation at his disposal directly provided by the gestalt theory does not suffice.   These are the cases in which, in spite of very strong configural coherence (not as with the findings hitherto cited), a displacement does not occur when meaningful figures are regarded. Here, too, he introduces a new explanatory principle. He assumes that here something supervenes as a condition which he designates (following an earlier terminology of Wertheimer's) an *anchoring moment*. He believes a new determining factor for localization to be represented by the concept of " anchoring ". He takes it as the starting point for his explanation, when upon presentation of meaningful figures (the butterfly figure) no displacement occurs. He talks of a complete " victory " of the localization of the section falling in the sound half of the field, and suggests that " a butterfly whose body passes through the fixation point, for example, is apparently (psychically) relatively firmly anchored to it, so that a displacement is not so easily possible ". And on this basis he proceeds at once to the formulation : " The displacement of a gestalt extending into both halves of the field only occurs when too powerful anchoring moments in favour of the correct position do not counter-act it."

When this principle is examined in regard to its explanatory value from the viewpoint of scientific theory, it is immediately evident how such a way out of the difficulties is entirely precluded. Such concepts as " anchoring moment ", and likewise, " unit character," in so far as they are designed somehow to enter into the analysis of the conditions, possess no demonstrable meaning whatsoever. Köhler himself has set up as criterion of the utility of a scientific concept, as measure of its scientific-theoretical value, the requirement that in respect of every theory it must be possible to decide concretely whether it is justified in its existence or not. It must, therefore, in particular permit of taking negative instances into its purview as well, as being in principle possible. But such negative instances are, in point of principle, not possible, if any significance is attached to concepts constituted like these anchoring moments or unit characters. Thus, let us assume a case where, in a certain example, a con-tradiction between concrete observation and theoretical expectation arises. Then a loophole for explaining this discrepancy would be at hand without ado, by simply incorporating *ad hoc* in the definition of the physiological basis, a corresponding " moment ", according to need ; and thus every difficulty would be at once disposed of. But no scientific derivation of concepts has been accomplished by means of such *ad hoc* principles.

Once we have made it clear, in relation to our previous considerations, what the psychological facts of the matter directly underlying these questionable " moments " we have cited may be, the inference is quite plain. Special conditions of apprehension must be involved here, and nothing more ; and the modes of localization at issue must be made intelligible expressly in terms of these very conditions of apprehension. That this holds can be seen even more directly from a final discovery of Fuchs, one at first sight contradicting all that has hitherto been reported. Fuchs found that, under certain circumstances, a displacement can ensue even in a direction towards the impotent side of the visual field as well. It is not in every case merely a matter of the displacement's either not occurring at all, or else always occurring in such a way that the gestalt appears to be extruded from the damaged zone. Numerous cases occur besides these in which the *displacement* of the centrally exposed objects ensues in *the direction towards the damaged side*, e.g. in a case of amblyopia of almost the whole right hemi-field. In this last case Fuchs has specially established, as a condition of it, that such a displacement, e.g. of circles towards the damaged side, occurs particularly easily " when the *attention* . . . was set towards the *cognizance of the right* (i.e. the damaged !) *side*. The circles, in spite of their objectively central position, were often localized to the right, alongside the fixation point, commencing $1\frac{1}{2}$–2 cm., as the case might be, to the right of it, and extending relatively far into the amblyopic zone ".

This and similar cases show unequivocally, that in point of fact a condition that cannot be interpolated, when the gestalt-theoretical context is the starting point, is crucial for the nature of the displacement—the " attentional attitude ", the " location of the fixation point ". The displacement ensues, quite as a general rule, in the direction towards the " centre of gravity of the cognizance ".

We can see how Fuchs himself is constantly and ever more inevitably driven to the problem which we have already elicited, in our discussion of the phenomenon of

figural structure, to be indeed the core of the whole complex of problems—the *problem of " attention and gestalt "*.
All the more must it be regretted that Fuchs himself—in
consequence of his bondage to the gestalt theory, in his
thinking—constantly brushes this problem aside, with
the remark that up to the present no positive researches
upon it are available. This conduct of Fuchs is the more
amazing, since actually his lines of argument finally
converge more and more upon the significance of the
" attention factor ", and eventually issue in a " theory
of attention ", which seems calculated to assemble all the
observations upon hemianopics into a rounded-off and
indeed genuinely psychological picture.

In his concluding theoretical considerations, Fuchs links
up with certain discoveries made with normal people,
which can be brought into relation with his own findings.
These are the findings of Lipp, 1910, in which noteworthy
facts about *localization in peripheral vision* came under
observation. In order to check a research of Wirth,[1] Lipp
carried out the following experiment : Upon a homogeneously illuminated perimeter surface, divided into
ring sectors (84 fields) and extended conically before the
observer, he presented a brighter supplementary stimulus
(fixation in the centre of the surface), in the
most varied peripheral positions, and investigated the
brightness threshold. In the experiment he varied the mode
of cognizance, while keeping the fixation point constant.
For instance, he caused a peripheral ring sector of given
size, a peripheral half-ring, and a peripheral full ring to be
discriminated through cognizance. The investigation
showed that the mode of cognizance also had a decisive
influence upon the localization of the selected ring. False
localizations thus occurred, and this patently in a regular
way, such " that the displacement ensues in the direction
towards the field emphasized by the attention ".

Starting from this, and on the basis of his own incidental
checks, Fuchs draws the conclusion " that a tendency
exists to assimilate the localization of a visual impression
to the localization of the area which is discriminated with
relatively greatest attention in the visual field, and hence

---

[1] Cf. Wirth, Wundt's *Phil. Stud.* 20, p. 487, or his *Analyse der Bewusstseinserscheinungen* : " Zur Theorie der Bewusstseinsumfangs."

appears with relatively greatest clearness ". And moreover,
this assimilation is the stronger, " the greater the degree of
clearness of the discriminated area " (p. 306). Fuchs
proceeds to bring these findings into direct relation with
his own discoveries. He establishes that in his own
observations upon hemiamblyopic and hemianopic vision
the very same set of conditions is evinced as in the
work of Lipp. And he accordingly views his results as
being theoretically explicable, through their incorporation
into normal psychological contexts.

In consequence of this organization of his results, he
regards himself as being over and above this actually
enabled to go further and present certain of the most general
peculiarities of hemianopsia in quite a new light. Commencing from this, he discusses generally the question of
how the field of vision of the hemianopic is constituted ;
and he attempts to explain how it happens that his halved
visual field does not appear to the hemianopic in the same
way as a hemi-field of vision is wont to be apprehended by
the normal person, that is, as a half field.[1]

The decisive fact for this discussion, he holds to be
that a displacement of the median axis, and with it of
the total visual space, towards the side, can be established
as characteristic for all hemianopics (according to Best,
1917). This displacement, moreover, can ensue towards
the blind as well as towards the sound side, as is evident
from the way the patients miss their aim when grasping at
things proferred to them.

For this fact, too, Fuchs finds a direct psychological
explanation, by again having recourse to Lipp. In nearly
complete hemianopsy we have " in an extreme degree " the
same circumstances as are present with normal people, when
half of a field of vision is discriminated with fixated regard,
as in Lipp's experiments. Lipp has reported " that in this
discrimination ' the apperceptive mid-point ' or ' centre of
gravity ' lies not in the boundary line running through the
fixation point, but to the side of it, within the semi-circular
shaped field ". The latter, as Lipp remarks, here following
Lipps, becomes " something ' stretching out from that

---

[1] Visual field = " the simultaneously visible portion of external
space "; field of vision = " what is for the time being psychically given,"
the field actually contemplated at a given moment—according to Fuch's
usage.

centre and coalescing in it ' ; it becomes as it were ' a centre emanating from itself ' " (Fuchs, p. 314).

From these observations upon the intra-configuration of this sort of hemi-field which is selected by cognizance, the mode of appearance of the hemianopically seen "half field " permits of being forthwith understood ; and the errors of localization manifested in the patients' failures in grasping become explicable without straining.

To this end we must needs pursue the phenomenal analysis of normal vision somewhat farther, with Fuchs. The analysis presented above is correct for the usual case. In this "the attention is 'distributed' over the whole of the (contemplated) area of the half field. *One* region, however, has gained a special character in this hemi-field, in virtue of the fact that it has become the *main anchoring point* of the attention ", in such a way "that the *half field ' organizes '* itself with *reference to it* ". In spite of the *fixation point's* lying unaltered, straight ahead, in *the boundary line, the optical presentation* organizes itself *with reference to a region in the interior of the hemi-field* (1).

Besides this there is also (2) a quite new structuration which the hemi-field organizes for itself in another way, namely with reference to the boundary line. " The boundary line can become the 'line of gravity' of the hemi-field, inasmuch as the hemi-field is something extending out of it sidewards, or even built up on it as it were ".

Both occurrences, the latter very rarely, have parallels in the vision of hemianopics. For them, in the ordinary course of events (cf. 1), " the field of vision is, just as usual, something extended upon all sides, a field of vision organized analogously to the normal one. It has . . . a left side as well as a right, a top no less than a bottom, apprehended with reference to a definite centre (midpoint). The patient believes himself to be ' regarding ' this new mid-point. For him it forms the direction ' straight ahead ', ' straight before me ', and thus defines the ' *subjective* median axis '. The consequence of this is that, as Best found, the *objective* median axis is displaced into the blind area ". The patients miss objects they are grasping at in a corresponding way. However, by means of a special mode of cognizance, arising from a knowledge of the objective circumstances of their deficiency, the patients can also on occasion maintain another centring of their

o

field of vision, one in which the boundary line more or less acquires the main emphasis (cf. 2). The " midpoint " of the area of vision which has been preserved loses its former significance ; the line dividing the disabled from the normal region becomes the anchoring place of the attention. Hereupon this median line gradually recovers the significance it had before injury—that is, the displacement of the median axis is now cancelled, while simultaneously the field of vision appears more or less definitely bounded as a half field. Indeed, a displacement in the reverse direction ensues : the median axis appears to be shifted into the undamaged zone, as Best has noticed. Fuchs explains this by the fact that with regenerating hemianopsia the hitherto absolutely blind half gradually becomes only amblyopic. The impressions now arising on this side, just because they are " bad ", bring about a special " direction of the attention " to this region. But with this new allocation of attention a new organization of the field of vision comes about, this time starting from a " centre of gravity " transferred to the disabled region.

Thus the phenomena of hemianopsia seem indeed to be quite satisfactorily explained on the basis of the viewpoints furnished by Lipp's work. We are ready to admit without reserve that Fuchs has contributed something of value to theory by pointing out these connections—even if we must declare ourselves to be incompetent to pronounce a final judgment upon it.

But apart from this one, certainty remains—that Fuchs actually forgets entirely, throughout these theoretical discussions, that he desired to provide confirmation of the gestalt theory. It is perfectly plain that he has lost every link with the gestalt theory in this part of his work. It does happen, to be sure, that the gestalt theory is superficially invoked, in that findings actually secured in other ways are again dressed up in the terminology of the gestalt theory, and this without any special nuances. For example, when he says, " from the position of the gestalt theory one would say : another gestalt is in consciousness now." As a matter of fact, however, his bonds with the gestalt theory seem to be completely severed in this work. All the concepts and lines of reasoning which enter into the interpretation here, are also possible and reasonable without any reference to gestalt-theoretical thinking.

In one place only does he somewhat more seriously
endeavour to link up with the gestalt theory's means of
thinking. Fuchs is of opinion that he can define still
further how the organization of the field of vision takes
place. He connects it with " structure functions " of the
field of vision, that is with " gestalt conditions " ; for he
declares (p. 321) that what is here present is nothing other
than a " structural reaction ", in Köhler's sense. He
emphasizes that " the patient reacts in a compulsive
manner to the residue of the visual field which remains for
him ". " Only because the visual field of the hemianopic
has such a peculiar form, does the corresponding field of
vision organize itself in this singular manner. Herewith is
displayed a definite allocation of the attention."

We are nevertheless incapable of perceiving that anything bearing upon the gestalt theory has been achieved in
this. At all events, nothing is " explained " by it ; for
when one simply talks of " structural reactions ", obviously
nothing definite is being made out in respect to the underlying body of facts. At bottom this is nothing but a verbal
solution.

Whether processes are here involved which can be
exhaustively defined in purely physiological terms, or
whether we must not go beyond the bounds of this
characteristic framework of the gestalt theory—this term
tells us nothing in regard to such matters. If Fuchs
intends to express by means of it " that the attention
is not a *deus ex machina,* a crucial creative factor ", this
might be justified. Taking it in this sense, one might be
allowed to emphasize that " as soon as some or other gestalt
is presented, the discerned area determined by it organizes
itself towards us of its own accord, so to speak ". But in
regard to the significance of the attentional attitude as a
condition for the manner of this organization, it must
not, after all, be forgotten, simply because of this one fact,
that this attentional attitude itself can perhaps arise by
derivation from the mental contents—as expressed by the
concept of " involuntary attention ".

Holding firmly to this main point, that Fuchs' theory
is, when all is said and done, nevertheless an attentional
theory, one must at least retain complete freedom of opinion
in respect of a theory purely physiologically orientated.
The very findings Fuchs quotes, in order to give his thesis

of the formation of a new "attention centre" with hemianopics a still more definite material structure, are able to make it clear, in the most obvious way, that one cannot in any case do justice to the facts with a purely physiological orientation.   For example, he discusses tachistoscopic reading experiments with hemianopics (p. 325 ff.) and thus shows, to begin with, that "those letters [are] clearest . . . which lie in the attention centre of the moment"; and furthermore that, in particular, this attention centre appears to be shifted more or less towards the periphery "in accordance with the object given".   Here the position of the "attention centre" appears throughout to be fixed not by the preserved residue of the field of vision as such, in the anatomical sense perchance (pp. 329–30) ; but the extension of the area in which letters, dots, etc., are at all seen with tachistoscopic exposure, is throughout dependent upon the size and position of the exposed object—the gestalt which is present.

Fuchs believes this to be further evidence that the gestalt-theoretical orientation alone is truly adequate to the facts of the matter.   He also finds in this a further example of the fact that a *structural* reaction is here involved, i.e. one dependent upon a gestalt coherence. But it becomes manifest in this very connection how necessary it is to free oneself from the purely physiological context.   It is not the objective gestalt, the one conforming to the stimulus which is critical for the organization of the field of vision, but " that gestalt which ought to be apprehended in conformity with the *Aufgabe* ".   Thus, whatever the physiological processes which could be presumed on the basis of the stimuli, they play no rôle at all here.   If we should wish to conceive this influence of the *Aufgabe* as somehow physiologically represented, in the form of " gestalt dispositions " for instance, no explanatory value whatsoever could be ascribed to such a venture.   There remains no alternative but to analyze these manifestations in terms of genuine psychological categories, if one desires to avoid sinking into total indefiniteness.

When all is said and done we must draw the conclusion that Fuchs, because he chose the gestalt theory as the framework for his investigation to begin with, has landed in a distinct difficulty.   With reference to this framework, he should have regarded the significance of attention to be merely secondary for his findings ; but with reference to the facts, he himself eventually arrived at actually placing it in the centre of his whole discussion. That in spite of his energetic profession of the gestalt theory he eventually liberated himself from it—though, to be sure, without himself noticing this—deserves to be recognized. It testifies to the stringency with which the facts in this field of research, so rich in results on account of the special pathological conditions, imposed the line of discussion so foreign to the gestalt theory. Hence it is not surprising that Fuchs' work has remained entirely devoid of unity in its theoretical import. The attention theory stands in fundamental detachment beside or on top of his original gestalt-theoretical orientation.

In view of this, it follows that the original gestalt-theoretical standpoint must be abandoned as being too narrow. The gestalt theory is not capable of providing any approach to the phenomena we have discussed. Here too, as in all the previously considered facts about figural structures, it proves to be inadequate.

CHAPTER III

THE GENERAL CONCEPT OF THE " STRUCTURE " : COLOUR AND TONE GESTALTEN

On account of an interesting conceptual elaboration, the gestalt theory's line of approach shows itself, as we have seen, not to be confined to figural structures, " gestalten " in the narrower sense of the word ; it is extended to the " mutual relatedness " of qualities, inasmuch as it makes *the conditions of simultaneously perceived qualities in general* a topic of enquiry.

I. THE EXTENSION OF THE GESTALT CONCEPT BEYOND THE PROVINCE OF FIGURAL STRUCTURES

The question of the phenomenal and functional singularity of simultaneous perception only becomes significant to one with a particular theoretical conviction, that is, only upon turning away from the synthetical outlook. A psychology proceeding synthetically would in this case simply establish a " here and there " of two qualities, each of which would be held to be independent in its so-being and unaltered by its concomitance with the other. With an anti-synthetic orientation one is bound, instead, to come upon the question of whether something other than a mere " juxtaposition " of the two colour qualities being regarded is present or not. The possibility of enquiring whether " gestalt phenomena " do not in some way play a rôle here too, arises—and indeed Köhler did interpret the facts of the matter along these lines in 1918.

§ 49. *The " mutual relatedness " of qualities as a phenomenally ultimate datum*

The experiments which Köhler carried out in connection with the problem posed for consideration here, as to the nature of the qualities as phenomenally given, developed in virtue of a purpose which was, at first, independent of them. Köhler's object was to study the psychical achievements of anthropoids, and he did this by arranging tests of functions similar to the achievement experiment. Thus he set out, for example, to test the optical functions of the eye in the chimpanzee (crossed disparition, visual size, colour, 1915 ; perception of colour and size differences 1918), and generally carried out, in addition, " intelligence tests upon apes " (1917) making use of the methods which Hobhouse and Thorndike had established in animal psychology—generally by the method of selective training, or alternatively that of free reaction in reference to a complex situation.

Köhler's lines of thought in these successive works may be followed up with an eye to the question of how specific gestalt-theoretical principles are either expressed or upheld or substantiated in them. A picture then emerges that is germane for us, as we have already stressed.

Up to 1917 Köhler is to a considerable extent straight-forwardly empirical. In 1915 he is testing for the facts only. He considers his main theoretical result to be, above all, that " transformation through experience " cannot be accepted as a valid explanatory principle in such reaction-achievements. His work is thus actuated by the problem of nativism versus empiricism. Similarly, in 1917, in the *Mentality of Apes*, the word "gestalt" does not in any way whatever appear as a theoretical principle. Admittedly there is some talk of the "handling of forms", and the names of Wertheimer and v. Ehrenfels are in this connection mentioned side by side. But a "gestalt theory", in the form of an acceptance of its principles, does not, at any rate, lie behind the whole work—even though here and there a similarity of the "unitariness" and "closure" of the chain of action manifested, to what is superficially established (e.g. p. 228), and even is understood by the "whole" in the gestalt theory, though certain terms and views already appear, which subsequently acquire a markedly gestalt-theoretical character (cf. p. 189 ff.). [English Edition.]

Only in 1918, basing himself on the selective training researches of 1915, does he work out the problem which is important in the present connection. Köhler sets himself the task of for once "considering the *general* problem as to what kinds of processes in the animal participate in such selective training, setting aside the special questions of sensory physiology". Hence our discussion need only start off at this point. Indeed here the basic orientation of the gestalt theory is quite sharply underlined from the outset ; and the problem is elevated to a question of principles by the fact that Köhler develops his own evaluation of the experiments, in contradistinction to a pointedly synthetic manner of interpretation.

Köhler trained chimpanzees, as well as barnyard fowls, to choose the lighter (*a*) of a pair of given brightness qualities (*a*, *b*). Looking at the matter synthetically, one would interpret the processes appearing here as showing that in consequence of the training the establishment of a definite "reaction value" for each of the qualities is achieved—a positive one for the bright colour, and a negative one for the dark colour. It would be of such a nature that this result of the training is co-ordinated to each colour in its own right, that the mode of reaction (positive or negative) is directly bound up with the presentation of one of these colours—quite independently of the rest of the perceptual field.

Köhler refutes this manner of interpreting the facts. After securely establishing a training for colour (*a*) of the pair (a, b) he presented a new pair of stimuli (b, c), in which the (b) of the practice experiment occurs together with a still darker colour (c). Hereupon—as indication of the results of the training—the lighter colour (b) of the pair (b, c) is selected, the very colour, that is, which had become " negative " in the pair (a, b).

What does this signify ? That the choice on the part of the animals investigated is directed in the main to the " mutual relatedness " of the objects learned. " The effect of learning pertains to the structure of the pair," it is a " structure function ". Thus in the result of the training it is " characteristically not the single colour by itself, but the 'mutual relatedness ' of the two, which is determinative ".

With this interpretation—plainly anti-synthetically orientated—Köhler introduces an entirely new functional principle into the psychological treatment of the problem, which is intended to be made responsible for the outcome of the reaction, namely the " structure moment ". The behaviour is held to be specifically " structurally orientated ". Köhler is here thinking along a perfectly definite line, that of the gestalt theory. He assumes that, under the stimulus conditions in question, the *perception itself* is already constituted in a definite way ; in fact the perception is already supposed to evince " as pre-eminently characteristic not the single colour wholly in its own right, but the mutual relatedness of the two ".

How this " mutual relatedness " is to be conceived must be more exactly developed out of Köhler's formulations.

The framework of these animadversions is given in the statement : " The phenomenology of human consciousness distinguishes two ways in which the mutual relatedness of colours (just as of other phenomena) can appear become effective, *colour gestalten* and perceived *colour relationships* " (p. 14).

In the conception of the colour gestalt lies the special note of Köhler's pronouncements, the new significance which they have as permanently productive, primarily for the problem of selective training, but also for the theory of gestalten. Köhler does not venture to delineate the meaning of this concept of *colour gestalt* more closely. This alone is clear : The " mutual relatedness "—in the sense of the colour gestalt—represents itself to him as a quite specific, original datum of perception, in contrast to the traditional interpretation which takes cognizance of such " mutual relatedness " only in the form of a (thought-like apperceptive) apprehension of relation. But the import of this concept obviously seems to him to be adequately settled by the mere fact of using the term *colour gestalt.* The gestalt character is the only positive defining moment which Köhler offers. All other theoretical points of definition to be found are not given directly on the basis of the facts, but are deduced from this statement ; simply because Köhler believes that he may now forthwith attribute to the data under consideration all those peculiarities which seem to him to be characteristic of gestalten in general.

Thus he brings forward a very significant argument in order to prove that in colour gestalten we are throughout dealing with primary data. He contends (having in mind the contrast alleged between " colour gestalten " and " colour relations "), " Every attempt to reduce the first group to the second, to explain gestalten as relations or, if need be, as multiplicities of relations, must come to grief upon the fact that maximally characterized gestalt effects are possible and frequent, when there can at the same time be no question at all of consciousness of relations." And he substantiates this more exactly by saying, " One will be the less able to deceive oneself about this, the more one is accustomed to banish constructions without compunction in favour of true phenomenology. In the realm of spatial gestalten, one should not, for example (as has recently happened) regard the perception of a circle as essentially given in the constant, equal distance-relation of the peripheral elements to the centre. Phenomenology shows that a circle can be perfectly characterized, perceptually, even without a centre being given as well ; that the perceptions of relations which thus vanish are therefore inessential for the constitution of the perceptual circle ; that, finally, the centre could not ' by supplementation ' become in the least exact enough to permit of founding the very sharply defined (and extremely sensitive to variations) percept of the circle in such a roundabout way."

To the question here adumbrated, that of the relation of

gestalt impression to consciousness of relations, we should undoubtedly reply to the same effect. When Spearman, for instance (1926), endeavours to trace the entire phenomenon of gestalt and configuratedness back to the apprehension of the relations existing between the single elements of the unit of perception, one would, as against this, inevitably draw attention to the merely secondary rôle of the consciousness of relations. It is not Köhler's demonstration alone that would lead us to this, for equally definitive is, for example, Benussi's emphasizing, in 1914, that " the perceptual apprehension of a gestalt in no way presupposes a clear, thought-like apprehension of the relations of its components. The gestalt as an object is of course impossible without those relations, but the presentation of the gestalt is in nowise bound to the notions of relation " (p. 281, corresponding to p. 188) ; and also his (Benussi's) remark (*Archiv* 17, p. 91) that even in respect to the æsthetic effects of a (figural) gestalt the apprehension of relations as relations is in fact not involved.

As regards the question of *colour* gestalten, however, Köhler's statement contributes nothing of course ; for, to begin with, it has not yet been made clear whether and how " gestalten " are really present in this case. Equally little is contributed when Köhler proceeds from this to attempt to expound how the consciousness of relation is, conversely, based on the "having" of gestalten. He says : " When confronted by pairs of colours (under certain conditions, pairs of colour groups) a person can bring his gestalt perception into the state which we call perception of relation. The original and naïve meaning of this word, which should be retained for it, contains somewhat of ' active evocation ' of the pair, somewhat of a making explicit of the special ' mutual relatedness ', the like of which is otherwise not at all requisite for the seeing of a colour gestalt. Even what is designated a judgment of comparison upon the two colours of the pair—' they are different, the right hand one is redder,' and so forth— likewise appears, irrespective of the linguistic expression, essentially to emerge in this ' intensified manner ', which the experiencing of a two-colour gestalt takes on during the perception of relations " (p. 14). But this too, at bottom offers nothing more than what was already terminologically expressed in his contrasting of colour gestalten and colour relations. As to what the difference consists in, nothing is directly brought out about it.

The one mark of distinction which remains is obviously that in *colour gestalten* we are dealing with *primary processes, directly given with the stimulus situation,* which directly—and, ultimately, with physiological representation—portray the relationship of the qualities, on the phenomenal side. This moment, at any rate, is present in the background, when Köhler subsequently proceeds to lay emphasis on the fact that, in the structurally orientated behaviour of chimpanzees and fowls, truly "natural" modes of behaviour are involved. He may not hold the phenomenological distinction between gestalt and relation perception to be definitive, in connection with the investigation of animals ; yet the use made of these very observations on animals in subsequent contentions shows plainly which way the verdict eventually falls. None other than the animal is held to show how the complicated reactions are not dependent upon any sort of special "higher psychical functions", but follow simply from the gestalt characteristics of the perceptual datum.

How Köhler comes to bring the gestalt category to bear here deserves to be more closely followed out. Köhler summarizes the essential points of his empirical discoveries briefly in two statements :—

(a) "The single colours which enter into a pair, acquire an *inner bond.* Their rôle here, no matter whether it is gestalt or relation which is concerned, they owe not to their *absolute quality,* but *first and foremost to their correlative position in the particular system,* that is, their position in relation to each other in the colour entity, or, when it so happens, in a qualitative series. The character of the bond corresponds to this correlative position in the system."

(b) "In the case where the correlative position of the colours is preserved while the absolute qualities are altered, the gestalt and the perceived relationship become *transposed.* The most important example, in which the stated condition is fulfilled, is found *when the colours within a qualitative series are displaced* " (p. 14).

In these two pronouncements we find again those two features which we previously found enunciated in the theoretical part, as criteria for the gestalt character of a process—firstly, the factor of "closure" (see (a)), and secondly, the criterion of " transposability " (see (b)). It is true that Köhler himself has not established this affiliation with the gestalt criteria in this explicit form.[1] Nevertheless, only from this starting point does it seem possible really to see, as positively substantiated, how a classification of the findings in question under the concept of gestalt can be held to be permissible or requisite. It is clearly evident how the essence of the mutual relatedness is supposed to lie in this closure, and that it is the transposability which expresses Köhler's idea that this mutual relatedness of a " bright-dark gestalt " is something autonomous, contrasting with the absolute qualities of the two colours.

In this "mutual relatedness" Köhler perceives the manifestation of a specific gestalt function, or, putting it physiologically, a specific gestalt process, of the same sort as the functions or processes enunciated by the gestalt theory in connection with the spatial gestalten in the narrower sense. Here, in order to denote what is special about the instances now adduced, he talks of " structure functions " or, physiologically, of " structure processes ".

The theory of such structure functions, or structure processes, assumes that *gestalt processes* are present in what is perceptually given, not only in so far as the single elementary contents coalesce into unities, forms, in spatial organization and articulation ; but that they *already arise purely in reference to the qualitative relation of* (say) *the colours*. It follows as a matter of course that in this case, too, they are physiologically directly represented in the same way as the spatial gestalten are believed to have been proved to be. Indeed, they are supposed ultimately to possess a primary significance even at the biologically most deep-lying stages, one of greater importance than the absolute presentation itself. This *absolute presentation* as such is taken to be *utterly devoid of significance for the natural reaction*.

It is plain how radically Köhler carries through his extension of the gestalt-theoretical doctrines, in these pronouncements. It is furthermore evident—and this only amounts to a reinforcement of his position—how he has arrived at these enunciations entirely from the starting

---

[1] Probably because at the time the conceptual clarification was not so far advanced, especially in regard to the gestalt criteria (cf. above, Book One).

point of concrete experimentation, that is by an inductive route. In fact it appears as if, in these training-experiment findings advanced by Köhler, a direct *experimentum crucis* has actually been discovered, one which reveals how a non-gestalt-theoretical interpretation does not do justice to the facts of the matter. Obviously it is a relevant question as to how these facts of the matter present themselves upon critical analysis, primarily in regard to the functional significance of the concepts Köhler has propounded.

§ 50. *The functional import of Köhler's concept of " mutual relatedness ", and the structure of the selective reaction*

The crucial point about Köhler's concept of " mutual relatedness ", is obviously the *thesis of the primary significance of the structure function,* which is implicated in that concept. This thesis has as its basis the fact that, according to Köhler's observations, the single components, the absolute presentations, entering into the mutual relatedness, are held to play no rôle, even at as lowly a stage in the animal kingdom as the barn-fowl.

However, there are experiments (Köhler, too, alludes to them) in which it is shown that, in point of fact, with certain forms of selective training the single presentation does indeed possess direct biological significance, and that there is no priority of anything like a structure function—the experiments of Pavlov.[1] When these findings are taken into account, it necessarily follows that the structure function should not be erected in the absolute form in which Köhler does so, as exclusively decisive. The question will have to be considered as to whether the issue of the experiments was not in some or other sense determined by the conditions of the experiments.

The correctness of this view is vouched for by Köhler's own material. As his investigations progress, he is led to note that, actually, in his experiments too, an absolute colour training must be admitted besides the operation of structure functions (p. 24). And this is not enough. Definite conditions can even be stated, according to which the reaction arises either in the shape of an " absolute " or else

---

[1] In training to a tone as a food signal, the co-ordination of the reaction to the *absolute* quality was so striking, that no reaction occurred even with tones deviating only to a very small extent.

of a "relative colour training". The outcome of the
reaction depends essentially upon the way in which the
critical choices are planned ; the more the test-choices
are distributed among experiments upon the former
training-pair, the less does structure function come
decisively into question. There can therefore be no doubt
that the conditions in these experiments are much more
complicated than appears from Köhler's "explanation".

What the *special psychological features* which constitute
this complexity consist in, cannot be more closely
envisaged from Köhler's account of 1918 ; it could at
most be deduced from the findings quoted. Nevertheless
these lacunæ can also be filled without such deductions.
The description of the behaviour of chimpanzees in making
such choices, given by Köhler in his earlier work (1915),
can lead us to the features which are from this viewpoint
crucial for the understanding of the experiments. Köhler
has himself reported, in 1915, what constitutes the really
crucial achievement of the animals in these experiments.
For one thing, it does not consist in the bond between
structure and reaction in general. When this connection
does not seem to arise, either swiftly or only gradually,
it should not be attributed to the corresponding
difficulty or ease with which this connection as such has
come into being. Köhler emphasizes that actually the
essential achievement of the animals lies in a somewhat
different direction, that it consists in the *discovery of
the actual training material.*

This opens up a quite definite line of enquiry.
Unfortunately this line of enquiry is no longer incorporated
in the discussion of 1918, in connection with the idea of the
structure functions. We are of opinion, however, that it is
nevertheless of the utmost importance. When it is taken
into account, the question of the predominance of the
"relative colour training", the question of how it happens
that the animal, on the other hand, sometimes chooses in
accordance with the absolute presentation, acquires an
entirely new and substantially wider framework. In
this connection, the essential problem is this : How does
the animal manage at all to select, from amidst the totality
of situations presented to it, just that particular absolute
colour value as such, for instance, to which the reaction
in conformity with the absolute presentation is, according

to Köhler, co-ordinated. The question is whether, in regard to such "discovery of the training material" under the experimental conditions of Köhler's training methods, it is not perhaps possible to understand, without the imputation of a primary significance to the structure functions, why the reaction appears to be co-ordinated rather to the mutual relatedness of the colours than to the absolute colour value as such.

We shall only understand these circumstances, when we take note of analogous instances, in which such discrimination of a "training material" can be traced out directly *in human introspection.* "Training" of the sort under consideration, designed for humans, and in which the genesis of the achievement is bound up with correctly discriminating the "training material", have been reported by Ach, in his ingenious experiments with the *"searching method".* In these, a series of objects differing in shape, size, weight, and colour are presented, and a co-ordination between the properties of these and designations attached to them must be apprehended from the actual situation. The picture of the situation in Ach's experiments has very great affinity with that of Köhler's training experiments : A " field " of objects is given, of intrinsically greater multiplicity, to be sure, than that which is to be found in Köhler's work, and it is necessary to discriminate a single, definite feature of it, to apprehend it in its relationships, if the test-period is to be successfully negotiated.

The results Ach was enabled to bring forward on the basis of this experimental method, have been confirmed, in the connection in which they are of interest to us at this point, in a work by Hüper (1928), who also amplified them in regard to the inner processes involved, on the basis of the direct statements of his subjects. These provide material which seems calculated to enable us also to appraise, at least approximately, the state of affairs really present in Köhler's experiments.

The very beginning of the experiments is worthy of note. To begin with, a complete incertitude on the part of the subjects as to "what is actually in hand" appears, an incertitude which may sometimes be retained for a very long time, even right through the experiments. Apart from this, a definite apprehensional picture of the total situation is already associated with the entry into the experiments. This is at first purely optical, but is, from the outset, concerned with the total situation, with the " mutual relatedness " of the " things " in the field, their groupings, their inner organization by form and shape, with spatial distribution.   It also proves to be critical as an orientation again and again in the course of the experiments.   The crucial achievement which supervenes in the course of the experiments and under the urge of the special experimental conditions, here, too, consists in the fact that something definite is discriminated as being essential in this total situation.   Certain specific properties of the objects exposed must be apprehended and brought into relation with generic names.   But this achievement takes place by an exactly observable, gradual genesis. Under certain circumstances it is not accomplished till very late.   It is always bound up with definite ways of directing the apprehension—a point which turns out to be fundamental in the evaluation of these observations ; and these are the first to lead the subject to regard those specific properties as substantial in their own right, and to grasp them in their co-ordination.

The crucial point is the fact that only thus is the " viewpoint " gained from which the given situation can be fully brought into relation with the test *Aufgabe*.   In these experiments a gradual " becoming " is involved, the consequences of a building-up of the experiment by stages, as Ach himself has brought out with the greatest clearness, when he talks of a " *successive* determined abstraction " and also of " *successive* determined attention ".

When all this is taken into consideration, the essential features presented by Köhler's choice reactions appear in quite a different context.   One will needs try to bring the occurrence of absolute or relative reaction in Köhler's selective training experiments into direct relationship with these findings, especially when Köhler's communications of 1915 which we have cited, are borne in mind.   And this relationship can be discerned without difficulty.   Even the very simplest experimentation with similar choice reactions of humans, reveals that here too the individual reaction-colour need not by any means be apprehended as a colour, as a quality ; that here too the position of the particular constituent within the whole is noted to begin with ; and that the reaction as a rule follows from this point, without change, until an error steers the cognizance in a different direction, so that the colour is also thereupon discriminated. So far Köhler's empirical discoveries are, therefore, substantiated. But even if, according to this, the " mutual relatedness " is acknowledged as a special form of the presentation, or even as the " natural " foundation of the reaction under normal circumstances, a direct *primary* significance is not thus attributed to it. To us the " mutual relatedness " as such appears to be by no means as directly determined by the stimuli as Köhler would have it. On the contrary, it proves to be fixed in its " so-being " only on the basis of just those special " determinations ", " attitudes ", " directions of apprehension " with which the subject approaches the experiment, or which institute themselves in the course of the experiments, to some extent " coming over " the subject.

The crucial factor in the issue of the reaction is the intra-articulation of what is given. Only when this has been accomplished in reference to the elements concerned can a corresponding co-ordination of the reaction to the " correct " relational moment ensue—the correct " viewpoint " for the judgment has been attained. But this intra-articulation is not made intelligible by simply hypostasizing structure processes, or colour gestalten. What is critical for the nature of this intra-articulation is, characteristically, the direction of the mode of apprehension (cf. Ach's successive attention). This, at times controlled by the course of the experiments, determines the nature of the intra-articulation and is accordingly an essential condition for the issue of the reaction.

There is no doubt that we can readily correlate Köhler's observations on animals with these.[1] The more so, if with

[1] The fact that for these achievements special " higher functions " which may not be taken for granted in the case of animals, have to be supposed in the case of humans, is no refutation of what we are saying. For the above-mentioned intra-articulations are in nowise bound to such functions. This is proved by experiments occurring in a somewhat different connection, which were carried out by W. Hansen at the Kiel Institute. They show that such a differentiation, such a transformation of the reaction in its co-ordination to what is given, to the complex stimulus situation, actually ensues at times without any " conscious " reflection about " goals " and " means ". It comes about in the simple re-articulation of what is given in its dependence upon the apprehensional attitude, as this in its turn evinces itself more or less fortuitously, or else is induced by the intrinsic circumstances of the experiment.

P

Volkelt (and Krueger) we assume that the apprehension of animals does not grasp objects in their intra-articulation, as they are presented to our developed consciousness ; but rather that the differentiation of the " world " of the animal takes place solely in the direction of definite " vitally significant " moments, in such a way that only total- or complex-qualities are relevant. From the point of view of what is biologically significant, the discrimination of one single quality, of a colour as a colour, would indeed hardly deserve to be reckoned among the vitally significant facts in the life of animals. Hence it is intelligible why the training achievement in the normal course of events at first does not take place on this basis. On the other hand, the very fact that other kinds of training are also feasible —that is to say, in so far as the animal is led in the course of the experiments to discriminate the individual object in isolation—this fact proves that we are here concerned with special conditions, which essentially transcend what is determined purely perceptually, that is by the objective stimulus, and which refer to the animal's " state of being set " in regard to the situation.[1] From this point of view, Köhler's drawing attention to the possibility of such a " mutual relatedness ", which is as yet free of actual " apprehension of relation ", must furnish the point of departure for extraordinarily important investigations in the future. But the idea that the reaction could be intelligible simply in terms of a " context-", or " mutual relatedness-", or " structure-" process of direct physiological nature, *primarily* engendered by the stimulus-pairs, appears far too narrow when taken in conjunction with all the phenomena. The " mutual relatedness " can by no means be acknowledged as a primary datum, in Köhler's sense.

Nor can this position be altered by the fact that Köhler's opinion as to the primary character of the " mutual relatedness " can possibly be further supported from the starting point of the conceptual system of the gestalt theory.

---

[1] Our view receives particular support from the fact that (as Herr Volkelt informs me) Bierens de Haan, found *quite specific, absolute reactions in bees*, which corresponds to the fact that here—e.g. in searching for feeding places—*the colour appears as absolutely vitally significant.*

§ 51. *The structure process in Köhler's physiology*

Köhler's thesis that the "mutual relatedness" of qualities is a primary fact of perception, is found to be incorporated in the conceptual fabric of the gestalt theory in virtue of the fact that it seems possible to bring it directly into connection with his gestalt physiology. Thus the theory of "mutual relatedness" receives some reinforcement; for the objection we have developed, that it is a secondary phenomenon which is involved, is naturally thrown open to question, as soon as an immediate representation for this "structure phenomenon" can be successfully furnished from the starting point of physiology.

To be sure, one cannot, to begin with, discover any thorough enquiry along this line, in the gestalt theory. Köhler does mention "structure processes" in this sense in 1918, but nowhere does he make a definite statement as to how these are to be conceived physiologically. Koffka also, in 1921, only emphasizes that the mere admission of the occurrence of "structure uniformities" does not yet imply the renunciation of an exact physico-chemical explanation e.g. in the case of colours (on p. 266, note to Dittmers); but on the positive side he too did not indicate any physiological deduction with reference to a thoroughly worked-out example. From this one could infer that the available physiological apparatus of the gestalt theory was not yet adequately adapted for this task; and one could perhaps from this standpoint regard our foregoing position as strengthened.

However, this gap is filled when we return once more to Köhler's general pronouncements upon gestalt physiology, in 1920. Here an example forthwith offers itself which, even though not thus evaluated by Köhler himself, must undoubtedly be entitled a "structure phenomenon" in our connotation; and this is an example in which Köhler's physiological theory actually appears to prove extraordinarily productive. The example we refer to is found in the phenomenon of the difference threshold (Weber's law), where the problem at issue is—to formulate it in terms of structure theory—what are the conditions under which a "mutual relatedness of stimuli", say in the optical sphere, phenomenally leads to a genuine "mutual relatedness" of different quality, and what are the further conditions under which the stimulus field has a homogeneous structure at the time.

With Köhler, the foundation for the direct physiological treatment of this question is given by the particular manner in which he in general conceives the difference of the colours to be represented. According to this, different physiological " reaction types " are at a given time associated with the different colour stimuli in the optic sector : " Different molecules, more particularly ions, enter at least partially into reactions of unlike types, in such a way that regions of unlike kinds of reaction differ from one another not only because of the concentration, but also by reason of the chemical nature and the mobility of their ions." The qualitative difference of two fields is thus represented physiologically both by differences in *kind* of ions and by differences in the *concentrations* of ions. This occurs in such a way that a two-dimensional variability is physiologically possible, corresponding to the phenomenal variability according to colour *quality* and colour *intensity*.

To begin with, Köhler develops these considerations for the simplest case. On the physiological side, he assumes only variability of the ionic concentrations of the participating electrolytes, but takes the kinds of ions to be alike. I.e. on the phenomenal side, he lets the brightness alone vary and not the colour quality. For this instance of a brightness-threshold there then emerges, after the utmost further simplification of the assumption, the following basis for subsequent deductions. " In both of the contiguous areas [let there be] one and the same (and for simplicity's sake) univalent pair of ions, but having those unequal concentrations of ions on the two sides . . . which correspond to the two different speeds of reaction."

Starting from this, Köhler then deduces the fact of the limen, by investigating the potential difference which arises in the physiological sphere, in accordance with the stimulus conditions. But this potential difference readily permits of mathematical derivation from the conditions governing the state of the ionic system, on the basis of Nernst's theory of galvanic chains ; that is on the basis of the amounts of diffusion. Here Köhler makes direct use (pp. 212–14) of Nernst's deductions :—

" Let us consider a surface-element q at the surface of

contact of two areas of unequal ionic concentration ; let us call the direction of the normal to this element n, and imagine the concentration and osmotic pressure not as unsteady but as extremely swift in the direction n, and constantly varying. Let the velocity of the positive ion under the influence of a force Λ pro grammion (i.e. the mobility) be U, and that of the anion V. The osmotic partial pressure of each ion we shall call p (and this therefore is a quantity varying with n) ; and we shall call the electrostatic potential (referred to one grammion as the unit of the quantity of electricity) ϕ. The ions underlie the actions of forces which go back, on the one hand to the spatial variation of p, and on the other hand, to that of ϕ. But since movements with enormous friction are involved, the velocities are proportional to the acting forces. If c is the ionic concentration at the cross-section q ; and if the force Λ pro grammion acts throughout the very short interval of time dt vertically to q ; then the following quantities of the substances travel during this time through q and in the direction of the normal : $-Uqc.dt$ and $-Vqc.dt$ (that of the cation, and that of the anion). In reality the force of osmotic origin is $\frac{1}{c} \cdot \frac{dp}{dn}$ for a grammion, and the electrostatic force is $\pm \frac{d\phi}{dn}$. Thus the amounts travelling away become, under the influence of the two forces acting together :—

$$-Uq\left\{\frac{dp}{dn} + \frac{d\phi}{dn} \cdot c\right\}dt \text{ and } -Vq\left\{\frac{dp}{dn} - \frac{d\phi}{dn} \cdot c\right\}dt.$$

A separation of the two ions can only take place in imponderable quantities. For a stationary condition must ensue in a very short time, in which the electrostatic force generated between the two so strongly restrains the ion which hastens ahead and so strongly impels the ion which remains behind, that both take on the same velocity. Thus the two quantities of travelling ions we have just defined represent the same amount. From this emerges the equation :—

$$\frac{d\phi}{dn} = -\frac{U-V}{U+V} \cdot \frac{1}{c}\frac{dp}{dn}.$$

But in dilute solutions the equation for the conditions in ideal gases holds, viz., $p = cRT$, where R is the gas constant, T the absolute temperature, and p is the osmotic pressure instead of the gas pressure. If then, c is introduced as an independent variable instead of p, this equation follows for the potential discontinuity between partial fields of ionic concentrations, c_1 and c_2 :—

$$\phi_2 - \phi_1 = \frac{U - V}{U + V} \cdot R \cdot T \cdot \int_1^2 \frac{dc}{c} = \frac{U - V}{U + V} \cdot R \cdot T \cdot ln \frac{c_2}{c_1}."$$

Up to this point we have simply Nernst's derivation of the law of mass action. The result permits of being more briefly summarized in the formula

$$\phi_2 - \phi_1 = \text{const. log } \frac{c_2}{c_1}.$$

Köhler now evaluates this formula for the case of the conditions obtaining with thresholds. That is, he carries over the concept of threshold to his physical picture, under a special assumption. "An electrostatical displacement, the course of which is adjusted to the electromotive force, is held to become manifest wherever the potential discontinuity attains at least a certain liminal value, which is equal to a definite quantity, for example e, of microvolts."

From this follows the inference : " Hence log $\frac{c_2}{c_1}$ must likewise rise to a certain liminal value $\frac{e}{\text{const.}}$; or else, the ratio $\frac{c_2}{c_1}$ can be brought down to a minimum value." The increment $\varDelta c$ which makes c_1 into c_2 is according to this, fixed in such a way that $\frac{\varDelta c}{c}$ must always be a given quantity : $\frac{\varDelta c}{c} = \text{const.}$ But this signifies nothing else than that Weber's law holds for the required potential discontinuity, dependent as this is upon the concentrations ; or that the relative difference threshold for the ionic concentrations, determined according to the behaviour of the electrostatic displacement, has a constant value (pp. 215–16).

زالمال عة ოთხกิ

This final result thus shows most impressively how the uniformity of the Weber-Fechner law appears to be exact on the physiological side.

There can be no doubt that this represents a positive theoretical achievement. But it must nevertheless not be forgotten that this achievement was ready to hand long before Köhler and before the gestalt theory, at any rate in the form of the idea. Nernst himself, in his day, not only put forward the theory of electrolysis in general; he also did not omit to observe the possibility of directly applying it to nerve physiology. Indeed he himself derived the threshold phenomenon, especially that of the absolute stimulus threshold, from such premisses. Hence the success achieved in the above-mentioned elaborations of Köhler cannot in any way be lodged to the credit of the gestalt theory. Its roots lie not in specific gestalt-theoretical presuppositions, but in more general ones, in the ideas of G. E. Müller and Nernst, which Köhler borrowed for his own physiology, but which are in themselves much less narrow than the specific gestalt-theoretical principles. These neither include the gestalt theoretical principles, nor is the gestalt theory so constituted that it, on the other hand, of necessity implies these electrolytic premisses.

In regard, therefore, to the problem of the gestalt theory, this physiological-conjectural treatment of the threshold problem can furnish no decisive standards.

As regards the quite general problem of "mutual relatedness" however, the question is far more complicated. It is true that Köhler can also invoke the formula from Nernst's law of mass action, in order to "found" certain peculiarities which he asserts for the "togetherness" of colours, physiologically, for the case of the threshold phenomenon. Thus he is able to interpret the formula to mean that the amount of the potential discontinuity depends not upon the absolute concentrations, but upon their relationship. For example, if the concentration on both sides is tripled—which corresponds to totally altered velocities of reaction and, hence, "absolute colours"—the electromotive force still remains the same. In brief, "it can be transposed, in the precise sense [of psychology]," p. 215. Hence transposability, at least, is physiologically represented if, with Köhler, we base it upon the Müller-Nernst theorems. But this holds, to begin with, only for the threshold phenomenon, and it holds only in virtue of a definite, special assumption of Köhler, one in itself not at all contained in the general theorem, namely, the assumption about the concentrations, which the translation of the threshold phenomenon to the neurophysical system signifies.

It can therefore by no means truly be said that the threshold phenomenon and its transposability have been deduced directly "from the starting point of physics". Without the tacit recourse to the phenomenal findings, Köhler would never have arrived at his view. Thus here, too, we have at bottom a case of *ad hoc* adaptation.

This, moreover, settles the question as to what significance it would have if one were to attempt similarly to deduce the " mutual relatedness " and its transposability, for any colours whatever, by a direct approach from physiology, thus to demonstrate the " mutual relatedness " to be something primary. This question is a simple generalization of the analogous question in the case of the threshold phenomenon. If, as we have just shown, in Köhler's deduction of the Weber law the premisses of the " deduction " already involve the tacit transference of phenomenal moments to physiology, naturally the state of affairs is in all respects necessarily the same for the more general case of mutual relatedness of colours. Should Köhler make an attempt really to build up this mutual relatedness in the physiological sphere, it can be stated from the outset that nothing is thus proved in regard to the character of the phenomenal " mutual relatedness ", or its theoretical import. For if a " deduction " from physiology of the primary existence of a " mutual relatedness " should emerge, then that " mutual relatedness " would already from the outset be presupposed in the deduction, in the specific phenomenal character attributed to it by the gestalt theory. Accordingly, the results of such physiological constructions can, in point of principle, supply no information in regard to the above-mentioned problems of interpreting the mutual relatedness. For any direct knowledge about the physiological side itself is denied to us. Hence a solution to the question as to whether the fact of the " mutual relatedness " must be interpreted according to the viewpoint of the gestalt

theory, or whether it does not demand quite another interpretation, must certainly be sought only within the bounds
of further directly empirical findings.

To be sure, the empirical findings in connection with
which Köhler's attention was first drawn to the " mutual
relatedness ", do not appear to be suited to this purpose. We must emphasize that they involve conditions
which are much too complicated and too difficult to
envisage for anything to be proved by their means. The
task therefore arises of pursuing the problem in simpler
instances—a task for which other contributions from
the side of the gestalt theory are available, even though
they do not, in the publications concerned, appear directly
incorporated in this context of thought.

2. SPECIFIC EMPIRICAL FINDINGS IN REGARD TO THE
    GESTALT THEORY OF " MUTUAL RELATEDNESS "

Factual knowledge pertaining to the principle of " mutual
relatedness " is more extensively at our disposal in the
province of music. Here " mutual relatedness " is something that has long been familiar. In every melody one
is confronted with a " mutual relatedness " of tones ;
and when melodies came to be designated gestalten, this
itself—even though in a different terminology—quite
explicitly implied the problem of " mutual relatedness ".

Alongside this more extensive province of " mutual relatedness " in psychological acoustics, specific, elementary
findings of Koffka in optics can also be adduced, which
may be invoked in support of the notion of " mutual
relatedness " (1923). We shall turn first of all to these
latter.

§ 52. *Structure phenomena in optical perception. Koffka's*
conception of boundary contrast

Attention has, for one thing, been drawn to optically
experienced structure phenomena by Koffka, inasmuch as
he endeavours to re-interpret the threshold phenomenon
along these lines, while simultaneously extending the
conception to acoustics (1922 ; indeed, even in 1917). It is

evident from the outset that such re-interpretation can of course never be regarded as proof. At the most it can indicate that the thesis is not already refuted by the facts under consideration. It cannot supply evidence in positive justification of the new interpretation. Apart from this, Koffka's way of treating the threshold problem exhibits a certain ambiguity and vagueness of statement which will not conduce to the strengthening of our faith in the points he develops. On the one hand, he commences with the distinction of "figure" and "ground", to which he subordinates the gestalt problem, thus conceiving it in relation to the theory of figural structures. On the other hand, however, he treats it much more along the lines of a genuine "mutual relatedness", taking his stand not so much upon the configural "relief", but upon

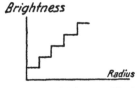

Fig. 16.—Brightness distribution in Hering's boundary contrast discs.

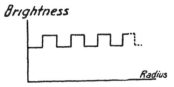

Fig. 17.—Brightness distribution in Koffka's ring discs.

the colours as such; and he deduces the threshold phenomena from the fact that when the difference between the stimuli is slight "an assimilation takes place, whereas by contrast, when the differences between the stimuli are greater a law of 'relief' holds good"—exactly after the style we discussed when considering the threshold findings of Gelb and Granit. Thus we cannot expect any further clarification from this starting point, however instructive these pronouncements may be individually, in respect to the aims of the gestalt theory and the ideas of its adherents.

Much more definite, and very closely linked with the facts are communications Koffka published in 1923, which seem able to lead up to the notion of a structure principle in a very precise way. These are Koffka's observations on boundary contrast and its gestalt-theoretical interpretation.

Koffka   proceeds   from   Hering's   experiments

demonstrating boundary contrast. For this demonstration Hering made use of a staircase disc (cf. fig. 16). Koffka establishes that " the characteristic mark of this disc is that each ring lies between a brighter and a darker one ". Under these conditions, the result is that each ring correspondingly possesses one darker and one brighter edge ; " in fact it exhibits a brightness gradient across its whole extent," although objectively it is homogeneous.

Koffka now puts the question, how far is this characteristic mark of the Hering discs essential for the arousal of boundary contrast ? It *facilitates* the effect, but " is it *constitutive* of it ? " Koffka investigated the mode of appearance of another kind of disc (cf. fig. 17), so arranged that bright-dark-bright-dark follow alternately upon one another by equal steps.

He establishes that no boundary contrast can be observed with these discs ; and he thereupon asserts that the presence of " brightness steps " upon *both* sides of the critical field is a necessary condition for the genesis of boundary contrast in general. " The boundary contrast depends upon the fact that *both* boundaries of the contrast field fulfil definite conditions, or better : the condition upon which boundary contrast depends involves *both* boundaries of the field." Moreover, " not only must the field lie between a brighter one and a darker one, but the two steps, that towards the brighter one and that towards the darker one, must also be mutually adjusted " (p. 202).

Thus the two brightness steps, as steps, are taken to be critical ; that is, a specific " mutual relatedness ", a " brightness structure " of a quantitatively definite order, is the essential condition for the production of the result. It therefore seems that in the Hering staircase disc the boundary contrast is produced by structure processes. Hence it would not be just to continue to designate the phenomenon boundary contrast, but one would have to say that, phenomenally, the critical surface in itself here once more exhibits a definite brightness structure. This brightness structure, this phenomenal brightness gradient, is the expression of forces which are borne by the structure process assumed to be bound up with the brightness steps in question. And these forces, moreover, must be, as Koffka states, " quite appreciable, else they could not fill up the configurally unitary, small field so remarkably inhomogeneously "[1] (p. 202).

We may well ask how far the introduction of a functional efficacy of the brightness steps, in the sense of Köhler's structure process, is in reality necessarily implicated by Koffka's findings ; how far a theory which does not take its stand upon such " brightness steps " is in this connection excluded.

Koffka, in his investigations, lays the main stress upon these particular instances of stepwise arrangement (Hering discs) ; and he asserts that the absence of boundary contrast in the case of his own disc compels one to admit that the forces underlying the boundary contrast are bound up with the brightness structures of the discs. The question, however, is whether it can really be inferred, from the

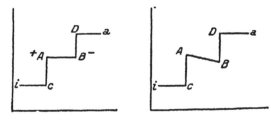

Fig. 18.   (After Koffka, redrawn.)

fact that boundary contrast is not observed with the simple alternating ring-disc, that the " forces " manifesting themselves in the boundary contrast of a staircase-disc, are not present at all in the other case. Now the operation of such forces on both sides of any ring induces an alteration in colour tone of a like sort ; and, on the other hand, the configural unity is very strong particularly in the case of small critical areas and, to use Koffka's expression, would have to act after the fashion of an assimilation. Hence there would undoubtedly be a possibility of " explaining " the phenomena in this way too. It follows, therefore, that such a functional operation of a " mutual

[1] The reason why he emphasizes this is because, in the very same brief communication, he quotes an example, based on the observations with the so-called pseudo-Masson discs which have already been mentioned (p. 178), in which the gestalt unity, despite strongest differences between the stimuli, determines a phenomenally homogeneous colour distribution ; and this is the more conspicuous the smaller the stimulus-field involved.

relatedness " can by no means be cogently deduced from this experiment.

But one is especially hard put to it upon discovering how Koffka thereupon attempts to define the mode of operation of the structure process assumed by him, physiologically, in terms of the forces involved. To quote him verbatim : " As to the nature and mode of action of this force, the following hypothesis may perhaps be erected, by resorting to *Köhler's* theory. Let Fig. 15 [here Fig. 18a] represent the objective distribution of brightness in a three-ringed disc. At each boundary a potential difference will then be generated, in such a way that m becomes positive towards i in A and negative towards a in B. Under these conditions, if certain other assumptions are satisfied, a potential difference can also arise between A and B. On the ground of the condition demonstrated by us to be constitutive, we now assume that these special presuppositions are fulfilled when boundary contrast takes place. Conversely expressed, boundary contrast arises when the conditions are so constituted that a compensable potential difference arises between A and B too. This in turn must be so constituted that A deviates in reference to B in the same direction as it does so in reference to C. The phenomenal brightness distribution will then correspond to Fig. 16 [here 18b]. The influence of the breadth of the ring can now be understood—the broader the field, the greater the difficulty with which the tension between A and B can become effective. It can similarly be understood why it is a constitutive condition that the field undergoing boundary contrast should be embedded between a brighter and a darker one " (pp. 202–3).

And yet, how does all this come to be intelligible ? Well, the premisses are sufficiently broadly selected to accomplish this—and for that matter the opposite, too, with exactly the same feasibility. Everything depends upon those " certain other presuppositions " subject to which a potential discontinuity " can " also arise between A and B. Nothing is known about the special " presuppositions " referred to, but it is " assumed " that they are fulfilled when boundary contrast occurs ! But what is the instigation of this assumption ? Simply that it fits the phenomenal facts so smoothly ! In brief, the phenomenal findings are thus bodily translated into physiology. Not "from the starting point of physics", as the scientific ideal of the gestalt theory demands, but on the contrary, from the starting point of what has to be explained, are the premisses derived which assimilate the physiological circumstances to the phenomenal ones.

Hence this example of a "mutual relatedness" cannot satisfy us either in regard to the functional analysis, or in regard to the gestalt theory's physiological facilities for interpretation.

More may be expected from a "mutual relatedness" which played a part as far back as the earliest enunciation of the gestalt concept, that is, the "mutual relatedness" of tones.

§ 53. "*Mutual relatedness*" *in tones : The apprehension of melody and harmony*

In the apprehension of melody and harmony we are faced with a precise example of the gestalt phenomenon, one which was already described as typical by von Ehrenfels. To test the gestalt theory by this very example must therefore be especially attractive.

The gestalt theory would have to assume that in the case of a given tone-sequence, it is not only the individual tones which come into effect physiologically, but on the contrary that a special total process, the "melody process" in fact, does so too ; and this in such a way that the single tones represent only dependent "moments" within the whole, whereas the total process—independently of the single tones involved—determines the impression of the melody (transposability).

Two features must be regarded as characteristic of the gestalt-theoretical interpretation. Firstly, the absolute transposability, warrant for the assumption that the total process is primary as against the individual moments ; and secondly, the direct control by the stimulus, in so far as the objective tone-relations are critical for the coherence of the melody.

Both premisses seem to be valid, according to the usual knowledge drawn upon in problems of melody. But then further notable findings have emerged, from closer experimental analysis, as essential in the matter.

The interpretation of the nature of melody which the

gestalt theory has developed, following von Ehrenfels, first lays itself open to critical opposition when certain observations of Juhasz, *Zur Analyse des musikalischen Wiedererkennens*, are taken into account. These experiments, which were concerned, as a rule, with melodies of three tones, produced noteworthy results with reference to the problem of the transposability of melodies.

Throughout these experiments doubt seems to be thrown upon the thesis of unconditional transposability which was already used as a basic one by von Ehrenfels. It is true that in the case of transpositions of familiar tone sequences the impression frequently arose that the transposed form was experienced as a known one. In other cases, however, it is evident that the subjects did not, under the same circumstances, describe the transposed form as a known one. This happened even when the original sequence was throughout correctly retained, as was revealed by repetition of the original tone presentations. Thus "transposed sequences are often confused with the original sequences, but in other cases they are not" (p. 151).

"The confusion of the transposed sequence with the original one . . . depends upon the *degree of transposition*" (p. 153). The majority of confusions occur with those tone sequences which are transposed by one octave. Sequences transposed by a fourth or a fifth are also frequently confused with their originals, but less so than those transposed by an octave. The least amount of confusion occurs in the case of sequences transposed by a major third and a major sixth. Triads given transposed by the other intervals are confused with the originals less often than those transposed by a fourth or a fifth, but more often than those sequences transposed by a major third and a major sixth. It must consequently be concluded that the absolute musical transposability which is held to be self-evident by von Ehrenfels (following Mach), and provides the basis for the excogitation of the concept of gestalt quality, can in point of fact not be admitted. A transposed tone sequence does *not* appear to us as instantaneously the same tone sequence as its original! On the contrary, in many cases we apprehend the transposed tone sequence as quite different to its presentation in its original pitch. "The tone sequence thus seems to possess a specific character which alters when the tone sequence is transposed."

Juhasz' results are in agreement with the conclusions of a number of other investigators. Revesz had already suspected the existence of a definite "characteristic of a key". Von Kries reported that violinists with absolute hearing find it impossible to play upon a violin tuned even a single semitone too high. Helmholtz, too, noted the existence of a characteristic of a key, and related its more or less marked emergence to the timbre of the musical instruments employed. Above all, Krueger (1907) emphasizes that : "The whole of a chord of a third by no means retains the same properties, as a whole, no matter how I may transpose the third ; but the complex-qualities are always only more or less similar".

It follows, therefore, in connection with our gestalt enquiry, that the Ehrenfels theorem which was at first made the foundation of gestalt theory, that is the transposability criterion, leads to difficulties in the realm of the experience of melody. Two possibilities, which Juhasz also submits, follow from this. Either the melody is in point of fact not so independent of the elementary "absolute presentations" —and then it cannot be regarded as an exact example of gestalt phenomena ; and/or, transposability is not a decisive criterion for gestalten—and then the fact remains that in these very "gestalten" the individual elements retain their specific significance, that the melody as such to a certain extent builds itself up upon these single tones, and is dependent upon them in a much closer way than would be anticipated from the gestalt theory.

The gestalt, therefore, is not so absolutely represented in its own right, but exists only in the concatenation of the single tones. The "mutual relatedness", as it is phenomenally given in melody, proves not to be either functionally or physiologically primary in the same sense as the single tones.

However, a still more pregnant instance opposing the gestalt theory follows from certain experiments by Heinz Werner (1926). These experiments deal with some very remarkable facts.

Werner maintains that : "We can produce intervals and harmonies of the same character as in our 'normal system' within very small ranges of tones. Thus we

must revise the assumption that intervals depend upon
relations between frequencies of vibration, which are
fixed once and for all (Octave, 1 : 2) " . . . " There are
'micro-melodies', as well as 'micro-harmonies', which make
the same impression, under certain circumstances, as our
normal intervals and harmonies, in spite of the totally
different physical fundaments " (p. 78). Furthermore,
" any possible ratio of frequencies of vibration can denote
a definite consciousness of an interval, since the interval-
characteristic depends upon the *system* in which the interval
is experienced."

The noteworthy point of all this is the following :   The
tones of these micro-intervals acquire their musical
qualities by a characteristic *process of development*, more
exactly portrayed by Werner, only one factor of which
need here receive attention.   This course of development
proceeds in the form of an increasing definiteness of the
tones (and intervals) in the system, " beginning from a
very complex and diffuse tonal constitution," continuing
to quite " specific and unequivocal tonal characteristics ".
" Initially every tone has a very complex timbre, in which
the real tone quality, that is, what a high and a low *a*,
for instance, have in common, does not yet display itself.
Instead of it, something else is very insistent, namely
the brightness and the hollowness of the sounds.   At first,
especially, every tone has its own timbre, every tone
stands alongside of every other one as an equally complex
though diffuse individuality, which prevents any musical
relationship between the tones.   *At the start we are not
dealing with music, with a system.*   For the tones really to
become musical bricks, every particular tone should not have
its own individual tonality, but all must take on an identical
being ; every tone must, up to a point, be the exemplar
of a class, that of the musical quality.   This metamorphosis
of the tones from single complex timbres into musical
qualities soon ensues in the course of the investigation.
Everyone who has once completed the experiments is
amazed to find how insistently *qualities which were previously
not there at all unfold themselves through relational
apprehension.*   By bringing into relation with one another
tones which previously appeared to be little or not at all
differentiated, they become differentiated in specific
qualities " (p. 79).

Q

Thus the tone-intervals of musical character *arise only in virtue of relational apprehension*, the " mutual relatedness " of tones is *not* inevitably physically fixed in physiological *structural reactions*, but it is the result of a special process, which can be traced out in the study of micro-intervals.

In a micro-system of this sort, according to Werner, genuine micro-harmony is to be found. And it is possible to demonstrate that here, too, the same general laws of development are to be met with as in the case of micro-melody (p. 85). For example, if we take the two micro-tones *a* and *d* which determine the interval of a fourth, we at first hear the not very pleasant buzz of the beats. Gradually, however, one learns to hear through this buzz, as if through a fence, . . . but herewith the consonance of the fourth, which in the normal system would have the character of a major semitone, emerges with ever greater distinctness. In addition, the consonances of the fifths, thirds, and sixths, up to the octave, can also be apprehended.

Here, too, a specific developmental process is involved. The harmony as a " simultaneous mutual relatedness ", a simultaneous gestalt, takes shape in its so-being only within a quite definite developmental context. The " mutual relatedness " either in the harmony or in the melody, is not primarily given with the stimulus situation of " togetherness " or " sequence ". On the contrary, the very same objective stimulus situation gives rise to entirely different experiences on the phenomenal side, which, in their so-being, are essentially dependent upon specific processes of formation. These processes of formation, it is true, have not been more exactly investigated by Werner. But they indubitably no longer permit of being comprehended in terms of the simple copy-schema of physical and psychophysical gestalt processes ; they should be defined, rather, in terms of apprehensional interrelationships.

In Heinz Werner's findings, therefore, we discover a quite conclusive control which—especially if they should be substantiated by subsequent and perhaps more thorough experimental checking—has the greatest significance in reference to the refutation of the Köhler-Wertheimer gestalt theory.

When we reconsider the discussions devoted to the

problem of " mutual relatedness ", as a whole, from this standpoint, it must be admitted that they can in nowise be positively drawn upon for the founding of the gestalt theory. Nowhere do we meet with a really valid finding which necessitates explanation exclusively by gestalt-theoretical doctrines, and which would thus cogently commend acceptance of the theory. Just where the facts seemingly stand in definite relationship with the theory, closer scrutiny shows that an unbiassed consideration of psychological experimentation on a wider scale calls for a much greater complexity in the interpretation of the problem in all its bearings, than has been relied upon in the interpretation of the experiments at issue (Köhler's selective training experiments). With other findings, by contrast, it emerges, either that a logical error was present in the interpretation itself, or else the experiments furnish material which quite plainly compels a conclusion opposed to the gestalt theory. From these facts, therefore, the gestalt theory can expect no support for its position.

SECTION TWO

THE NOTION OF A DYNAMICS OF GESTALTEN

From our foregoing exposition, the gestalt theory seems to be by no means so well founded, even in its earliest domain, that of perception, as to deserve to be called a theory in the genuine sense of the term. It is evident in numerous places, that the doctrines of the gestalt theory do not, upon more exact interpretation and keenly pursued conceptual analysis, do justice to the facts; they do not correspond to the richness and abundance of the implications of the problems, which are really comprised in the facts. In other instances a direct opposition between the theory and experimental findings is displayed. Nowhere, however, is an example to be found, where the observations could really cogently lead one to accept the theory.

After what we have thus far established, there still remains, in the scheme of our critique of the gestalt theory, a further task. We have to investigate how the gestalt theory fares in respect of its achievements in those psychological provinces which extend beyond the study of perception in the strict sense.

In our expository part we have indicated the lines of thought by means of which the gestalt theory was able to expand its scope so far. These lines of thought are determined in the last resort from the starting point of the world of physical concepts. Analogously with a distinction which is fundamental in that domain, a dichotomy is discerned among gestalt processes too : " relatively independent of the time factor "— " temporally variable " ; " resting in itself "—" developing temporally " ; to the " statics of gestalten " is opposed a " gestalt dynamics ".

Gestalt dynamics also includes gestalt phenomena which are not temporally relatively invariable ; that is, phenomena of the arousal, transformation, and elaboration of gestalten, in brief every concatenation evolving temporally. It is supposed to enable the entirety of so-called " higher psychical processes " to be interpreted in terms of the gestalt theory. It is, however, supposed to manifest itself equally in the province of perception. In fact it was in this very province that the first notable evidence for the dynamics of gestalten was believed to have been found. Our discussion will, to begin with, deal with this original evidence, or perhaps premises, for a gestalt dynamics, and will then turn to the utilization of these modes of thought for the interpretation of the higher functions.

CHAPTER ONE

THE DOCTRINE OF GESTALT DYNAMICS IN THE REALM OF THE PERCEPTUAL GESTALTEN

The notion of gestalt dynamics in perception is just as old as the notion of gestalt conformance to laws in general.

It is a special case of the latter. That indeed is how Wertheimer already conceived it, when in his search for gestalt laws he was brought to ascribe definite " tendencies " to gestalten, the tendencies towards a " good gestalt ", towards a " precise gestalt " and so forth, which are supposed to determine the inner gestalt organization. Before he himself made any communications on the matter, Köhler—without more pertinent experimental work, but purely on the basis of his gestalt physiology—also set out to lay the foundations (1920) constructionally, " from the starting point of physics," for gestalt dynamics, at any rate in a tentative way, thus to assure it a framework of principles. Only later did particular experimental analyses endeavour to collect material intended to give empirical support to the idea. Our criticism will turn first of all to Köhler's general observations.

I. KÖHLER'S DOGMATIC FOUNDING OF GESTALT DYNAMICS AND ITS CONFORMANCE TO LAW

§ 54. *Köhler's deduction of a fundamental gestalt-dynamical uniformity " from the starting point of physics "*

At the end of his book of 1920, Köhler sets himself the question, what statements could be made about physical gestalten which do not already have the character of an equilibrium in the physical sense. He links this up with the question as to what else characterizes those physical processes which are not independent of the time factor, which do not have the character of an equilibrium ; and from this point of departure he very easily arrives at the premisses for a solution of his problem. The issue, in his opinion, is only this : How can we carry over the corresponding fundamental principle of general theoretical physics to gestalten in general, and to the psychophysical-phenomenal gestalten in particular—that is, the *principle of minimal energy*, of entropy, which in physics distinguishes the states of equilibrium of every system from its other possible states, and on the basis of which the transformation of a state from the labile initial stage to the stable position of equilibrium can be envisaged.

To carry this over, only one thing is necessary, according

to Köhler. The question must be answered, " *What do gestalten* which correspond to minimal energy values *look like* ? " For the principle in point is of practical value for the treatment of psychological gestalten only when we can supply " *purely structural* viewpoints " corresponding to the direction of the transformation, since there is no possibility of making direct statements about the energy contents of these gestalten, as would be necessary for the direct application of the line of thought.

Köhler now believes that the very same characteristics which Wertheimer considered himself to have discovered in his investigation of phenomenal gestalten, will suffice him for dealing with this problem in physics. He believes it possible to demonstrate " *tendencies towards the arousal of simple gestalten* ", and towards " *precision of the gestalt* ", in physics too. As evidence for this he (and also his interpreter Becher, in more concise, and conceptually clearer form) develops an *example*, in which the physical side of this whole problem can be made concretely intelligible. " Let a strong electrical current be passed through an inelastic, easily flexible metal filament of given length, which forms some sort of closed figure, and lies on a smooth surface. At the moment of closing the circuit, the filament, as the theory of electricity shows, will, if the strength of the current and the mobility are adequate, commence to move, and continue until the figure formed by it has taken on a circular shape. The metal filament, the course of the current (and the field surrounding it) thus dispose themselves as simply and symmetrically as possible in the space. If this disposition is achieved, the filament traversed has then reached a position of equilibrium ; the conducting-filament gestalt (as well as that of the field) has become independent of the time factor " (Becher, p. 42). But the direction in which this rearrangement takes place, according to Köhler, plainly shows itself to be structurally determined in a characteristically pure way ; and this—independently of the energy factor—is taken to be specific for the end gestalt. It is to be regarded as a " tendency towards the arousal of simple configuration ", towards " precision of structure " (cf. p. 43).

Thus a basis for a chain of inference is created, which *legitimates*, with one stroke, *the idea of gestalt dynamics*,

and at the same time its essential, in fact sole, principle.
For,

1, there is complete correspondence between the dynamic processes in general physics and those in the province of physiological and phenomenal gestalten. In both they run their course—structurally described—in the direction towards precision of the end gestalt. But now,

2, the physical processes of this kind are, described in energetic terms, the expression of the principle of the minimum energy of the system. Consequently,

3, the tendency towards precision of gestalt, abstracted by Wertheimer as determinative for the phenomenal, or alternatively, neurophysical happening, does actually hit upon a fundamental uniformity. It is none other than the principle of entropy, deviating from this only as regards the criterion, but intrinsically identical with it.

Thus the principle of gestalt precision is elevated to a quite high level. At the time it was palpably still very indefinite with Wertheimer—did he not hesitate a considerable time before publishing the work in which he reports his evidence for it? Here it appears at the outset incorporated in a context of imposing scope, from which its foundational significance seems to be impressively deduced.

§ 55. *The inadequacy of Köhler's concepts and lines of reasoning*

Whatever the pretensions of the context in which, as shown above, Köhler finds a place for gestalt dynamics, his lines of reasoning actually cannot at all satisfy one. Upon closer inspection they prove to be nothing other than a beautiful illusion. Köhler himself may have felt this, when he puts forward his animadversions as at bottom suggestive rather than anything else ; when, above all, he does not himself explicitly formulate the precise claims which we have just developed as the immanent consequences of his view.

It will suffice if we briefly enumerate the individual difficulties in his contentions.

Even in its form the line of argument is faulty. For in its first major premiss it rests upon a mere analogy, and its conclusion tacitly includes an inadmissible extrapolation.

As far as its purport is concerned, it is entirely beyond discussion, even on the physical side :—

1. The concept of *structurally distinguishable* simplicity, the notion that one can *perceive* by inspection whether a physical system is stable or not, and in what direction it is bound to change, *is totally absurd, from the standpoint of physics*.[1]

The "simplicity" from which physics starts, the greatest simplicity of the energy conditions in accordance with the principle of minimal energy, has a quite definite meaning in physics. It is a matter of strictly quantifiable ascertainment of facts. But nothing can be made of structural simplicity in Köhler's sense. There is no possibility of sensibly constructing a rank order of degrees of "structural simplicity". We thus discover ourselves in a sphere of absolute conceptual vagueness and arbitrariness, which is intolerable from the point of view of physics, accustomed as it is to rigorous theoretical thinking.[2]

2. *The co-ordination* which Köhler believes himself to have established *between the principle of energetic and that of structural simplicity*, is in no way intrinsically sustained to a satisfactory extent. It is wholly arbitrary, firstly because it is based on a generalization from only a few examples that is unwarrantable from the point of view of scientific theory ; but above all, inasmuch as the exposition of these examples only leads to the desired goal through the fact that Köhler, quite heedless of what signification his statements should have, simply inserts the appropriate *words*. Physically, "simple" can only have a definite meaning when it is interpreted in accordance with the principle of minimal energy. Köhler, moreover, sets out to distinguish degrees of simplicity both in physics

---

[1] What justification has Köhler for asserting that the circular form of the current filament is structurally the simplest one? He would, correspondingly, have to assume the circular form to be critical, e.g. for the gestalt of the lines of force of a magnet. At any rate he must admit that the form of a "catenary", the equilibrium figure of a chain of fine links hanging freely from two supports, is in nowise thus made intelligible. Anyone, provided he is at all concerned, as to this example, with problems of this nature, would regard the parabola, for instance, as a structurally simpler form than the actual curve, whose inner complexity is proved by its equation.

[2] Even the authority of E. Mach cannot help to establish the position of Köhler (see above, pp. 122 ff.).

and in the phenomenal findings, on the basis of the formal constitution of the structure ; but at the back of this lie the ideas of a very remarkable teleology—none other than that which impelled the Greeks, for example, to regard the sphere as the most perfect body and circular movement as the ideal movement.

However, to set up an identity between the simplicity of the seen circle, as phenomenally given in immediate impression, and the physical forms of " simplest construction "—the simplicity of the path of a circular current—this amounts either to foisting upon the physicists speculative ideas, such as are to-day hardly intelligible to us, as we find them in the thinking of the Greeks ; or it means accepting an empty analogy, which at bottom refers merely to words, as a substantiation.

3. And finally, it is already evident from a remark of Becher that, somehow, the analogy cannot pass muster for the example quoted by Köhler. Becher asks, " how does it happen that this tendency asserts itself with perceptual configurations just when a ' certain weakness ' of the corresponding factors is bound up with the stimuli and excitations ? Quite contrariwise, in the case of our loop of metal filament through which a current is passed, the tendency towards simple structuration, that is towards the circular form, arises the more strongly the more powerful the current " (p. 43). And here undoubtedly lies a conclusive negation of Köhler's thesis that the same uniform law underlies both cases.

It is accordingly quite impossible to arrive at a dynamics of gestalten in the manner proposed by Köhler ; or, as a special matter, at all to deduce the principle of gestalt precision, which is supposed to play a critical rôle in regard to what is given in our phenomenal perception, " from the starting point of physics "—even if, as we have done in our discussion, one goes so far as to grant Köhler's general gestalt physics to be justified.

The assumed laws of gestalt dynamics can receive substantiation in no other way than on the basis of direct phenomenal analysis. This was where Köhler actually took them from, in reliance upon Wertheimer's theorems ; and to this we must now turn our criticism. We must enquire to what extent the *facts* can in truth be so interpreted.

In this connection it must be noted in advance that the facts as a matter of course appear hitched to a fixed *theoretical framework*. The first approach to a gestalt dynamics, established with the facts as starting point, is in any case most intimately related to the erection of general gestalt laws.

To be sure, these gestalt laws, as we have seen above (§ 38), at first referred only to the question of what general characteristics pertain to the static phenomenal gestalten as expression of the " inner structure principles " inherent in them, in so far as the happening was held to shape itself " not because of blind external factors, but because of an intrinsic ' inner exigency ' " (cf. Wertheimer 1922). Now these principles do not appear merely as bare, general definitions of a formal sort. They are interpreted quite specifically as the principles of the underlying uniformity of action.

Thus the possibility is provided of at the same time defining the dynamic gestalten in terms of the static ones, in so far as these very static gestalten—being end products of that dynamics—also express the uniformities of the dynamic ones.

The result is therefore, characteristically, that the *gestalt dynamics need not actually be newly created* or founded upon special experimental research. In point of fact, no really new theoretical moment is introduced into the conceptual apparatus of the theory through the empirical material which has in the meanwhile been brought into relation with it. From the expositions of its adherents, the theory appears to be holding its own everywhere. How far this is indeed so we shall now proceed to put to the test.

From the approach we have sketched, we can predict that the endeavour to demonstrate empirically the efficacy of the principles of gestalt dynamics, would be made in *two ways*. On the one hand, the attempt would be made to determine this efficacy from the *phenomenally appreciable end effect* at a particular time, *from what is achieved through it*; and on the other hand, the enquiry would be undertaken as to whether the action of this dynamics could not be followed up *directly as it occurred, immediately in the process*.

We shall, to begin with, turn our attention to the findings falling under the first line of enquiry.

2. INDIRECT EMPIRICAL SUBSTANTIATION OF THE IDEA
OF GESTALT DYNAMICS—FROM THE END RESULTS OF
THE DYNAMIC PROCESSES SOUGHT FOR

§ 56. *Fuchs' explanation of the phenomena of " gestalt
completion "*

The problem of *gestalt completion* became a vital one for
the gestalt theory in a quite definite empirical connection,
namely in connection with Fuchs' analyses of the seeing of
hemianopics. It is interpreted in such a way as to make
the phenomenally discoverable effect appear as a *result of a
dynamic gestalt activity*. Suppose a circle (circumference of
a circle or filled-in circle) is centrally presented, by means
of a tachistoscope, to a hemianopic who has been shown by
perimetric or campimetric investigation to have a distinct
hemianopsia, say, to the right. Now according to Fuchs
(1920) " in spite of strictly fixating the centre of the circle,
some of the patients profess to have seen not a semicircle but
a whole circle.   The paradoxical result thus revealed
is that the patient apparently still sees with the blind
half of the eye " ; and this happens " even with hemianopics
who are completely blind on the defective side " (p. 422).[1]
And in fact—to express it in the categories of present-day
gestalt dynamics—a form actually does appear which is
in every respect consonant with the principle of the
precision of gestalt. A total form arises along the lines
of the " simplest possible configuration ".

Fuchs himself does not make use of the categories of
gestalt dynamics.   Yet he interprets the phenomenon
exactly in accordance with the general conception of gestalt
dynamics, and we can perhaps for this very reason see the
more clearly to what extent theory and facts agree ; for
he is nevertheless thus led to go into his theory in greater
detail.

Fuchs aims at explaining the phenomena to the last
detail in terms of the gestalt theory—dispensing with
the assumption of " ideational completion ", in the sense
of a psychological production theory, made by Poppelreuter
in interpreting exactly similar findings. He prefers to
start directly from the stimulus conditions, basing himself
on general considerations as to the mechanism of

---

[1] Cited from the reprint in Gelb and Goldstein, *Psychologische
Analysen hirnpathologischer Fälle*, i, 1920.

physiological gestalt processes. In his opinion the term
" completion ", by which Poppelreuter characterized the
phenomenon, is theoretically misleading.

In his findings he perceives simply the operation of
that distinctive inner closure which the gestalt theory
ascribes to the physiological processes. For his
explanation he requires only the single presupposition
that the neurophysical basis of our phenomenal gestalt
experiences already possesses specific gestalt character ;
that it is not a mere aggregate of single excitations which
is involved, but that definite inner relationships are
physiologically concurrent. He proceeds to assume
the following : In virtue of this very inner, dynamic
coherence between the single parts of the somatic field,
the total process which corresponds, say, to an image
of a circle can be initiated in two ways. It can be initiated
not only through the presentation in the objective stimulus
of a manifold of points having a real circular distribution,
but also when only a certain part of such objective fundaments for the gestalt process is present, and this then
appears to be sufficient by itself to " arouse " the total
gestalt process. Hence he explains the observed
phenomena by means of a " totalization " mechanism [1]
according to which a definite " gestalt excitation " seems
to be sufficient to set the total process going.

It is Fuchs' opinion that in these circumstances the
phenomena of so-called gestalt completion, for the very
reason that it is, more correctly stated, a matter of " gestalt
totalization " where they are concerned, can be looked
upon as specific evidence of the applicability of the gestalt
theory. The assumption of characteristic total processes
is held to prove exceptionally fertile in the case of these
phenomena. According to his experiments they do indeed
appear to be amenable to this assumption in every respect.
However, upon critical scrutiny this impression proves
to be far more a consequence of the deductive manner of
his exposition than the product of the immediate facts
in his empirical findings. When these facts are clearly
sifted out, and the means of explanation utilized by
Fuchs at the same time put to the test more exactly,
an essentially different picture emerges.

---

[1] This word being used in the sense of *gestalt* mechanics.

The inadequacy of Fuchs' view follows at once when we analyze the nucleus of his actual findings, his reports upon the *conditions* which underlie the mechanism of gestalt totalization.

According to his observations three factors must converge as a necessary condition for the genesis of a genuine gestalt totalization.

(1) " Adequate gestalt excitation " from the sound side.

(2) A definite degree of " surveyability " in connection with the size of the object (p. 430).

(3) " Avoidance of a critical attitude " on the part of the subject (p. 436 ff.).

The difficulties commence immediately, with the concept of " gestalt excitation ". How does this excitation function ? And upon what does it act ? Gneisze justly says, in regard to this concept, in the course of coming to terms with Fuchs, " I cannot think of anything in the domain of physiology to which the gestalt excitation could reasonably be referred. Gestalt excitation can only occur in respect of psychical forces ; but these could not have any relevance for Fuchs, since according to Wertheimer's theory mental gestalten arise in consciousness in a finished form as soon as the physiological cross-functions have run their course." For indeed, " is it possible to speak of a gestalt excitation if the gestalt forms itself in the physiological sphere in accordance with the laws of mechanical causal nexus ? Is it to be conceived that the cerebral excitations caused by the action of an incomplete circle are stimulated to influence it in a particular way ? Or is it to be thought that the brain is stimulated to engender out of itself further excitations or physiological processes of a different sort, in addition to the excitations which arise in it on account of the stimuli emanating from the incomplete circle ? " Purely from the starting point of physiology, without knowledge of the actual phenomenally observed occurrences, it would in no way whatsoever be possible to arrive at such ideas. The concept of gestalt excitation forthwith appears to be a purely *ad hoc* means of explanation. But with this the concept of the " totalization " mechanism also falls to the ground. If the observed " totalization " is explained by means of an underlying physiological mechanism of this sort, it has no value at all as knowledge, now that we have seen that this mechanism cannot be interpolated directly from physiology as starting point. Fuchs' viewpoint that all these questions are settled simply with the word " total process " fails to gain our assent.

As little satisfactory is the way Fuchs' second condition, that of *surveyability*, appears to be incorporated into the gestalt theory. Fuchs' manner of coming to terms with this so pre-eminently psychical a factor is typical of the way in which inconvenient problems are simply disregarded in the gestalt theory. Fuchs gives a remarkable " reduction " of the influence of surveyability, in terms of gestalt-theoretical principles. He presents the matter in such a way that it is a question merely of the " factor of gestalt excitation " (the legitimacy of which is simply assumed), being dependent upon the surveyability. He thus makes it seem as if the question of surveyability is no longer at all germane in its theoretical significance, since everything appears to be " configurally " controlled. And by this artifice he causes the concept of surveyability, which also expresses in so eminent a way a subjective conditionality of the phenomenon in question, to appear to be fitted into the context of the gestalt theory without any closer elucidation.

In the whole problem of gestalt completion, such an elucidation of the subjective conditions which play a rôle in the phenomenon is in fact unavoidable. This is at bottom explicitly conceded when Fuchs puts forward the " avoidance of a critical attitude " as the third necessary condition.

It is clear that very far-reaching questions, which are bound to be of the greatest importance for the understanding of the facts, are involved in this designation " critical attitude ". It would have been to the point if Fuchs had from this entered upon the task of really investigating more exactly the influence, and the psychological singularity of this " attitude ". He does indeed observe that a cognizance or attentional factor is here concerned. He reports that " the descriptions ' duller ', ' thinner ', ' worse ' . . . were rendered by the patient when, in response to the experimenter, he specially regarded the side " which corresponded to the damaged half of his sight (p. 18). But he has not thought it necessary to follow up more closely the problems here implicated.

In this connection he could have noticed, from his own protocols, that the manner of cognizance was in fact an essential condition for the mode of appearance of the critical parts of the gestalt. Indeed, he himself reports that very different possible experiences could arise in respect to the phenomenal characters of these parts, depending upon the manner of cognizance, from the impression of an altogether unitary total gestalt, through cases in which what was declared to be seen in the blind half of the field appeared " worse " than what was seen in the sound half, up to cases where, finally, nothing positive could any longer be reported about the constitution of the " perceptual field " in the blind zone. All these numerous findings he dismisses by simply speaking of a " disturbing effect " of the attention in these cases. Instead of this, he should have formulated the problem in such a way as to indicate that it was incumbent to investigate what conditions of apprehension in general have an influence upon the configuration of the contents, in the case of the perceptual circumstances at issue.

He has himself stated that, in point of fact, even in those cases where the totalization effect presumed by him to be normal arises, special conditions of apprehension are critical for what is generated. He expressly says : " For the part exposed in the functionally sound half, which is sufficient for completion into a whole gestalt, the bare objective fact that, being a part, it has the constitution indicated, is *not* enough to elicit the totalizing gestalt apprehension. It is, on the contrary, *necessary that it should also be apprehended* (!) by the subject *as a part thus constituted* " (p. 79).

A discovery of this sort does not fundamentally fit in with a theory according to which this effect is supposed to arise directly as a result of the dynamic moments of action inherent in the purely physiological gestalt processes. For —to take Gneisze's just criticism of this point (1922)— this suggests that " the image of the gestalt of the incomplete circle becomes *a determinant of the physiological event* in consequence of which the arc lacking to make the figure a complete circle is seen. . . . But according to every consistent physiological theory the conscious phenomena are always only the *consequences* of physiological events, never their *determinants* ".

Fuchs often lapses into this sort of inconsistency in regàrd to the essential basic ideas of his own theory. One finds many places in his work where he believes himself to havè hit upon something of direct gestalt-theoretical import, but where the facts themselves lead him, in the natural course of the exposition, actually to go beyond the framework of the theory. Thus, in order to elucidate his concept of gestalt excitation, he says that an incomplete gestalt " under certain circumstances forthwith subjectively provokes completion " ; an " urge for completion " is, for instance, associated with an adequately large portion of a circle (p. 433).

Gneisze justly remarks (p. 314) : " A portion of a circle strives for completion. Surely this can only mean that when we *become aware of a figure as a portion of a circle* we feel ourselves impelled to see or to imagine a complete circle. This impulse arises in us because we have become aware of the law regulating the formation of the portion of the circle, and our reason demands that a law be completely satisfied. The impulse cannot possibly be operative in the cerebral excitations ruled by causality, nor in the field actions, nor in the reciprocal effects of the cerebral excitations which develop on the basis of the field actions. It can, moreover, not operate in direct union with the becoming aware of the gestalt of the portion of the circle, but it can only supervene when this displays itself as fully developed and proves to be incomplete. Thus here too we have an event—according to Fuchs' own statement—which is associated with the physiological events, and the conscious events which are their necessary reflection. The supplementary gestalt, the arc completing the imperfect circle into a whole circle, thus, at any rate, owes its arousal to an activity of the percipient which has nothing to do with the physiological events of Wertheimer's theory."

The case is not much different with another theoretically important formula of Fuchs. This, it is true, in conformity with the theoretical framework, is throughout supposed to be interpretable in terms of physiology ; but finally, in the analysis of the facts, it lands in the same difficulties— viz., the *formula of the " compulsive gestalt "*.

Fuchs utilizes it in those cases where he cannot achieve a full explanation by means of the concept of gestalt excitation. He introduces it, for example, when it is incumbent to explain why certain drawings, such as star and half-star figures, release no completion, by maintaining " that a totalizing gestalt apprehension is possible only with certain ' characteristic ' and indeed ' compulsive' gestalten " ; that is to say, with that sort " in which the part falling into the sound half of the field, and therefore really seen, already bears the law of the whole in itself " (p. 499).

We immediately recognize that this concept of the " compulsive gestalt " is identical with Wertheimer's *concept of the good, the precise gestalt.* It is clear that in Fuchs' work, too, in spite of his other, more detailed, theoretical suggestions, whenever a critical point arises, that same, single, great uniformity is invoked as a final explanatory measure, which we have previously distinguished as the essential one in gestalt dynamics, and have already discussed in its physiological and physical bearings.

We are here in a position to assess the discussion of this principle in reference to its validity in the phenomenal-functional analysis which commences directly from what is given. We can ascertain that in this connection, too, the principle fails to be satisfactory.

Even a superficial perusal of Fuchs' work makes it palpable that outright contradictions are involved in the application of this concept, especially if Fuchs' discussions of gestalt displacement (see above §§ 47–8) are also adduced. At one time—in the earlier work upon displacement—the fact that displacement of parts in figures of meaningful objects does not happen (p. 279) is traced back to such " compulsion ". " Apparently the figures of *known objects* (watering can, bicycle, butterfly, fish, etc.) are *too compulsive gestalten*, the parts of which are too firmly anchored to one another, by reason of gestalt and associative factors, for a disintegration and partial displacement to arise." On the other hand, such figures, again, do not seem to be " compulsive gestalten "—for gestalt completion is here absent. In fact, " even the knowledge and the *clear image* of the total object or of the part situated in the blind side, does not assist to complete this part in such a way as to admit of its being perceived " (in the case of hemianopics, p. 431, and in the case of hemiamblyopics, p. 495 ff.).

An explanation of the difference in the two cases, a reconciliation of these contradictions, can certainly not be found in Fuchs' work ; in fact the existence of a discrepancy here seems to have escaped him altogether. Naturally, too, where Fuchs' presuppositions form the starting point, and where the orientation is purely by the stimulus and the gestalt processes " controlled " by it, such variation when the objective situation is the same, cannot be understood. It can only be understood when the possibility of specific subjective conditions playing a rôle in the configuration of our perceptions is entertained.

At any rate, taking it all together, one cannot say that clear and valid arguments are to be discovered in Fuchs' work in favour of the elaboration of a gestalt theory, in the sense of Wertheimer and Köhler, even if Fuchs himself is of this opinion. On the contrary, one cannot obviate the impression that, on account of the orientation of his experiments by the gestalt theory maintained by Fuchs from the outset, essential problems have been passed over, indeed have not been noticed at all. A final consideration of the question of totalizing gestalt apprehension will of course only permit of being made upon the basis of such further experimental conclusions. It is certain, however—this can already be discerned from our considerations of Fuchs' observations—that this final theory will not be the gestalt theory.

§ 57. *The mechanism of gestalt transformation according to Wulff*

Observations undertaken by Fr. Wulff in the Giessen laboratory upon the relation between *memory and gestalt* (1922), can to a certain degree be placed alongside Fuchs' gestalt completions—in so far, that is, as they appear to be gestalt-theoretically characterized by the rubric *gestalt transformations*.

Objects in the form of simple figures drawn upon paper were given to the subjects to look at. After the elapse of an interval of time, they had to draw these from memory. The result, objectively determined by the drawing performance of the subjects, was characteristic. The figures drawn showed quite definite deviations from the stimulus figures. Deviations in two directions appeared : in the direction of " making precise " (fig. 19), of a more emphatic selection of the significant features of the gestalt in question ; and in the direction of a " levelling " (fig. 20) of the forms of the gestalt features, an attraction of parts relatively projecting from the " nucleus " of the gestalt, towards the nucleus. Wulff's interpretation of this result offers a specific example of gestalt-theoretical explanation.

Since, in these observations, it is a question of a deviation in the " structure ", of " structive variations ", the relationship with the gestalt theory is evident without more ado. The new contribution in respect to the gestalt theory which here arises, is the evaluation showing that the specific gestalt laws also preside over the memory, and the manner in which it is sought to make the dependence of the memory content on gestalt laws theoretically intelligible, in a concrete way.

The classification under the gestalt laws, those of the dynamics of gestalten, is readily accomplished : " We have detected two directions of variation," he says, " ' making precise,' and ' levelling ', which seem to be opposed to each other. But they have one feature in common. In both it is a matter of alteration along the lines of a ' better gestalt '. However much the distinctness and the inner articulation may diminish in the course of time, the inclination towards the ' good gestalt ' is not affected by it " (pp. 370–1). " The law of *precision* serves as the most general law regulating all variations. This states that every gestalt becomes as ' good ' as is possible " (p. 372). " In both cases we meet with the structuration of a more significant, ' perspicuous,' precise structure, be it by means of exaggerating some particular distinction, or through making a peculiarity more sharply conspicuous (making precise) or the reverse (levelling) " (p. 373).

Wulff is able to tell us somewhat more concretely how it happens that gestalt laws in this way " preside over the memory ", by having recourse to physiology in the shape of an engram theory. " Exactly as every gestalt whatsoever cannot be perceived, so every perceived gestalt whatsoever cannot be retained in the memory. That which remains behind in the memory, the physiological 'engram', is accordingly not to be conceived as an unalterable impression which only becomes more and more blurred in the course of time, like an engraved drawing on a paving-stone. On the contrary, this engram undergoes alterations on the basis of gestalt laws. In the place of those originally perceived, gestalten altered in certain respects arise in the course of time, and these changes involve the gestalten as wholes " (p. 370). Again, therefore, everything seems to be " explained " in the simplest possible way.

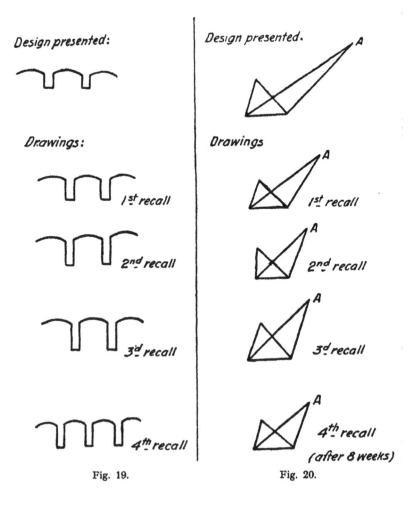

Fig. 19.   Fig. 20.

And yet to begin with, one can surely not avoid being greatly surprised at the remarkably slow manner in which the transformation of the gestalt engram comes to pass. The gestalt processes with which we have elsewhere made acquaintance as evidence for the operation of "gestalt tendencies", actually take their course in a characteristically impetuous and—compared with what is given, with the initial gestalt—reckless manner (see below, § 58, pp. 254–5).

But Wulff's interpretation makes it look as if a gradual transformation were arising in the course of time. There seem, however, to be no evident grounds upon which to explain why the mode of occurrence of the processes in question may here be assumed to be entirely different from that of other cases. At all events, as we have more exactly set forth above, we might if we cared, with Köhler trace these "tendencies" of gestalten back to the fact that physiologically we are here dealing with transitions from unstable to stable distributions in systems, transitions which signify the establishment of a state of equilibrium, and which ensue in conformity with a minimum of "structure energy"; but such a manner of occurrence will certainly not be intelligible forthwith. For all such processes in any way directed towards the establishment of an equilibrium, characteristically take their course "impetuously" throughout physics; unless some sort of obstructing factors modify the process in such a way that it ensues by gradual stages of a quasi-stationary character. Such inhibitory factors—always on the physiological side, be it noted—could, however, in this very matter of engram formations, not readily be made intelligible. Let us assume that, as a fact, with a given stimulus situation, gestalt dynamics can be operative in such a way as to prevail here in the determination of the phenomenal gestalten, and, moreover, in an extraordinarily impetuous manner, over-coming the retinal topography set up by the stimulus situation. Then, under the circumstances to which Wulff's "gestalt transformations" are subject, it must actually be expected that the process will ensue much more impetuously, since all constraint by a retinal topography is absent, and the gestalt dynamics can thus work itself out quite freely.

Setting aside these difficulties in the physiological

interpretation, however, the description of the experimental material should also perhaps be somewhat amended in its phenomenal bearing. Wulff is of opinion that we are here dealing with structure changes in the " memory image ", that therefore the regarding of the figures involves purely perceptive registration. But the question nevertheless arises whether we are really still in the purely perceptive sphere here. And there is the further question, whether what is reproductively present to the subject when he is making the drawings is indeed purely a matter of memory images. Wulff himself says that " non-optical presentations " explicitly play a rôle, above all the " awareness of the rule ". " In the awareness of the rule, relations play a big part. The subject ' knows ' of definite ' relations '. It is these relations which in recall often furnish the firm frame for the gestalt in which they occur. This is true sufficiently frequently for the highly visual subjects as well . . . . " (p. 358). But this amounts to a criticism of himself. In the face of such unequivocal observations it is incomprehensible how Wulff could ignore the rôle of the psychology of thinking in his experiments. There can be no doubt that one does not do justice to the facts with the statement that it is a matter of structure alterations of the " images " which are to a certain extent preserved in memory.

It makes no difference to this when Wulff falls back upon Köhler, for whom, as we saw above (p. 33 ; p. 202 ff.), " the perception of relation is to be counted not as something specifically new in comparison with the gestalt perception, but as one of its special modifications " (p. 158). By thus referring to Köhler, Wulff obviously wants to meet the objection that one should have to relegate the awareness of the rule, the knowledge of relations, to a different level. But Wulff himself has no proof to offer in this connection. When he says that his protocols comply best of all with Köhler's view, the question arises, firstly, whether he is in possession of sufficient material obtained by systematic introspection to settle this point (nothing in regard to it can be seen from his work) ; and secondly, it has to be borne in mind that apparently his subjects comprised solely colleagues of his at the Giessen institute, who were obviously more or less versed in the gestalt theory's mode of thinking and speaking.

The problem can only be settled if one enquires whether in point of fact all the work that has been accomplished by the modern psychology of thinking in the elucidation of the special nature of the thought processes, must be set aside in the face of what the gestalt theory has to tell us about thinking. This question can only be cleared up when we have dealt more thoroughly with the " thought gestalten ". Apart from this, however, it may at any rate be said, that if the same work had been carried out with a basic orientation towards the psychology of thinking rather than towards the gestalt theory, it would certainly have yielded a picture essentially richer on the descriptive side. Because of the gestalt-theoretical attitude, an impoverishment is here produced even in the descriptive results. But the very same applies equally in respect to the functional problems which are involved in the experimental findings. For it can readily be perceived how the adherence to the gestalt-theoretical categories has caused a certain essential issue not to be noticed at all.

The only explanatory principle Wulff entertains is the " tendency towards precision of the structure ", and he affirms that he has made both the transformation in accordance with " levelling " and that in accordance with " making precise ", comprehensible by means of it. Even if we willingly grant him this, another question still remains open, namely when does " levelling " and when does " making precise " occur ? This question must certainly be admitted to be of some importance. When this question is posed, we see that on the whole, nothing, absolutely nothing at all, is told us in Wulff's communication about the psychical functions manifesting themselves in these performances. It is true that he speaks of the conditions of apprehension playing a part even at the time of first seeing the figures, when they are stamped in ; but a thorough-going analysis of this fact is completely lacking. Wulff is satisfied with being able to introduce the formula of the precision of structure. Thus no answer is given to this question.

The further problem will also arise as to the perceptive and the apperceptive-intellectual participants in the stamping-in achievement. One will enquire whether and how the process of gradual genesis of the figure in the reproduction by drawing, influences the result ; how, quite generally, the relation between the drawing and the memory object must be envisaged. Upon all these questions Wulff can give us no information either. But the reason why the work was so narrowly conceived in regard to the problems posed by it, lies in its bondage to the gestalt theory, which here explicitly acts as an impediment to pure empirical research.

The notion of gestalt dynamics here proves to be by no means fortunate. The question is whether it will appear in a more favourable light when we consider those findings in which the operation of this dynamics is held to be susceptible of being followed out directly in its course of development.

3.   DIRECT SUBSTANTIATIONS FOR THE DOCTRINE OF GESTALT DYNAMICS

When we are faced with the task of following out dynamic gestalt activities directly in the process, material towards this end can only be expected in the field of the seeing of movement ; and this, moreover, only in connection with the findings about apparent movements. These are movements which are not directly founded upon the stimuli, but are relatively free from them, and can therefore be brought into relation with the inner dynamics of the gestalt processes involved. These phenomena are thus incorporated into an entirely new context. They are not of interest in so far as they exemplify noteworthy movement phenomena, but rather on account of the fact that they can serve as " analysers of the gestalt process " itself. In this way the γ-movement first became significant for the gestalt theory in a new sense.

§ 58. *The γ-movement as expression of gestalt dynamics*

The γ-phenomenon was for the first time interpreted specifically in terms of gestalt dynamics, by Lindemann (1922). In his work the γ-movement appears as an example of those cases in which the datum of perception is determined not directly from the stimulus as starting point, but on the basis of an inner configurational dynamics. It makes the " becoming and subsiding of gestalten " which has to be deduced from this dynamics, accessible to direct observation. " A resting stimulus-configuration is not under all circumstances immediately paralleled by a resting gestalt. On the contrary, there are conditions under which the gestalt phenomenally appears to be in movement, and this movement represents a development towards the end state of the gestalt which persists in a state of rest, that is, its genesis " (p. 51).

The γ-phenomenon is thus *from the outset* interpreted as a quite *specific gestalt effect*. And as a matter of fact, it actually occurs only when a well-articulated gestalt is experienced in the end state. This is sufficient guarantee, for Lindemann, that genuine gestalt processes underlie the γ-phenomenon. He believes this to be more impressively substantiated, when he discovers that the more detailed findings as to the direction and course of the movement, permit of being traced back to those very, specific laws of gestalt dynamics which we have hitherto encountered.

This holds, to begin with, in regard to the most general gestalt-dynamic uniformity. Here, too, according to Lindemann, we find a tendency towards precision of the gestalt ; for the movement can be quite generally characterized in such terms as "that parts of figures betook themselves to positions or tended towards positions, which corresponded not to the single stimulus belonging to them, but to the whole ' good gestalt ' ". " Thus a point in the periphery, on the chord, always sprang to the centre of the circle (see p. 42 ff.) when the stimulus situation was such that a good gestalt could not forthwith accompany it ; when a point fell out, it moved *in the direction of a good end gestalt*" (see especially p. 46 ff.). And further : " If there are small *gaps* in the objective figure, the free ends make a *most violent movement in order to close them*, especially so in the case of the circle, the ellipse, and the triangle (see p. 28)—in exact *correspondence with Fuchs' statements* about gestalt-totalization tendencies." " Figures which were borrowed from Wulff's work, showed γ-movement along the lines on which alteration had taken place in the reproductions in his investigations, and the same dependence on apprehension evinced itself " (pp. 51–2)—thus *confirming Wulff's findings*.

Thus the γ-phenomenon does indeed seem to stand in the closest relationship to the findings mentioned, and

Lindemann sees in this justification for bringing the idea of gestalt dynamics to bear here too. He takes this agreement as the starting point for his own theoretical considerations. As far as we are concerned, this correlation will certainly have little power of conviction in reference to the theoretical verdict. We will indeed concede that, in essence, one and the same psychological phenomenon is at the bottom of all these various findings of Fuchs, Lindemann, and Wulff. But in view of the result of our enquiry into the work of Fuchs and Wulff, we will assuredly not admit without more ado, that one has of necessity to resort to the Wertheimer-Koffka-Köhler gestalt theory in the interpretation.

Lindemann, to be sure, has attempted directly to prosecute this reduction of his findings ; and indeed he places them in relationship with Wertheimer's original physiological theses, as well as with Köhler's psychophysical ideas. Yet neither the one nor the other attempt at explanation is satisfactory.

The *reduction to Wertheimer's theory* which Lindemann gives, follows Koffka. He identifies the γ-process, inasmuch as it is " a dynamic expansion process " " which only leads up to the finished persistent gestalt ", directly with Wertheimer's field-process (1912). For, as he says, " this dynamic event in a whole area is the nucleus of what Wertheimer at that time designated radiation, and what he meant by field-action."

However, this identification, upon closer consideration, involves an essential discrepancy. The γ-phenomenon is characterized not merely as an " expansion process ". This process ensues in a special manner, in the form of a differentiation of the figure, specifically so that the figure appears " to be organized on the basis of a centre of gravity ". With Wertheimer, however, the field-action manifests itself in that a multitude of single excitations is there, to begin with, and then, through field excitation, these single excitations to a certain extent become welded together into a unity which we experience as figural unity. Wertheimer's field excitations could therefore only appear phenomenally represented in their successive operation by the fact that, starting from a " plus-stage ", in which what is given appears atomistically as a pure juxtaposition of sensations, a transition to a " gestalt stage " is experienced—a state of affairs which has nothing in common with what is met with in the γ-phenomenon.

Köhler's theory of gestalten seems to be in a somewhat different position. His way of thinking seems to be able to hold its own splendidly with Lindemann's empirical facts. According to Köhler, " in the theory of physical spatial gestalten . . . an element of current which commences in definite retinal elements does not proceed necessarily and always to the same, once for all fixed, point of the visual cortex " ; " where any of them issues in the critical fields, is in every case determined in accordance with the total conditions of the system " (p. 57). For : " As every interference in a stationary state (in a physical system) leads to a ' *precipitate process of displacement* ' which can only then issue in a new stationary condition, so also the sudden stimulation of our sense organs leads to a specific event which in its turn brings with it the resting end gestalt. What we have called γ-processes is nothing other than this very event " (p. 55).

And yet, though the general fact of γ-movement here appears to have been made physiologically comprehensible, one must nevertheless deplore the absence of any *concrete detailed definition*. But above all, the same difficulty with which we have so often been confronted comes to the fore again. Lindemann expressly establishes that " the movements arising always depend upon the gestalt which comes into being " ; but not directly upon the stimulus gestalt. They are, in a marked degree, " a function of the *apprehension*, when the stimulus-configuration and fixation are constant." But the gestalt processes, if they are at all to have any degree of definiteness, cannot be thought of in conjunction with this.

We must therefore conclude that Lindemann's findings, just as those of Fuchs and Wulff, bring to notice a characteristic dynamics. We must state, too, that it has reference to phenomenal gestalten ; but we cannot admit that it is explicable to the last detail by means of Wertheimer's, or alternatively Köhler's gestalt processes.

§ 59. *Stroboscopic apparent movements as gestalt-dynamical processes*

Only one set of facts in the study of perception still remains, for which an explanation through gestalt dynamics has been sought—the province of stroboscopic apparent movements, as these have been interpreted by Hartmann, and, following him, Köhler.

It is specially noteworthy how the position of the movement phenomena in the gestalt theory has, with this interpretation, altered in correspondence with the transformation in the theory itself. Whereas previously—in Wertheimer's physiological approach—the seeing of movement provided the foundation for the understanding of the seeing of gestalt, now, after Köhler has developed an autonomous gestalt physiology, the seeing of movement can conversely be deduced from the gestalt process.[1] Hartmann and Köhler accomplish this task, by attempting to represent the movement effect as a direct manifestation of the gestalt dynamic processes. They believe themselves thus to be reducing both the β-movement and the γ-movement, as well as the "fusion" investigated by Hartmann, to a unitary basis of explanation. We shall follow out, as an example, Köhler's account of the explanatory principle for the β-movement.

To begin with, Köhler defines the task of his theory as having to make comprehensible the *specific unitariness* of the state of movement which sets in phenomenally, and which—in accordance with his basic view—must be functionally-physiologically represented. Furthermore, the theory should accomplish two things. It should equally explain, firstly, the "*pure movement*" introduced by Wertheimer, i.e. a movement without "carriers", as, according to Wertheimer, it is supposed to arise under certain circumstances; and, secondly, movement with "*qualitative induction*", as is the normal result in the optimal stage, i.e. the fact that the qualities of the two phases appear effective for the mode of appearance of what is moved (e.g. the coloration).

Köhler accounts for the necessity of in his turn providing a new approach, going beyond Wertheimer's short-circuit theory, by establishing that Wertheimer's theory does not in fact prove equal to this very phenomenon of qualitative induction.

Köhler's thesis presents itself to us in an apparently

---

[1] Cf. in connection with Wertheimer's original interpretation our own appended considerations.

very simple form. The only presupposition is the " free propagation of elements of current ", as Köhler assumes it in his physiological theory. According to the gestalt theory's conceptions, " the *course of the elements of current from the retina upwards* as far as the physiological level, is in no case rigidly fixed in detail, so that the retinal point of departure determines point by point the further path or whereabouts of an ascending line of current. If it is true that the optic sector, like so many physical systems, forms its states as wholes, in reaction to the total stimulus-constellation of inner and outer conditions, then the path of a line of current is also determined according to these total conditions " (p. 398).

From this emerges the approach (p. 399) for the building up of the physiological event in the case of *successive stimulations*.

The physiological process obviously runs its course by two different stages. There is nothing of special note in regard to the first. " As soon as stimulus *a* acts, a sort of " column " of elements of current in any case ascends from the retinal surface concerned up to the higher regions of the optic sector. The peculiarity arises only when the second stimulus supervenes. Köhler says : " My hypothesis is, that under these circumstances the grouping of forces in the whole system diverts the two columns of current in a direction towards each other, even below the psychophysical level ; thus they unite, and instead of two processes *A* and *B*, only one reaches the psychophysical level. If at the beginning the first column of current is already fully formed, while the second is only in the course of formation, one could expect, from the example of similar cases in physics, that the union will be achieved essentially through the displacement of the second process ; that this process will be drawn into the path of the first one ; and that therefore the single column ensuing will reach the psychophysical field approximately at that point where the process *A* would have arrived by itself (without the action of stimulus *b*). While, however, the stimulus effect from *a* (the *A* portion of the column) is subsiding, the effect from *b* obtains the ascendancy, and the column from *b* tends towards its state of equilibrium ; therefore the process arising through the union will be shifted towards this position of equilibrium, that is, in the direction of the point which B, if stimulus a had been absent, would have reached."

One sees that a very "lively" picture of the processes underlying the occurrence of the stroboscopic total effect emerges. This at the same time achieves a deduction of something else, besides unitariness and closure of the movement, viz. the "transition". It enables us also to understand how form and colour fit in with this movement; the problem of "qualitative induction" seems solved. Similarly, it renders intelligible : 1, the genesis of partial movements (that is, when no complete fusion takes place, but displacements and movements are nevertheless to be presumed, after the same principle) ; and furthermore, 2, the occurrence of pure "movement", as Wertheimer professes to have observed it (that is, when the process ensues so "impetuously", that the chemical reactions proposed in Köhler's theory to account for the genesis of the qualitative delimitation, which are conceived as tied to the electrical excitations, do not take place so swiftly, or with adequate strength).

On the whole it seems as if Köhler, as in the case of the physiological theory of the seeing of gestalt, has given a very illuminating solution to the processes underlying the seeing of movement, and one genuinely adapted to the thinking of the gestalt theory.

This theory has an even more convincing effect, when one gathers that, going farther than Wertheimer's observations, the theory has found a *verification* for them ; and, in particular, when one hears that direct experiments for testing the theory, inspired by Köhler, have led to the substantiation of the theory. To make the assumption—quite hypothetically inserted in the theory—of the attraction of two successive columns of current more plausible, Köhler himself has drawn attention to a series of *observations already previously known*, which seem to be evidence of corresponding alterations of position in the single excitations.

In the field of touch, von Frey and Spearman have demonstrated that the localization value of a given pressure sensation is influenced by other simultaneous or even preceding' pressure sensations ; and it has emerged that fusions could even be produced, in this case, with simultaneous stimulation. Furthermore, in investigations upon tactile β-movement Benussi has observed that the "subjective distance" separating the two main points of stimulation, becomes smaller and smaller, until eventually only one single, lasting contact can be discerned, which is stationarily localized in a fixed position at a point of the intermediate field.

On the whole, however, even Köhler could not impute too great a power of conviction, for the substantiation of his theory, to these findings. Consequently he has himself initiated *a more thorough experimental investigation*, the work of Scholz (1924).

Scholz made optical, tactual, and acoustical observations upon the phenomenal size of spatial magnitudes. In his experiments, a pair of continuous stimuli was presented at a definite distance apart, while a second pair was successively presented in such a way that the four positions of stimulation objectively formed the corners of a rectangle (with homogeneous background).

The main result is that, leaving aside the pauses, the phenomena are above all dependent upon the "*objective distance of the limiting points*".

Just according as this *distance* is chosen, the following phenomena appear :—

(a) When the distance is relatively great, *diminution* of the seen distance occurs—maximally so, with the movement optimum.[1]

(b) Conversely, with very small distances, an *augmentation of magnitudes* shows itself. (Again, as with (a), in all sensory spheres.)

As regards the *effect of the pause*, that is the speed of succession, no influence appears in the case of large temporal intervals. With increasing speed, however, the successively delimited magnitude, *to begin with*, becomes *smaller and smaller* until a maximal reduction is reached ; *but then* from a certain limiting value of the speed of succession—the same value at which optimal movement sets in—a *gradual enlargement* of the successive magnitude arises, until at last only a small reduction remains over at the simultaneous stage.

---

[1] When the distances are diminished a further subjective reduction of the distance appears in the acoustic and tactile experiments, going so far as fusion into a stationary impression. (In the optical experiments this stage is, by contrast, lacking.)

As regards the *rôle of the single points* in the displacement, it appears that in the optical sphere the light presented second is invariably displaced in a relatively more marked degree. With sound, however, intensity appears to have the critical influence. The tone of greater intensity shows the relatively more moderate displacement ; with equal intensities, both points are equally markedly displaced. On the tactual side, the circumstances are too labile and too uncertain subjectively, to allow anything definite to be said about particular localizations.

The *theoretical evaluation* given by Scholz for these results moves wholly in the tracks prescribed by Köhler. The " minimum inference " that emerges, according to him (p. 269), is " that two excitations appearing after each other and in proximity, at an appropriate interval of time, enter into the strongest functional relationship or culminate in this ". Like Hartmann and Köhler, Scholz perceives this relationship in the " impulsion of the excitations towards one another ", in such a way " that the dynamic total situation in the optic sector impels the second excitation which arises towards the first, even before the ' psychophysical ' level is reached, and in the optimal case causes the fusion of the two, so that only one column of current supervenes in the psychophysical field ; but this is in movement towards the ' normal locality ' of the second excitation, consonantly with the subsidence of the first and the predominance of the second stimulus effect " (p. 270).

Then the observed *reduction* of the path of the movement follows immediately " because of the impulsion of the excitations towards each other, and also because the second stimulus effect in general subsides so rapidly as not quite to reach its ' normal locality ' ".

Equally good agreement between theory and fact seems to exist in reference to the *magnitude of the displacement* of the two limiting points.[1] The *first point* is not so strongly displaced as the one appearing *secondly*. For, as Köhler says, " it is to be expected, from the analogy of other occurrences, that the union of the two processes is attained

---

[1] When Scholz here speaks of " stimuli " which are " displaced " (cf. p. 271), this is a confusion of thought, both psychologically and physiologically. Psychologically speaking, surely it is the *impressions* which undergo displacement; but in terms of gestalt physiology, one would have to talk of the displacements of single " gestalt processes ", " columns of current ", etc.

essentially through the shifting of the second. The latter is drawn into (!) the path of the former, and the single ensuing column reaches the psychophysical level approximately at the place where process A (without the effect of B) would also have arrived by itself."

As regards the *augmentation of magnitudes with small distances*, the result is, it is true, not from the outset accounted for in the theory ; but here, too, Scholz at any rate, is able to manage very readily (p. 271) : " If the reduction of the end of the path of movement rests upon the fact that the B-process fails to reach its position of equilibrium, it is from the outset conceivable that the reduction *must* (!) relapse when the positions of equilibrium of a and b lie very near to each other, and b therefore has a shorter route." Furthermore, " it is even possible that the B-process *in consequence of the already present dynamics* (!) shoots out beyond its position of equilibrium."

Accordingly, this phenomenon appears to fit in completely with Köhler's theses, and to verify them.

However, the question may not be disposed of as easily as this. The peculiarity of the situation in which we find ourselves here once more becomes clear, as soon as we measure it up against the general requirements of scientific theory. So judged, can it be admitted that a genuine verification is to be found in Scholz's experiments ? And what is the significance which can at all be justifiably attached to Köhler's way of regarding this " dynamics " of elements of current ? The two questions receive an answer in closest interdependence.

Commencing from Scholz's observations, we can, to begin with, establish that in those very facts in which Scholz's investigation takes us farther than what was known to Köhler, all sorts of difficulties are nevertheless concealed. This is so, even assuming that we in the first instance take our stand upon the Scholz-Köhler point of view. More than anything else, the augmentation of the magnitudes with short distances of the points produces difficulties. Let us grant that one can rest satisfied with the explanation of the " shooting out " of the second stimulus. Let us, that is to say, for argument's sake make the concession, that one can have something definite in mind when one traces this result to the " already present dynamics " ; then it is at any rate still impossible, up to the present, to deduce from the hypothesis how an augmentation at the *beginning* of the path of movement can come about.[1]

Similarly, it must be admitted that the *characteristic form of the optical curve of diminution*, the graphic picture of the dependence of the reductions upon the various objectively presented distance values, is *by no means comprehensible without further question*. If the theory were able to deal with the question perfectly, the occurrence of a sharp and high maximum of reduction at a quite definite distance value, would have to follow from it. Such an explanation, however, can undoubtedly not be achieved by the theory. It is quite impossible to comprehend why the " dynamics already present ", because of the " overshooting "—by this remarkable word is obviously meant what the physicist designates by " kinetic energy "—why this dynamics does not become noticeable in far greater measure when the space traversed is larger, and the quantity of energy involved stronger. If an " overshooting " of *B* with small distances must indeed be thus explained, then the effect here conjectured should not simply be forgotten, when the cases with bigger distances are considered, even though one runs the risk of perceiving for oneself that an explanation is not possible in this way. The theory here proves to be unequal to the facts.[2]

But the reasons for this inadequacy lie deeper down. They lead us once again from the empirical, and more towards the side of principles.

It is when we attempt to explore more exactly what the absence of any standpoint whatsoever for deriving a

---

[1] The experiments are concerned not with a persisting " forward-backward " movement, but with the transition $A \rightarrow B$.

[2] The similar inadequacy of Köhler's theory seems to be displayed especially well in the acoustic and tactual fields. Scholz himself here rejects the theoretical attempts at interpretation, with the characteristic justification : " The results . . . of the experiments appear on the whole as yet too lacking in perspicuity for any theoretical interpretation to come into question." If one should wish to approach these observations while retaining the schemata of Köhler's theory, this would indeed be difficult, for the experiments here show conditions essentially more complicated. If the optical curve of diminution was fundamentally indeducible, this most decidedly holds for the complicated conditions of dependence found here. One would hardly manage with the simple " dynamics " of the psychophysical processes, as such.

"curve of diminution" from the theory is due to, that we rapidly discover the crucial point. It lies in the way in which the second principle, that of "overshooting", is introduced, in the way in which it is related to the original explanatory principle. This introduction obviously takes place *ad hoc*. Furthermore, no relationship between the two principles can be at all tangibly indicated ; no material ground can be furnished "from the starting point of physics" which would determine, in a concrete case, whether the "overshooting" occurs or not. The only possibility of arriving at some connection of the second principle with the first, obviously lies through the expression "the already present dynamics" ; but this, certainly, would in no way provide a line of attack upon our problem of the curve of diminution.

When we pass from empirical matters to an appraisement of principles, it appears that the decisive viewpoint which becomes critical there, has already been distinguished by us. For what applies to the principle of "overshooting", applies fundamentally also to the principle of the "impulsion of the lines of current towards one another".

Whence does Köhler obtain his knowledge of this sort of reciprocal action of the elements of current ? What, actually, is being stated when such terms as "dynamic coherence", "impulsion", and the like are used? Scholz, significantly enough, says that "*only conjectures* are as yet to hand, as to the nature of the assumed ' impulsion ' ". We believe that in point of fact *nothing, absolutely nothing is directly* known about this "nature". And yet the position taken up by Scholz altogether suffices to justify even the very sharpest criticism against Köhler ; for it is evident from it, that Köhler's explanatory principles are themselves the most obscure factors in the whole theory. Köhler's whole train of thought suffers through the fact that here an attempt is made to explain "the known by the unknown".

Actually, of course, Köhler's pronouncements, as well as those of Hartmann, certainly comprise nothing other than a construction prepared purely *ad hoc* ; and it becomes competent to interpret what has to be explained, simply because the facts of the matter which are at issue are already taken as a basis for the premisses.

Thus it is not to be marvelled at that Scholz's experiments led to facts which had of a certainty not been expected by the theory; Köhler's "explanatory procedure" can of course directly reach only as far as the facts taken into account hold. However, the remedy which presents itself for the difficulties arising with Scholz out of the fact of "augmentation", again shows plainly how one can very readily manage to find a way out, in the framework of such a vague construction, by simply knowing how to adopt *ad hoc* analogous "supplements" corresponding to the altered empirical findings—taking it for granted, to be sure, that one does indeed venture to operate with constructions of this sort.

One has to conclude that in such somewhat adventurous constructions, the realm of science is, in the last resort, being deserted—in spite of the seemingly erudite, but as to import certainly unintelligible, terms in which Köhler's theory makes its appearance.

We cannot say that the notion of a dynamics of gestalten has gained anything through all these discoveries. The word "dynamics" appears, as a result of all the hitherto considered observations and disquisitions, to be only still more nebulous and indefinite. Its meaning is limited to a few general formulas such as the "tendency towards a good gestalt", and the like, as well as to unusual physiological inferences. A real clarification of the concept is still to be sought.

CHAPTER II

GESTALT DYNAMICS AS THE EXPLANATION OF THE HIGHER PSYCHICAL PROCESSES

The idea of the dynamics of gestalten finds a quite special field of application, in addition to that of the facts of the study of perception discussed above, in the "higher psychical processes". Whereas in the "old psychology" these were treated as contrasting with perceptual processes, that is, as truly "higher" processes, the gestalt theory endeavours to deduce them from the same basic conceptions as those from which the perceptual processes are deduced.

The peculiarity of these processes manifests itself only in the fact that the processes which are in general here concerned are of a dynamic sort. We shall follow up more closely how this conception has been elaborated, pre-eminently by Koffka, in the domain of intellectual and volitional happenings.

I. THE THEORY OF INTELLECTUAL LIFE

§ 60. *Thought psychology—the theory of "thought gestalten"*

The special attitude which gestalt psychology has towards the psychology of thought is characteristic of its line of approach towards all higher psychical events.

The general orientation is, to begin with, very straightforward. The special psychical units which are to be elucidated in thought psychology, are simply described as " thought gestalten " (Koffka, 1925, p. 573 ff.). They are, it is true, to begin with only designated thought gestalten " in order to distinguish them from straightforward perceptual gestalten ". The emphasis here explicitly lies upon " distinguish ", so as to indicate that " this distinction . . . is by no means of a fundamental nature ", that " intrinsically . . . perceptual and thought gestalten are most closely related, that in principle identity obtains between them ".

This assumption of identity, however, comes into effect in a very clear-cut manner, when the question subsequently arises of investigating the way in which uniformities permit of being determined in the sphere of the phenomena of thought psychology. There we find the point-blank statement : " Since we are dealing with gestalten, therefore all previously deduced gestalt laws hold good "—a very simple matter. It can be seen that at bottom the problem of thought-psychology does not exist for the gestalt theory. For, by thus simply establishing that gestalten are at issue, all further theoretical as well as experimental questions are fundamentally precluded. The establishing of this fact at bottom settles the whole matter.

It is true that Koffka has openly to admit that a closer definition of these " thought gestalten " has by no means at all been achieved as yet. " The task of working out the basic types of the thought gestalten in the same way as for the perceptual gestalten is one which still remains before us as a psychological problem." But this obviously does not disturb him in his pronouncements, although the justification for thus making that assumption of identity without more ado, could then perhaps appear decidedly questionable. The arguments which Koffka himself brings forward for this identity could, at any rate, hardly hold their ground before criticism.

Thus, for example, he perceives a substantiation for his thesis that thought gestalten and spatial gestalten are akin " in the spatial schemata which many people utilize in thinking ". He says " the fact that thinking tasks of themselves evoke such schemata, proves that their gestalt properties conform to those of the thinking task itself ". If Koffka had, however, taken more carefully into consideration the well-known works of G. E. Müller, he would have been bound to notice that in many cases there is no sense in talking of a " conformity " here ;   moreover, if he had adopted a critical standpoint, he would have had to observe that such a " conformity ", if it existed, need by no means be reduced to " identity ". He would also hardly have avoided a closer consideration of this " conformity "—i.e. definite logical questions about it.

The very same applies to a second argument. He is of opinion that " with many gestalten it is not at all clear whether they should be designated perceptual or thought gestalten ", and from this he infers their identity. This assertion is of course only possible when one takes one's stand, from the outset, fundamentally upon the gestalt-theoretical " identity standpoint ". If one reviews the results of research impartially (cf. Bühler, Ach), one will have to admit that at any rate the *distinctive* forms of " perception " and of " thinking " are very clearly differentiated ;   and that it is the task of psychology to achieve, from these precise instances, and on the basis of an analysis of the facts, a definition of the characteristics of both phenomena, carried through to a point where the possibility of *in principle* differentiating the two aspects seems secure.

But the actual motive behind the characterization of thought processes as gestalten, has not yet been touched upon in what we have said.   It is the question of the meaningfulness of the course of thinking which comes decisively to the forefront here. Only this question reveals the real reason why Koffka is able to consider the gestalt conception appropriate to the facts. By means of the gestalt concept, the meaningful as something original is intended to be embodied in the basic premisses from the outset.

Indeed, this brings quite new relationships into the discussion. The psychology of thought appears simplified and susceptible of application in a singular way. From the standpoint of the gestalt theory, one cannot regard the fact that rational relations obtain between concepts, when investigated by logic, as an unprecedentedly new and fundamental problem ; but the " identity standpoint " can be still further extended. The logical relationships are relationships of the gestalt ; they are subject to gestalt laws in the same sense as the realistic thought processes are subject to gestalt laws. " We can no longer be content with the old antithesis between thought processes subject to chance, arbitrary laws of reality and the concepts subject to the rational laws of reason." On the contrary, "here, too, there exists at bottom an identity, for real life is not irrational, units of thought at the level of reality themselves arise according to laws which are rational in their own right " (p. 574).

Koffka is particularly proud of this conclusion. He is of opinion that here, for the first time, a way has been shown by which one can fully comprehend the fact of meaningfulness from the starting point of " explanatory psychology " ; and he believes that he has thus achieved a concordat between " interpretative psychology " and " explanatory psychology ".

It remains a question nevertheless, as to whether one can do justice to the problem of the rationality of our thinking through establishing that it is no problem at all, that it has to be resolved into final and self-evident facts of the structure of our mental life. When we base ourselves on this interpretation, it signifies nothing less than that we at bottom altogether eliminate from consideration the problem of meaning, of rational relatedness. The concatenation which we designate rational is then simply accepted as something given and not further to be understood. In everything we experience it is then simply a matter of a direct copy derived from the physical-physiological side.

However, if we consider what is primarily meant by the concept of gestalt in the original construction of the theory, the question arises whether one can really, from the starting point of those theses, regard as substantiated this notion that meaning is directly explained. If we commence from the physiological theory, in the way in which Köhler attempts to build up gestalt coherences " from the starting point of physics ", we shall have to declare that from this basis a way to what one signifies by the words rational coherence cannot be found.

Such a transition is equally impossible from the starting point of Koffka's and Wertheimer's descriptive-functional gestalt concept, the criterion of which, the principle that " the whole is more than the parts ", *in the first place merely establishes a formal relationship* of an ontological or alternatively, logical nature between the whole and the parts. Even if this criterion is re-discovered in what we call a rational coherence, this by no means in any way provides the possibility of thus completely exhausting what we entitle a rational coherence. *In the problem of rational coherence* we are, in fact, concerned not with formal questions, but essentially with *questions of content.*

To believe, therefore, that the problem of meaning has at one stroke been solved with the aid of the gestalt principle, constitutes nothing but an outright evasion. And this evasion only becomes possible through the fact that in our present-day thinking a great deal more is actually associated with the word gestalt, in an unformulated way, than was to begin with covered by it within the framework of the gestalt theory. A plain equivocation has wrongly led to this interpretation.

Accordingly, Jaensch justly insists (1923) that in point of fact the gestalt concept of the gestalt theory here proves to be thoroughly inhomogeneous, and that its import must be sought along two quite different lines. " Physics is supposed to legitimate the gestalt scientifically," while its " luminous lustre emanates from a quite different sphere of life " (Jaensch, p. 166).

Hence we are bound to maintain that the problem of rationality, of mental coherence, can by no means pass for solved, simply through being classified under the caption

" gestalt ". Jaensch (1923) has reduced the antithesis which *de facto* exists here to an amusing formula by pointing out " that a gestalt can e.g. also be ugly ".

When the gestalt theory goes so far as to be particularly proud of its ostensible solution of the problem of meaning, this can only be regarded as evidence of how unclarified it is in respect to its conceptual import. This obliteration of the boundaries between logical and psychological problems should not be accredited as a special achievement of the gestalt theory. It is far more a proof of what incompletely thought out conclusions one can be misled to by the gestalt theory.

§ 61. *The dynamics of thought processes, and their laws in detail*

Koffka's psychology of thinking, to be sure, goes further than the general definitions of " thought gestalten " hitherto considered, in a quite definite direction. It attempts to comprehend more exactly the thought *processes* in their conformance to laws, and thus deals with the problem which forms the real objective of modern thought psychology. It treats this problem by simply elaborating the gestalt-theoretical principles, and seems able, without more ado, to solve all problems apparently entirely deductively, on the basis of this doctrine. The uniformity of the thought processes in detail is subject, as we have established, to the presupposition that gestalten are here involved, and that, consequently, all gestalt laws as such must be valid here. Hence in principle there is concealed behind Koffka's pronouncements the attitude that the theory of the psychology of thinking already appears to be fixed, and that no new factors have to be taken into consideration in regard to the details.

When Koffka proceeds to detailed statements about the gestalt laws involved, it must be firmly borne in mind that he is concerned merely with illustrations. In this fashion, Koffka comes to the " law of closure ". He does so for the reason that, according to his theory, this law covers the crux of the general problem posed by thought psychology. He asks, " what makes the task a task, and the question a question," and he solves this problem by introducing the concept of the " incomplete thought-picture ". He talks of " thought gestalten with gaps " and then asserts that " strong tendencies towards the closure of these gaps emanate from the gestalt ".

The simplicity of the gestalt theory's method of thinking can receive no more striking illustration than this " explanation ". " What makes the question a question ? "—" The question demands . . . and in its own right impels towards the solution."

One must confess that surely nothing material has by any means been gained by these pronouncements. *How* it happens that a particular thought has the character of a task can of course under no circumstances be regarded as elucidated thereby. To those who are of opinion that scientific progress can be made in any such way as this, we must point out, as so often already in our critique, that, on the contrary, we have obviously nothing but a vicious circle here.

This situation is not altered when we observe how Koffka continues to develop his train of thought. A more specific theorem, which Koffka forges for the actual mechanism of the process of solution, takes us further than the concept of the " incomplete thought picture " characterized by the " tendency towards closure ". This mechanism of the process of solution, in the restricted sense of the term, is determined by the law of " gestalt completion ". " Every member of a gestalt has the tendency to complete itself into a whole gestalt, in which case the sharpness of the contour and the articulation still remain quite undetermined "—entirely analogous to the state of affairs with incomplete perceptual gestalten.

What is hereby gained, we may ask, and what does this prove in regard to the gestalt theory ? In reference to the second question, we need only point out that this law of gestalt completion is in fact entirely identical with the law of complex-completion propounded by Selz. Hence the import of this proposition can by no means be so intimately bound up with the gestalt theory, as to enable one to infer from its applicability anything about the validity of the gestalt theory—for this it is all too indefinite. Next we may, in connection with the question as to what is hereby gained, recall what we found it necessary to say in particular about Fuchs' disquisitions upon the mechanism of gestalt completion. We cannot, then, be satisfied with this simple scheme.

However, gestalt completion as the basic law of the psychology of thinking enables Koffka to bring out forcefully in an apparently precise manner, that the gestalt category (naturally in the sense of the gestalt theory) must in fact be applied to the processes of thought. " It should not simply be said that every ideational element has this tendency ; for the point is that the phenomenon from which the completion commences already in itself carries the character which it had as a member of the gestalt. It is from the first erroneous to ask, what reproduction will the idea (the word) *Holz* [*wood*] evoke ? For *Holz* is only unique as a sound ; phenomenally it can be different in innumerable ways, and the gestalt completion will become effective accordingly—either in the direction of *Phantasus* and the other works of the poet, or of *Johannes Schlaf*, or of the hearth fire, and so on. It is not, however, as if wood or heating material could reproduce the idea of *Johannes Schlaf*, however close at hand this idea may have been on account of other forces. If one wishes to influence a train of thought unequivocally, it is in the first place necessary unequivocally to fix a phenomenon as a member of a definite unit— certainly not to devise summatively a number of aids to reproduction."[1]

Does this in fact include a special moment that points cogently towards the gestalt theory ? To clarify this question, it is necessary to hark back to our foregoing discussion dealing with the problem of meaningful coherence ; for in the facts of the matter there at issue, the real question is just how it happens that the import of an " element " is defined only within the rational coherence as a whole.

We have had to conclude that it is only a quite superficial link which allows the fact of rational coherence to be confounded with the gestalt theory at all ; but we shall now have even more definite statements to make. One would hardly recognize the mere classification under the gestalt category as an adequate " explanation " of *how* the process takes its course at any particular time. A more intensive

---

[1] *Holz*, the German for wood, is also the name of a well-known German poet-critic (Arno Holz), who at one time collaborated with J. Schlaf. [Translator's note.]

analysis is required.   The problem of determination, of
the orderly process, should not simply be passed over in
silence.

If we now proceed to take account of the form in which
Koffka believes himself to be able to solve the problems, we
shall have to reach an even more conclusive position.   It is
significant that Koffka believes it possible to solve problems
with which experimental research has been preoccupied
for the past two decades, by simply introducing some few
theoretical categories.   In so far as the catchwords gestalt,
gestalt completion, gestalt conformance to laws, create
the illusion of a solution where in fact unsolved problems
are still involved, we must regard the introduction of these
categories as outrightly detrimental.   The transition
to gestalt dogmatism of this sort spells the end of
psychological research.

§ 62. *The position of productive thinking in the gestalt
theory*

In the hitherto considered theory of thought processes
the gestalt theory has presented itself as essentially
dogmatic ; but it seems as if an essentially more empirically
directed mode of treatment is to be found in the domain
where " productive thinking " is discussed.   Koffka's
deliverances upon this side of the matter take their
departure from Köhler's experiments with chimpanzees
and Wertheimer's accounts of the psychological processes
involved in simple inference.   The question is whether,
through this concrete way of dealing with them, the results
of this discussion are better founded.

In the first place we must once more, however briefly,
refer to Köhler's anthropoid experiments, which figure,
with Koffka, as precise examples of how " a new thought
gestalt is grasped ".   Koffka considers essentially Köhler's
" stick experiment " where the apes are required to
achieve the use of tools.   " A dry tree stands in a cage
before which, at a distance greater than arm's length, lies
some fruit.   We let a chimpanzee into the cage.   What
will he do ?   Well, as soon as he notices the fruit he will
run to the bars and reach out for it.   In vain.   What will
take place now ?   Animals accustomed to rake in fruit
by means of a stick will now run hither and thither,
seeking a stick ; this too is in vain.   What now ?   One

animal will give up the business, will perhaps sit down at the foot of the tree and gaze longingly at the fruit. Another, on the other hand, will suddenly rush to the tree, break off a branch, and draw the fruit in with it " (p. 578).

Koffka's interpretation of this finding is typical for all the facts of the matter. He says : " The achievement consists . . . in the fact that the ' branch ' becomes a ' stick ', that a thing which is a member of a very firm gestalt (the tree), separates out from it to leap into another gestalt (the bridge to the fruit). Here we have a typical new achievement." And furthermore : " An open gestalt, the route to the fruit, acquires its closure from another, closed gestalt, and this happens because a member of that gestalt undergoes a process of transformation. The main achievement here is the transformation process. If it has succeeded, everything else takes its course on the basis of the already existing gestalt (use of stick) of its own accord . . . . " The " new thought gestalt " is " grasped ".

What is attained by means of such an interpretation ? To us it appears to signify merely a purely formal description of the transformations which the units undergo in con- nection with the solution, in regard to their meaning- content within the whole concatenation. And indeed it is really *nothing more than a merely superficial, formal re-description* on the basis of contrasting the " meaningful structure " before and after the solution. This re-descrip- tion is, to be sure, so presented as if it could somehow have a direct and positive " explanatory value ", for the reason that the " process of closure " is referred to, and this is obviously in some way conceived as a dynamic process. But it is clear that the " how " of the thought process cannot thus be accounted for ; we cannot admit that anything is contributed by this.

As a matter of fact the crux of these contentions of Koffka lies elsewhere. He himself emphasizes that this closure ensues through the fact that " a member of the gestalt undergoes a *transformation process* ". This having been established, all is once more unfortunately done with, but in itself this does not really tell us very much. The questions actually at issue are surely very *definite* ones. *How* does this transformation process come about ? How does it happen that this particular transformation process arises and not perhaps anything else ? Or to put the question more definitely, in what way is this "transformation" process related to gestalten in general ?

Koffka's pronouncements contain answers of a sort even to these questions ; but they are, taken altogether, very characteristic and unusual. As regards the last two questions, the answer is contained in the term " open gestalt ". What can be accomplished by means of this concept, we have already sketched. For what is really the main question, *how* the arousal of the transformation process should at all be conceived, *how* it happens that this process at one time ensues and at another does not, a new answer is provided. In the one case or else in the other " the conditions of the system of the animal must themselves have been different " ! (p. 578). There can be no doubt that at bottom the explanation is of course hereby shelved. What does " the conditions of the system of the animal " mean ? Indeed the real task is to analyze these. But the analysis of these is completely precluded, in the gestalt theory. For to the gestalt theory they are either the " relatively variable conditioning factors in the nervous system . . .", as such never concretely definable, and/or they consist in the " readiness to carry out a certain structural process " in the presence of *those very* " gestalt dispositions " which correspond to the result, which must therefore from time to time be introduced *ad hoc*. They have thus no concrete explanatory value whatever, being invoked only to " plaster over " a gap in the gestalt-theoretical system, to retain Koffka's terminology (cf. p. 576). This vague reduction to the " transformation process " cannot therefore lead to a satisfactory theory of creative thought.

Perhaps an elucidation of productive thinking along the lines of the gestalt theory can be expected in a more precise form from Wertheimer, in his work of 1920, which actually concerns itself with enquiring into this productive thinking, in an analysis of the syllogism *in barbara* (SaM, MaP, SaP).

If we set aside all the accessories in the shape of examples, etc., Wertheimer's results permit of being summarized in a brief line of reasoning.

It is not " the mere simultaneous grasping of the two premisses that gives the conclusion ", as yet ; there is added to this "a remarkable snapping together", "a pitching into one another".

Wertheimer provides a schema for this "pitching".

"In S?P the object given as Sm_1 is taken as known; there is no direct way from Sm_1 to P . . . —I cannot answer the question of ?P;

But : the object proves to be "uncentralizable" in Sm_2 and from Sm_2 aP is established or better establishable" (p. 17).

And, furthermore, it is here a question of quite " definite formal moments "—exactly as with Ro.

" The decisive moment in many cases often occurs by way of an (appropriate) *extraction*—definite features in S are discriminated and shifted to the foreground. In other cases the decisive moment ensues in a peculiar *synthesizing* of elements. In still other cases we may with accuracy speak of *centralization*—where it depends upon the part from which the others seem organized. . . . And the centralization leads to penetration into the nature of the facts, to *a grasping of a definite, inner, structural coherence* of the whole, to the grasping of inner necessities" (pp. 18–19).

In this fact that characteristic *formal* moments seem determinative, lie the special features of Wertheimer's interpretation. From this as starting point, Wertheimer draws a contrast between his interpretation and the prevailing viewpoint, inasmuch as " hitherto such achievements have been essentially attributed to ' fantasy ', ' chance ', ' inspired intuition ' " (p. 18). This starting point, too, shows up the relationship with the gestalt problem. In all these cases, according to Wertheimer, it is a matter of " structure operations of the greatest significance " (p. 18).

But is this connection with the problem of gestalt or structure also a direct connection with the gestalt theory ? Even if the gestalt or structure category fits the processes and phenomena coming into question here very well, it cannot be conceded that the gestalt concept, upon which the gestalt theory must base itself with exactitude, should here be interpolated ; and that, therefore, a touchstone is here provided for the validity of the gestalt theory's contentions.

Wertheimer, at any rate, contents himself with the purely immanent analysis of the examples given by him and says no more than what has been quoted above, as to theory. He obviously perceives a connection with his gestalt theory in the very fact that the word " gestalt ", or " structure " is susceptible of application here ; but he does not attempt to link it up with the concepts propounded in the gestalt theory ; indeed it was impossible for him to attempt this, seeing that the decisive development had at that time not yet taken place at all.

When we for our part put this connection to the test, as to how it fares in the light of the present position of the gestalt theory, we find we are not able to admit that these formulations really fall within the scope of the gestalt-theoretical doctrines. At any rate, neither from the starting point of gestalt physiology, nor on the basis of the laws of gestalt dynamics, is it possible to furnish an approach to these phenomena.

One could, of course, imagine that perhaps a possibility of linking up theoretically exists, by starting from the latter, inasmuch as the gestalt laws, as elsewhere to be found, do not raise a claim to perfection and finality ; and inasmuch as here new examples of gestalt uniformities are discovered.

But one cannot fail to recognize that the situation is then exactly the same here as with our testing of the gestalt laws erected by Wertheimer in 1923 (see above; p. 147 ff.). Here, too, one has to ask how, under what conditions, such and such formal determinateness of structure arises ; what circumstances are responsible for the results' shaping themselves in such a way or in this particular direction. Wertheimer's formal results do not even scratch the surface of the problem. If, for instance, the way in which Selz presents his analyses in the sphere of thought psychology is compared with these results, one will be bound to say that the gestalt theory surely disposes of the real problems exceedingly rapidly.

If Wertheimer, directly in virtue of the fact that " structure operations " do appear to be met with here, should consider these problems solved simply by incorporating them into the scheme of the gestalt theory, this would involve a lack of clearness in the import of the gestalt theoretical doctrines—the same lack of clearness which we were able to reveal above, apropos of the general question as to the problem of meaning—however serviceable in other respects Wertheimer's observations might be in detail.

2. THE PSYCHOLOGY OF REACTIVE BEHAVIOUR

The gestalt-theoretical psychology of reactive behaviour represents, in a specific manner, the elaborations of the idea of a dynamics of gestalten. If we explore in detail, following Koffka (1925), the approaches made to this—one can certainly only speak of approaches in this connection—the necessity emerges of concentrating the discussion upon a number of main problems.

These problems are defined chiefly by the way in which the attempt is made to present the contrast between the gestalt theory and the " old psychology " in this province of psychology. The characteristic conclusion is already ordained in a general orientation which establishes the relation of the perceptual side to the volitional one.

" We have hitherto almost all the time spoken as if the organism consisted merely of a sensorium, sense organs, and a brain. If this were the case it would be irretrievably exposed to the onslaughts of nature. But the organism also has limbs and muscles which are governed by the central organ, and which constantly effect changes of the individual in relation to his environment. I can run away or attack. What I do depends upon what takes place in my phenomenal world " (p. 583).

" Action depends upon perception and thought, but also, conversely, perception depends upon action ; for through my actions I alter my perceptions. Here there is the closest mutual interaction. It is an artificial dismembering to separate these domains from one another. In reality they belong together, not like two beams one has bound together with a string ; but like arms and legs, i.e. they all belong to the great whole " (p. 583). And further, they have as a whole, in their interrelatedness, quite specific gestalt character, that is to say in the way they cohere."

How the interpretation of the relationship along these lines is arrived at becomes most thoroughly intelligible by returning to Köhler's physiological theory. This permits that harmonization of action with perception which Koffka desires, to be developed from the hypothesis in a characteristic manner. For if we think Köhler's hypothesis

T

through to the end, the following state of affairs is, in my opinion, disclosed : A physiological gestalt excitation, activated by the objective stimulus situation, extending as a unitary physical system from the retina through the entire " optic sector " as far as the visual cortex, need not be taken to cease in this area. On the contrary, the extension of this gestalt excitation can proceed farther, right into the " motor sector ", where it issues directly in action, in such a way that one ought to interpret the whole excitation process as a single physiological gestalt, cohering in itself, and extending as a unitary structure-event, governed in itself by gestalt laws, through the optical-motor total sector (not that there is actually any sense in separating the optical from the motor sector).[1]

Herewith, of course, the " unity " of perception and action is postulated in the most radical manner—in a manner which at the same time makes it plainly discernible, that in the gestalt theory's way of thinking what is phenomenally experienced in the course of a volitional process is intrinsically insignificant and must be looked upon as a pure epi-phenomenon.

In the analysis of real action such a schema naturally yields nothing concrete. It will, as happens exclusively with Koffka, have to commence at a point closer to the concrete instance. Always, however, this conjunction of perception and action, as we have just laid it bare in respect to its deeper roots, remains of the most central significance, even when it does not become directly conspicuous in this precise manner. It acquires function here, inasmuch as it covers a special factor of the relationship between stimulus and reaction, which, in the opinion of gestalt theoreticians, was not embraced by the " old " theory—the fact of meaningfulness in this relationship. And the very fact that this configurational nexus appears fully to cover such meaningfulness, impels Koffka to ascribe palpable superiority to his gestalt-theoretical interpretation as against the " old " interpretation.

In the " aggregative " interpretation of all the " old psychology ", he contends, as compared with the foregoing citation, the conjunction " as if by means of a string " plays an exclusive rôle. He emphasizes that " at any

---

[1] Cf. specific examples in the succeeding paragraphs.

rate this assumption was throughout generally made for the reflexes, and, in the strictly mechanistic theory, eventually for all, even for the highest, activities ". Whereas on this view " the coherence must everywhere rank as extrinsic, lacking meaning, determined by innate paths or paths acquired as a result of repetitions ", for Koffka the great achievement of the gestalt theory in the field of volitional problems appears to be that no difficulties exist for it in regard to the meaningfulness of the co-ordination of stimulus and reaction. He sees in this a quite special result, a decisive advance in psychological theory in general. For he is of opinion that the scientific situation has in this way been basically altered in psychology, inasmuch as he believes the cleavage between an " interpretative psychology " attempting to do justice to these rational relations, and an " explanatory psychology " which cannot in its own right accomplish a transition to the phenomena of meaning, to have been fully overcome by him. He has recourse to the assertion that the facts of meaningfulness offer no special problem whatever to the gestalt theory, but that, in its view, it is a universal characteristic of gestalten in general which is here met with.

There can be no doubt that by thus assigning to the special question at issue a place within the general framework of gestalt considerations, the total problem, as well as all questions of detail, is basically re-orientated. As for the way in which the stimulus-perception gestalt and the reaction here hang together as a process, this must again emerge from the theorems of gestalt dynamics—following the same schema as in the psychology of thinking : " Gestalt with gaps → closure process ".

We must investigate in more detail how this schema is utilized in the concrete interpretations of particular basic forms of the reactive life. Only then will the singularity of the whole account, its inner sterility, become evident.

§ 63. *The reflex mechanism and its substitution by something better, in the gestalt theory*

With reference to the reflex complex, Koffka's theory presents a very sharply-focussed standpoint. We shall content ourselves with indicating, by means of an example, the extraordinary results to which his line of approach leads. Of course, the reflex concept is to be entirely expelled from psychology ; let us therefore see how it is replaced.

Koffka develops his conceptions in connection with the observation that children very early *turn their heads towards a source of sound*, and this with a certainty that is reflex in nature.[1] Since the reaction appears with children of only $1\frac{1}{2}$ years of age, he believes he may exclude the possibility that the child perhaps at first hears the sound, and then voluntarily turns his head to it. In his view, the sound must be counted as " itself the cause of the move-ment " ; the movement is taken to be directly brought about by a definite " property of the stimulus ". And furthermore, the very same property of the stimulus is held to bring about the turning of the head, as is responsible for the impression of direction. This we know exactly enough from the discovery of v. Hornbostel and Wertheimer, as far as localization to the right and to the left of the median plane are concerned. If a sound impinges from the side, it reaches one ear earlier than the other, and this temporal difference is the stimulus for the acoustic impression of direction. This can be most simply proved by sending the sound through a forked conductor, the two branches of which can be altered in length, and lead to the right and left ear respectively. As soon as one conductor is shortened relatively to the other, the sound migrates to the corresponding side. A sound coming directly from in front (or from behind) strikes both ears simultaneously. Thus when I turn my head towards the sound in the direc-tion of its source, I change the stimulus in such a way that the ears, which before my turning were stimulated at different times—it is a matter of extremely small temporal differences, measurable in hundred-thousandths of a second—thereafter receive the sound simultaneously. The excitation process which runs its course in the cerebral area stimulated from both ears, is therefore undoubtedly simpler after the turning of the head than before ; for now the single excitations to the right and to the left, upon which

---

[1] The following interpretation is an example of the fact that the physiological orientation has indeed a veridical meaning in the gestalt theory of volitional processes (see above, p. 278, note).

the total excitation depends, are in perfect congruence, whereas previously they were temporally displaced in relation to each other. The head-movement in the direction of the sound (and similarly when in a direction away from it, as in escaping from a barely audible enemy) thus alters the stimulus conditions in such a way that the sensory processes become maximally simplified. When we consider the event as a whole, the sensory part and the motor part as a unity, we discover once again that tendency towards simplicity which we have previously made acquaintance with as a gestalt law (pp. 583–4).

Here we see what significance is attached to the tendency towards precision, and in what sense the sensori-motor happening is subordinated to this principle. Obviously Koffka has the idea that, as it were, in the direct physiological happening in the acoustic sector and in the sector of " bodily posture " (to designate briefly what we are here concerned with), that in the sensori-motor happening of these two sectors, a coupling of such a kind exists as to make it necessary for us to look upon the whole as *a single* gestalt happening, cohering in itself, and so organized. And he proceeds to advocate the view that the successive stages of this happening could be comprehended and explained by means of this very tendency towards precision.

Analyzing more closely what Koffka offers in this example, one is bound to conclude that even the establishment of the sensori-motor conditions important for the perceptual side of the event along the lines of the Wertheimer-von Hornbostel temporal theory of acoustic localization, can in nowise be accepted. According to the recent investigations of Klemm, and especially of Wittmann, we must regard as proven, that the temporal difference of the two partial impressions of the right and the left ear respectively does indeed play a rôle in the localization ; but that it by no means constitutes the decisive factor. An equally large rôle is quite indubitably played by the effects of the differences of intensity which subsist between the two impressions of the two sounds. It has been proved that both effects can cancel each other ; that under certain circumstances the intensity difference can equally well be the determinative one, since it dominates the time difference.

What is the significance of this conclusion in reference to the further possibility of applying Koffka's explanation of the " reflex-like " turning of the head in the direction of the source of the sound ?

To begin with, it seems as if even with this modification in respect to the perceptual side of the example, the explanation of the " mechanism " of turning the head by means of the " tendency towards simplicity ", can be applied without alteration. For one can obviously say that the physiological event existing within the " zone of functioning of the binaural-acoustic sector ", even under these conditions still attains its optimal distribution when the axis of the two ears stands at right angles to the direction of the sound ; since this " symmetrical " gestalt, which one must, with Koffka's way of thinking, assume here in regard to the intensity, can have the same advantage ascribed to it, as compared with an unsymmetrical one, which, according to Koffka, the simultaneous arrival of the sound has over its arrival with temporal differences.

However, the case here is nevertheless essentially different, inasmuch as one may not leave those complications altogether out of consideration, which arise as soon as a mutually antagonistic action of the two components— time difference and intensity difference—is taken into account. According to experiment, median localization can occur in spite of existing intensity differences and in spite of existing time differences with binaural sounds, as these permit of being produced in the laboratory— that is, experiences in which the position of the head and the experienced direction of the sound are supposed to be already adjusted in conformity with the principle of precision. There can be no doubt, of course, that in this case neither the process corresponding to the intensity factors, nor the one corresponding to the time factors has the requisite properties.

Naturally, the gestalt theoreticians are still able to abolish the difficulties thus raised, with one word. One has merely to say that here in point of fact the two factors do of course not act separately, but are significant in accordance with their total effect ; that, therefore, a single, total gestalt is present here, which, through the mutual cancellation of the two factors, represents a low degree of simplicity in comparison with what is appropriate to it, but, as a whole, represents the best state possible.

This itself, however, reveals what can be fundamentally urged against the gestalt-theoretical view of the reflexes. The fact emerges that the conscientiousness of the theory in regard to determinability is very low. For, naturally, if one maintained this principle of simplicity, one could justly preserve this same schematic, and in itself vague explanation, time and again, even in the face of all further complexities which empirical research may still possibly bring forward.

If we subject Koffka's contentions to the principle which played so large a rôle at the commencement of the gestalt theoretical movement, the principle of "fundamental determinability", we shall appraise these "standards" correctly. By such means one can in the long run "explain" everything. But it cannot be concealed that in truth nothing has thus been explained.

§ 64. *The founding of the doctrine of reactions upon the "dynamic characters" of perceptual data*

We have, with Koffka's analysis of the reflex phenomenon, already drawn attention to essential features of the gestalt theory's explanatory equipment for reactive behaviour in general. The remaining reaction phenomena, such as instinctive activities and volitional processes, rest upon the same ground in a substantial measure. They take on a special implication, however, through the fact that here the meaningfulness of the coherence between perceptual situation and reaction behaviour is elucidated in a more definite way.

The contrast in question between these and the hitherto considered simple reactions, can be most readily displayed in the manner Koffka treats the *instinctive activities.*

Koffka emphasizes, firstly, as fundamental : "The instinctive activities are *active.* The bird fetches the material for its nest ; the male woos the female ; the beast of prey lies in wait for its catch, and so forth ; and they only cease when a goal is reached. Should one not say : in instinctive activity the animal is *directed towards a goal* ? "

The " activity " here attributed to the behaviour in the

case of instinctive activities as contrasted with the reflexes, betokens a new and highly significant problem for the gestalt theory.

Koffka, secondly, here comes upon the problem of the relation between perception and reaction.   With the reflexes, the conception held was as follows : A definite part of the dynamic gestalt energy imposed upon the organism by the perceptual situation, in addition to the manifestation of this energy in the experience of the phenomenal gestalt coherence, simply " poured " itself, as it were, into the physiological sectors corresponding to the motor happening, in a direct manner.   Thus a direct transition from the perception to the motor side was here assumed, and with this was associated a configural closure of the whole process.   In the discussion of the instinct activities a new feature is added.   Now the attempt is made to conceive the bond between perception and reaction as represented by a specific aspect of what belongs to the perception ; a definite " *expression* " is ascribed to the perceptual situation.

The specifically gestalt-theoretical feature of this is, first of all, the interpretation, for which Koffka tries to invoke the support of Scheler, that " expression " is a *primary, ultimate* psychical or, in the gestalt theory, *psychophysical phenomenon*, originally bound to the perceptual situation.

How Koffka seeks to substantiate this interpretation from experimental findings, can best be discerned in his analysis of the " uncanny ", which he presents in connection with Köhler's observations on chimpanzees.   Köhler reports : " One day as I approached the stockade, I suddenly pulled over my head and face a cardboard copy of the mask of a Cingalese plague demon (certainly an appalling object), and instantly every chimpanzee except Grande had disappeared.   They rushed as if possessed into one of the cages and as I came still nearer, the courageous Grande also disappeared."   Koffka interprets this entirely after the fashion of Köhler, when he says :   " It is not the *unaccustomed* which leads to this outbreak, but the *specific object* which terrifies us, and which appeared gruesome to the Cingalese themselves, though they manufactured this mask.   There can therefore be no doubt about it ;   the expression arises phenomenally without any preceding experience, and similarly, a definite expression pertains to definite units independently of experience." "Expression" is therefore *a fact of our perceptions that is primarily determined.*

"Expression," however, according to everyday speech is nothing but the "affective content" of the object in question. Thus Koffka gives us nothing but a recasting of his last thesis when he formulates : "Among the properties of certain units of perception belong distinguishing marks, originally indeed constituting their core, which we are accustomed to call affective." The *affective* is accordingly —and this is a highly characteristic pronouncement of the gestalt theory—avowedly a *"distinguishing mark" of objects*, not in any way something that has to be understood by reference to the subject, as an expression of his vital modes of reaction. It is quite explicitly something determined with reference to the objective things as such, *a pure "gestalt moment"* of the real process of perception, in the same sense as one must, according to the gestalt theory, say this of a quality—"an object is uncanny in no other wise than it is black." The concept of affect thus appears to be completely remodelled. As regards its import, it is, in the gestalt theory, better replaced by statements about the "expression" of given gestalten.

All of this, however, comprises only preliminary remarks in reference to the theory of the instinctive activities ; remarks which are calculated to elaborate the conception of the perceptual side, in the way in which this becomes necessary for the actual consideration of the volitional problem at issue. The actual *nuclear concepts for the theory* are still wanting. They are found by Koffka in the *distinction between the initial, the transitional, and the end phenomenon* in the gestalt process inadequately called a volitional process in popular psychology. When these concepts are taken as starting point, all the obscurity previously clouding our knowledge of volitional life seems to him to be utterly dispersed.

For example, the old problem as to how one can talk of the animal's being directed towards a goal in an instinctive activity, the problem as to how this could possibly be since it is totally ignorant of the goal (see above, No. 1), causes no difficulties whatever. For the goal, in his view, need not at all in this connection be regarded as in point of fact

of such and such a kind, thus or thus defined in content.
" The theorem that the animal is directed towards a goal,
need only state : the animal is *forwardly directed*, and its
restlessness only ceases when the goal is objectively
attained."

And he proceeds to interpret this : " To be forwardly
directed therefore means to have initial and transitional
phenomena.   We need no longer add, with behaviour
that is relatively passive. For the most part this will be
more active forwardly ; it is not only the phenomena
which point ahead, but I myself intervene, act, in order
to get ahead. That is, initial and transitional phenomena
evoke action, my action is aroused by such phenomena,
whereas my activity is stopped by the end phenomenon ".

The question of the significance of the affective part,
or the expression, for volitional processes seems to him to
allow of general explanation in an entirely similar way. He
states, " Expression is an initial or a transitional or an
end phenomenon. We must therefore also *ascribe these
dynamic characters* to the most primitive phenomena, among
which we have had to reckon the expression."

When we thus regard an instinct as a whole of inner and
outer behaviour, it follows that " it starts with an initial
phenomenon, then proceeds by way of transitional
phenomena, and concludes with a final phenomenon.
To put it more specificly : the action inaugurated by the
initial phenomenon continues, with constant adaptation
to the conditions, until such time as the final phenomenon
appears ". And herewith, according to Koffka, the matter
is completely and thoroughly clarified.

The magical effect of the concepts thus propounded is
indeed astonishing. Everything seems so simple, so
entirely free from difficulties, every problem seems solved.
But alack and alas, that *this* question is not answered as
well—how does one know whether a given situation
has the initial, the transitional, or the final character ?
This question unfortunately is left wholly untouched. And
when one endeavours to answer it for oneself, by resorting
to the way Koffka could be expected to apply his
" explanations " practically, one undergoes a sad dis-
illusionment. It is amazing how it was possible for Koffka
not to perceive for himself, that in all his differentiations of
situations we have actually nothing but a pure schematism.

Every concrete definition, every detailed establishment of fact, can only be given *ad hoc subsequently*, after knowledge of the process and its results ; but not, as would correspond to a " physics " of gestalten, on the basis of the conditions. And it is still more regrettable that as little investigation is made of how a given situation comes to possess this very " dynamic character " appropriate to it in relation to the course of the activity. To be sure, Koffka has declared, as a point of principle, that his division into transitional and final phenomena is intrinsically present in the structure of the phenomenal datum, in the absence of closure (initial or transitional phenomena) or even in the closure (end phenomena) which is given out to be a gestalt factor within the sensori-motor total gestalt. Yet nothing is thus gained in regard to the concrete instance ; what is at the basis of this, what is intended by it, cannot be clearly grasped.

Another possibility, it is true, over and above the one we have been considering, exists, in the gestalt theory, for describing these dynamic characters somewhat more substantially—the possibility of characterizing them by means of *definite, very real physiological moments.* In fact an attempt is made to define the import of the dynamic characters in such a way that our former objections appear to be disposed of. This definition ensues in prosecution of the path trodden by Koffka, and before him by Köhler, in connection with the characterization of the reflex event. The reflex movements are supposed to occur in such a way that less simple psychophysical processes become maximally simplified, so that physically speaking " a disturbed equilibrium is restored again ". Transferring this point of view, it follows very simply that " *The initial character is the disturbance of equilibrium ; the final character is its restoration ; the transitional character is change in the direction of the equilibrium.*" Thus it seems as if we can now no longer justly maintain our objection that a merely schematic definition, quite empty of content, is compassed in the concept of dynamic characters. Conditions of equilibrium are of very real occurrence both in the physical and, of course, the psychophysical sphere ; and it seems as if, on this basis, the concept of the " dynamic characters " of the perceptual situation can also acquire a satisfactory meaning.

However, the unalterable truth remains that, in spite of

Köhler's efforts in connection with gestalt physics and gestalt physiology, we have no factual knowledge about the psychophysical facts at issue. And, especially, we must not fail to recognize that it will not be possible to progress so far with principles only, as to gain a knowledge of these facts which could suffice really to accomplish a material definition of the "characters" in question in this way and from this aspect.

To be able to advance considerations of equilibrium at all, in the concrete case as well as solely as a matter of principles, it is necessary to be in the position to make definite presuppositions about the energetic conditions involved. Indeed, it is necessary even to be able to employ these postulates quantitatively, since the only other alternative is quite vague and indefinite argument by analogy.

But the presuppositions which would enable those definitions of dynamic characters to be made on the basis of the gestalt conditions of the perceptual situation as such, are undoubtedly not to be anticipated. This is as much as to say that the concrete definition of content itself, as is the case elsewhere, with many explanatory concepts of the gestalt theory, must once more be derived from the phenomena in their sequence. Thus, however, it should be perfectly evident, the possibility of acknowledging these concepts to be genuinely explanatory vanishes.

The total situation in this case, then, is no different from that in the previously considered examples of gestalt dynamics, indeed from that in all the attempts whatsoever, which we have recounted, to supply evidence for the gestalt theory. The means of thinking which the gestalt theory has at its disposal for the purpose of conceptually threshing out the facts, are in nowise sufficient truly to master the facts theoretically, or indeed, even to do justice to the facts entirely in accordance with their many-sidedness. The gestalt theory cannot be accepted as a satisfactory picture of mental life.

PART THREE

TOWARDS AN APPRAISAL OF THE SCIENTIFIC APPARATUS OF THE GESTALT THEORY AS A WHOLE

In view of the results of our critical discussion, it will no longer be possible to agree that the gestalt theory is really capable of satisfying the requirements it has set itself. It fails wherever one seriously investigates whether it is proven.

In finally appraising the gestalt theory, it is not without significance to establish that this failure actually has its ground in quite definite obscurities of a sort concerned with principles ; that this failure is by no means so particularly grounded in an actual sterility of experimental and empirical work. For indeed, it can only be understood when one realizes that the gestalt theory, in its essence, is interwoven with characteristic metaphysical allegiances, and in what sense this is so. The opponents of the gestalt theory, as a rule, glibly pass these over; but they determine, in a fundamental way, all its thinking and research and steer it onto insecure territory.

That such allegiances exist, and that they do in fact come effectively into operation, even in the concrete and detailed conclusions of the theory, can be perceived without difficulty, when we once more recall, from this viewpoint, the considerations hitherto advanced by us in reference to particular psychological researches. For we need, at bottom, now only formulate, in a rounded-off synopsis, what is already to be found there, and thus develop, through a philosophical consideration, the characteristic inner relations which distinguish the structure of the theory. Even if we have, in this connection, to make an incursion into the realm of problems which are really philosophical, the discussion can nevertheless still be more than a subjective confession of faith in regard to the settlement of certain philosophical problems. For we shall readily be able to attain the goal we have in view by means of purely phenomenological reflection—

free from any actual adoption of a philosophical position, and, furthermore, independent of any limitations of bias— upon the conceptual structure of the gestalt theory in its entirety, as it stands before us both as an attitude in research and as a theoretical system.

§ 65. *The structure of the gestalt theory from the viewpoint of scientific theory*

The first question we shall put, in reflecting upon the grounds for the failure of the gestalt theory, is that of the relation of the theory to experimentation. For undoubtedly, it is just at this point that the critical circumstances must be sought for the fact that, in an empirical science like psychology, it was possible to erect and elaborate a theory which in the last resort neglects facts of this nature.

As regards the gestalt theory's position towards experimentation, the leaders of the theory have personally made utterances upon the subject in various places. The gestalt theory even comes forward with the claim that it desires to create new, and indeed healthier relations in respect to this.

Koffka, for instance, in 1919, characteristically expresses himself in this sense. As a standpoint for the appraisal of every theoretical endeavour, he places in the forefront the heuristic significance which can be attributed to it. An endeavour of this sort only has justification when it possesses heuristic value—i.e. when it leads to new problems which can be experimentally settled. " An hypothesis which is from the outset so constituted that it must either fit or allow of being adapted, no matter what new experiments teach us, is not a theory " (cf. p. 258). Now how does the gestalt theory in its contemporary state fare when measured by this standard ?

The above statement was published in 1919. Since then the visage of the gestalt theory has altered in a by no means inessential way in respect to the present issue. For under the pressure of the facts, explicit account has, in the interim, had to be taken—even though as a rule incidentally—of those ambiguities inherent in the influence of cognizance, of the mode of apprehension. These had not at all as yet been taken into consideration in the original doctrines of the theory, especially Koffka's

" mathematical attempt " of 1919 ; nor, as we have been able to elucidate *in extenso*, has the gestalt theory any place whatever for these facts in its original doctrines. The admission of these facts, even when it occurs in a concealed manner or without really due weight, accordingly amounts, strictly speaking, to a case where " new ", i.e. hitherto unconsidered "experiments" come into the context of the theory.

And yet, does the theory satisfy the requirements laid down by Koffka above ? That this is not the case should already be clear from our discussions, in virtue of numerous examples. We have seen that the extensions of the theory necessary on account of the newly included facts, were achieved by means of introducing appropriate auxiliary concepts, e.g. the concept of gestalt disposition. These auxiliary concepts, however, do not prove to ensue in a direct and rational way simply from the general conceptual doctrines of the theory. We were constantly made to conclude that they were from time to time imported *ad hoc* ; and that in respect of their actual import, they partly even stand in direct contradiction with the conceptual framework set up in the gestalt theory's doctrines. Taking all the facts of the matter into consideration, the gestalt theory can rank as a theory of the sort Koffka depicts as the ideal, only so long as it has not yet had recourse to these kinds of auxiliary concepts. But in admitting the facts expressed in these concepts it must needs invalidate itself. It thus forthwith relegates itself, in the matter of principles, to the ranks of those theories which are " from the outset so constituted as to allow of being adapted ".

Apart from this, however, the relation of the theory to empirical research appears to be by no means satisfactorily determined in an essentially more profound connection, at any rate when the practice of the gestalt-theoretical school is considered. Whereas one is in general obliged to regard psychology as a thoroughly empirical science, within the ambit of the present day standpoint of the gestalt theory, it seems to be at heart a theoretical science, in a sense which flatly abrogates the empirical character of psychology.

Indeed, if one has once clearly comprehended the essential nature of the gestalt theoretical viewpoint, one can have no doubt that it sets the theory above everything else in the science. Implicitly, there lurks behind the gestalt theory a general thesis about its content, viz. that a science exists only when there is a " theory ". With this attitude the theory at once becomes an end in itself. The object of scientific work is fulfilled in this propounding of a theory.

This stressing of the theoretical side, in the sense in which this is envisaged by the gestalt theory, retroactively leads to an internal attitude towards the empirical side and its facts, which is completely and utterly out of accord with Koffka's requirements as cited above. Under the spell of the theoretical attitude, it follows spontaneously that essentially only *those* facts in an experiment are perceived which stand in relation to the theory. And furthermore, the endeavour arises, quite generally, always to fit newly emerging facts into the entire body of the science in accordance with the preconceived theoretical views, at times by means of appropriate extension of the concepts and the explanatory viewpoints. A purely impartial attention to the facts as such, a genuinely existing interest in the purely empirical investigation of what is given, do not enter into the gestalt theory's line of orientation. True, the significance, from the point of view of principles, of the heuristic element in propounding theories has indeed been stressed, in the above-quoted explicit formulations on the part of the gestalt theoreticians. Nevertheless, the method of working actually met with plainly reveals how excessively, despite all this, the *pure theorizing attitude* asserts itself as the *truly dominant one* in the gestalt theory's orientation, and governs everything.

We could contrast another point of view with the general idea expressed in the practice of the gestalt theory—that in science theory is the crucial concern—by distinguishing, on grounds of principle, between " science " as a system of doctrine, and " science " as a body of research.

When one looks upon *science as a system of doctrine*, then indeed the theory as the final formula may be the essential matter, as establishing the content of the " known " in a definitive and exhaustive manner. But if we place *science as actual research* in the forefront of our considerations—and surely no one can doubt that in the present state of our young science of psychology this is the only point of view adequate to its situation as a whole—then the significance of the formula can certainly not be rated too highly. On the contrary, the crucial desideratum will be that the representatives of the science have sufficiently vividly in mind the real root of active research, namely the very great urgency of problematical points.

It can certainly not be admitted that the effect of the gestalt theory is to promote this. For not only is the interest of the gestalt theoreticians not directed immediately to the empirical side ; on the contrary, it is even necessarily diverted from it, since the magic word " gestalt ", conjointly with the theoretical apparatus which in the gestalt theory is directly attached to it, at bottom appears to solve all problems, and in fact does so to the minds of the adherents of the theory. However, an attitude which, as the evidence proves, leads to the result that in principle actually no problems whatever seem to be left unsolved, could bluntly be designated hostile to science. Any promotion of science as a body of research will, at any rate, not be expected from it.

It can therefore by no means be granted that in regard to its relationship to experimentation, the gestalt theory, as it exhibits itself in practice at the present day, in any way stands for an advance beyond the " old " psychology. On the contrary, it must confidently be stated that in many places in the contemporary psychology which is not gestalt-theoretically orientated, a truly unbiassed and genuinely empirical attitude in research obtains, whereas the gestalt theory is in these respects almost wholly deficient. Only *en passant* declarations—in Koffka's work of 1914—intended to emphasize abstractly those sides of the psychological approach found lacking by us, can be specified, in so far as a return to what is discovered in immediate experience is here consciously emphasized as a decisive principle. And similarly in practical research, only quite incidental examples, and these mainly in Wertheimer's own work (e.g. 1920), are to be found of the fact that, in spite of the theory, direct and more penetrating empirical analyses are arrived at. Freedom from bias palpably recedes more and more, in the attitude to research, in exact proportion as the gestalt theory consolidates itself as a " theory ".

But how does this excessive valuation of the theoretical come about, in spite of the fact that psychology in general,

U

since its submission to the experimental method, has long since won an entirely different position ? Its basis is the *peculiarity of the gestalt theory's theoretical thinking*, the manner and fashion of the development of doctrines and generalizations in the theory.

In order to describe this peculiarity we must commence with that part of the gestalt theory in which *gestalt-theoretical " explanation "* is systematically and most distinctly exhibited, namely Köhler's deductive treatment of the Wertheimer problem. Here, in Köhler's theory of psychophysical gestalten, we see quite unequivocally how the gestalt theory " thinks ". Here, on the basis of those architectural principles which Köhler believed could be discerned from the study of physical systems (distribution systems), the definition of physical and psychophysical gestalten is given ; and this precisely along lines such that the phenomenal gestalten, which are, in the last resort, the main issue in the psychological gestalt theory, seem to be directly " explained " in a *constructional fashion*. The fact that such a constructional procedure appears to be possible in the establishment, or alternatively elaboration, of the gestalt theory's conceptions, does not in the least degree condition the claims which the theory believes itself able to advance in virtue of its achievements. Hence derives the opinion that the gestalt theory offers direct and genuine explanations, in the sense in which one affirms this of physical theories. Thus is established that security with which the gestalt theoreticians thenceforth believe it possible to utilize the gestalt category. Lastly, from this follows the finality, ostensibly so extremely great, and on the other hand the multifarious applicability, extending both to biological and psychological problems, of the gestalt-theoretical way of looking at things. The real root of all is in essence the constructional attitude of thought characteristic of the gestalt-theoretical orientation.

It is not surprising that under these circumstances this attitude acquires great preponderance, in virtue of itself, in the total orientation of the gestalt theoreticians.

This constructional manner of thinking which developed, to begin with, in the field of psychophysical deduction, has effects beyond this territory, indeed upon the whole gestalt theory—even upon those enquiries which we have previously distinguished as psychological in the narrower sense, in order to delimit them from the strictly psychophysically orientated part.

The enquiries developed in empirical research and in general theoretical elucidations under the specific guidance of the psychological gestalt-theoretical conception, in fact continually give indications of this psychophysical substructure ; and they are, accordingly, essentially co-determined by its basic character, as seen from the point of view of scientific theory. The purely psychologically founded gestalt concept, too, always involves what seems to have been ascertained " from the starting point of physics " about the definiteness and certainty of the gestalt tenets.

Furthermore, this same constructional way of thinking is everywhere detectable in the manner in which " explanation " is in the gestalt theory directly subjected to this guiding conception. It is displayed in so far as the " gestalten " here appear as ultimate, effective factors, to be comprehended in their own right, as factors which, in their distinctive conformance to laws, determine the inner organization of what is psychophysically given, in accordance with quite definite " gestalt tendencies ". It is manifestly implicated, when the gestalt category and the derived concepts associated with it—such as gestalt completion, gestalt excitation, etc.—acquire direct explanatory value in the gestalt theory's body of conceptions.

But in this fundamentally constructional attitude of the gestalt theory's thinking, as could well be expected, lies the crucial barrier preventing the gestalt theory from impartially weighing-up the facts as they are. Moreover, this barrier is bound to arise directly as a result of fixing the essential nature of the gestalt-theoretical orientation, as a necessary and unavoidable consequence of certain ultimate convictions inseparably bound up with the basic postulates of the theory. It is based upon certain very general ties which we have now to discover in order finally to understand these circumstances.

§ 66. *The logical-ontological import of the gestalt theory and its metaphysical constraints*

The chief root of the gestalt theory's entire posing and treatment of problems is undoubtedly to be found in the singularity of its general orientation by the psychophysical problem. The psychophysical problem is held to receive a completely novel and essentially more profound treatment at the hands of the gestalt theory—this is its first and most general claim. And it is in connection with this problem that the specifically constructional standpoint in thinking, which we have just distinguished as a characteristic of the gestalt theory's attitude of thought, already becomes a first and essential method of approach. We have seen in what way the novel solution of the psychophysical problem developed in detail, and what significance is attached to the considerations advanced in connection therewith.

The claim Köhler thus raised was neither more nor less than that the psychophysical problem had ceased to be a problem ! The gestalt theoreticians are convinced that their theory has in point of fact solved the psychophysical problem in principle—and this, moreover, by directly building up from the empirically well-founded physical analysis, independently of any special line of argument of a purely philosophical kind.

However, the course of our criticism led us to show in detail how entirely unfounded this claim is ; and we were in consequence compelled to pass a very adverse judgment upon the methodological side of these reflections. At this point it is only necessary fundamentally to establish again how, purely in terms of principles, this claim affects the scientific structure of the gestalt theory.

We can state it quite tersely. The psychophysical conclusions which have a central position in the gestalt theory, are actually—far indeed as they are from deserving to rank as proven conclusions—nothing other than axioms of a purely philosophical nature underlying the whole system. They stand behind all the detailed discussions of the gestalt theory, as absolute presuppositions, as ultimate postulates. But the acknowledgment of them cannot ensue " from beneath upwards ", in direct reliance upon empirically determinable, immediate findings. It is based upon the simple acceptance of definite, very general, philosophical convictions. This radically alters the appraisal of the scientific import of the gestalt theory. It cannot continue to be rated as a straightforward theoretical formulation, founded purely on the basis of facts, genuinely and solely scientific, as is represented in its own claims. It must be regarded as philosophically burdened in a characteristic way. The fundamental establishment of the entire theory upon the so-called Wertheimer principle signifies nothing other than a simple and radical confession of a philosophical article of faith, nothing other than an indiscriminate re-interpretation of the entire facts in accordance with a preconceived philosophical conviction.

An even more far-reaching, basic philosophical pre-dilection, over and above this, and partly including this, manifests itself as a directive influence in the gestalt theory. The gestalt theory includes a radical *ontologization of psychology*. This ontological note in the gestalt theory's orientation still remains dominant even where the psycho-physical side of the theory gives place to a more psycho-logically analytical treatment (Wertheimer's direct analysis of phenomenal gestalten, 1924—see above, § 38). Here it is characteristic that the gestalt concept as such immediately acquires an explanatory function and this, moreover, on the ground of the idea of specific gestalt uniformity. What this idea leads to philosophically, is that an autoch-thonous ontological reality is attributed to the gestalt as such, in this sense : that any units of reality, so far as they are identifiable as gestalten, contain forces, tendencies, modes of action, directly determined in their own right, which must be ascribed to them just in virtue of their property of being gestalten.

The gestalten thus become primary realities, existential ultimates, in terms of which all events should be com-prehended. And, moreover, these ultimates are to be directly acknowledged as such, not, peradventure, to be first of all possibly indirectly established from the starting point of physics.

By this conclusion, the theoretical function of the gestalt concept is determined in a peculiar way—a way which makes it necessary to bring this concept into intimate relationship with the " element " concept so abhorred by the gestalt theory.

Hence we must in point of fact affirm that the structure of the gestalt-psychological system of science is by no means so radically different from the structure of the elementalist psychology as the latter appears to scientific theory. In

Wertheimer's system the gestalt concept is manipulated theoretically in exactly the same way as the element concept in the genuinely atomistic psychology. The gestalt concept covers a principle of an ultimate entity in the theory in exactly the same sense as the element concept was supposed to do. Its relation to what is " explained " is exactly the same as formerly, in the case of the extreme elementalist standpoint, the relation of the elements to what was derived from them. The phenomena appear as simple effects of an absolute, ontologically founded gestalt uniformity. In both cases, we are concerned with an endeavour to deduce the mentally " real " " explanatorily " from the starting point of some sort of (ontologically interpreted) *ultimates*, upon the basis of definite uniformities, tendencies, forces (either associative or of gestalt-like character) peculiar to these ultimates in accordance with their nature. And furthermore—this is the essence of their similarity—in both cases these ultimates are so singularly constituted, that a genuinely constructional derivation of what is observable, omitting nothing, is at the time conceived to be possible on the basis of them. This is so conceived that what we have said above, from our analysis of the gestalt theory's attitude in research, about the basic constructional orientation of its thinking, here directly appears as the necessary correlate to the ontological subservience of its explanatory apparatus. This strikes to the heart of its standpoint.

The ontological subservience of the gestalt theory to the ultimates we have described, betrays itself, in a very fundamental way, purely psychologically, in reference to the determination of the contents of what must be called the psychically real. It entails the imposition of *specific and utter uniformity on the entire range of psychological facts*.

The traditional classification of psychical phenomena, resting upon the qualitative multiformity of psychical data, is, as we have seen, completely abandoned in the gestalt theory. A single new distinction appears: that between static, or alternatively stationary and quasistationary gestalten, on the one hand, and dynamic gestalten, on the other. This distinction, which emerges from the systematic structure of the gestalt theory, that is, in virtue of the singular efficacies ascribed to those ultimates of the theoretical approach, has no connection with any classification of the old kind ; on the contrary, in principle all distinctions advanced in those " old " classifications are nullified, in the gestalt theory. For, as regards their import, all phenomena of psychical experience are without exception to be regarded as " gestalten ". Hence Spearman in his recent important paper on the gestalt problem (1925) justly describes the Wertheimer-Koffka-Köhler theory as a unitary one.

This has a very radical significance. The gestalt theory thus, in regard to fundamentals, does away with every distinction set up by the " old " psychology. It is of opinion that both a sensation and a thought content, as well as a volitional process, belong in their actual import entirely to the same context ; for each, however varying, is really apprehended and apprehensible only in so far as it is envisaged as an aspect, a moment, or a determinate part of a gestalt process. It believes furthermore, that the distinctions existing in the forms of manifestation are unimportant for true scientific knowledge ; for the understanding of the variously manifested phenomena concerned càn, according to the theory, solely be obtained by accomplishing the reduction to the single and universal uniformity, the gestalt uniformity, which stands behind everything phenomenal, and which is merely obscured in its purity through the variety of its forms of manifestation.

It is clear that this must have effects upon the pursuit of research, inasmuch as problems upon which psychological labour has hitherto been very assiduously expended become meaningless in this context. What, from this standpoint, can be the sense of striving to analyze in finer and finer detail the immediately detectable psychical data ? What significance, for example, attaches to all the laborious experimental work devoted by the Külpe School, in abundant and most painstaking researches stretching as far as the imposing works of Selz, to the investigation of the data of thought psychology, ever since the discovery of the singularity of " conscious attitudes " (*Bewusztheiten*) (Ach), and of " thoughts " (Bühler, Messer) ? We have been able to observe how all this work does indeed appear meaningless to the gestalt theory, for we saw how Koffka found a way of disposing of the problem of thought psychology in a much simpler manner. As regards the pursuit of research, therefore, we can from this draw the conclusion that an impoverishment is bound to arise in this direction, in the tracks of the gestalt theory. And indeed, we have seen that in this very respect a characteristic deficiency could be established in connection with definite researches of the gestalt theory (Wulff), in consequence of which the facts to be investigated had not been correctly grasped at all.

In regard to the product of its research, however, one cannot on this score avoid being led to a general affirmation which is substantiated by our previous detailed discussions. It is inevitable that, with this orientation in the gestalt theory, nothing should remain of the manifold of what is experientially given, save an extremely abstract and bloodless schematism empty of all immediate content. Hence, when the gestalt theory at times raises the claim that its enunciations have the special advantage of being largely close to life, as opposed to the products of the " old " psychology which referred solely to the false artefacts of the " laboratory ", this claim can hardly be admitted. The closeness to life claimed by the gestalt theory is certainly not attained through the peculiarity of its theoretical structure. It is attained rather through the fact that it embarked from the outset, with perhaps too rash a courage, upon those regions of mental life which appear essential for our life viewed as a psychical continuity. By contrast, we have hitherto in psychology ventured far more cautiously and with far less of the grand gesture, to deal with these psychological continuities, satisfied if we knew at least something with certainty, but not professing to have at once solved the whole range of problems concealed here.

The gestalt theory's claim that its enunciations link up specially closely with life, rests upon the fact that it seemingly has the means of forthwith mastering, un-equivocally, the problems of the meaning, of the purposive-ness, and of the internal organization of our stream of consciousness, in terms of its basic doctrine. But how does this mastery of these problems develop ? Once more, very simply : both the facts of meaningfulness, and those of purposiveness, as well as those of organization, are without exception correlated to the " structure " or gestalt concept. The concept of meaning, as well as that of purpose, is unhesitatingly identified with the gestalt concept, as conceived by the gestalt theory—and this settles the whole matter. The fact that thought sequences have meaning, that reactions " leap forward " meaningfully out of what is given in the outside world, is simply due to the fact that gestalt coherences are present, which, as befits their essential nature, from the outset far transcend the " intrinsic arbitrariness " of atomistic co-ordination, in their inner closure and complete organization.

But what is thus really achieved, when we take into account the reservations which must, in the light of our criticism, be urged against the conceptions of the gestalt theory ? The problem of meaningfulness and of purposiveness is obviously on no showing conducted to a true " solution ". It is, on the contrary, merely transferred to another level, that of the ontologically real, where the meaningfulness of the " gestalten " is constituted in its own right. The sole achievement here is that the problem is lifted out of the sphere of the scientifically tangible, and forthwith ceases altogether to exist as a problem ; so that appraisal of it is fundamentally and once for all renounced. For in the realm of the ontologically real one can naturally reach no concrete clarification in regard to all these problems ; it is simply a matter of acceptance or rejection, and not of any direct discussion of the problems. For indeed, here again the gestalt concept is an absolute concept of an ultimate, under which one can merely subsume the phenomena, but beyond which one neither must nor should enquire. The magical effect of the word " gestalt " stops all further investigation.

In the second place—and this is an even more damaging stricture—the gestalt concept which the gestalt theory has at its disposal, in its own right, appears from the first in no way whatever adapted for application to this problem at all. It is merely begging the question to believe that the word " meaning " can also be covered by the word " gestalt ", and this arises by way of a noteworthy equivocation. The term " gestalt ", as the gestalt theory is able to place it at our service, has its characteristic limitations. It acquires immediate content only from the starting point of physics. But if this strictly " physical " origin and import of the concept is retained, the question must be raised as to whether that which in the mental sense we designate " meaningful " is indeed directly comprehensible on this basis. We have already had occasion to touch upon this question, and, following Jaensch, to answer it in the negative. The actual mental world lies outside the sphere which is accessible directly from the Wertheimer-Koffka-Köhler gestalt concept. And if the gestalt theoreticians believe that they can nevertheless directly cope with the problem, this is due to the fact that the term " gestalt " possesses nuances of meaning, derived from quite other than genuinely gestalt-theoretical contexts—Jaensch talks of a " numinous glimmer "— which lie at the mental level.

In one connection only does the problem of meaningfulness, as the gestalt theory sees it, remain capable of further discussion, namely, in respect to the question of how we happen to experience a " meaningful reality " even in the continuum of perceptions ; for here the association with the " physicalism " of the gestalt can apparently be directly established. The position of this problem requires a more exact elucidation.

This elucidation is of special importance. It leads us back to a general philosophical presupposition of the gestalt theory, which is so debatable as indeed, in the present stage of the development of philosophical problems, to permit us to augment our reasons for rejecting the theory by one, and this a most important one, directly on philosophical grounds.

We can examine the matter by starting from the problem of how far one can do justice to the meaningfulness that can be demonstrated in perceptual reality by means of the gestalt theory. We then at once narrow the situation down to its crucial elements. The gestalt theory gives a very extraordinary reply to this question. " The receptor apparatus is in itself already so constructed as to be capable of achieving ' the apprehension of inner necessities ' ", those inner coherences which, transcending the " intrinsic arbitrariness " of the purely aggregative juxtaposition of elements, represent exactly what we mean when we speak of the fact of our perceptual world being meaningfully organized. In other words, the fact that our perceptual world is thus and thus structured, and in no other way, is directly due to the fact that the " objective " reality confronting our sense organs already contains these marks of definition within itself. The fact that our perceptual reality appears to be meaningful merely follows because, in this perceptual reality, we have before us a simple "structural reaction" of our organism to the objectively present gestalten of the real world, which must be admitted to be fraught with meaning.

Here we see, to begin with, that even in this special case the situation in regard to the problem of meaningfulness has not altered. Here, too, the problem is settled by simply relegating the set of facts to a higher level, in this case that of objectively real things.

Our survey leads us beyond this, however, to the major philosophical problem, as to how the gestalt theory does actually in general interpret the essential nature of the perceptual process, and what assumptions in matters of principle are involved in this interpretation.

First of all, the general point can be established that with the gestalt theory there palpably goes the direct assumption of a *realistic world-picture*, as regards the structure of "objective things". We can go further, and establish that the way the gestalt theory conceives the "apprehension" of real things in perception, on the basis of this realistic world picture, can be interpreted only in one sense : the gestalt theory, in this connection, is making use of a quite distinct *sensationalism*. For indeed, in the reality of "things", a multiplicity of definite gestalten, be it primarily of purely geometrical, or else even of super-geometrical, dynamical sort, underlies the perceptual process. In the action of these objectively real gestalten upon the senses there arises, through direct "control" from without, a physiological process of gestalt character directly corresponding to the real gestalten ; and on the phenomenal side, a parallel gestalt coherence is again directly co-ordinated to this gestalt coherence represented in the neurophysical sector—with the express retention of its defining gestalt characteristics. Furthermore, a co-ordination rigorous in every respect is vouched for between these different levels. Pervasive "gestalt identity" prevails, in such a way, that for this perceptual relationship the statement *nihil est in intellectu, quod non prius fuerit in sensu* does actually hold.

But this discovery that the gestalt-theoretical orientation involves a sensationalistic interpretation, permits of being further driven home in a characteristic respect—when we revert to the assertion, quite specially stressed by Koffka, that the gestalt theory is particularly adapted to overcome sensationalism. Clearly, in this assertion of Koffka the term must have a different meaning from what it has in our considerations. Koffka makes this assertion in connection with the demonstration that the gestalt-theoretical interpretation of the process of perception is far superior to the refuted interpretation (i.e. the sensationalistic one, in his sense) for this reason : The gestalt theory does not simply lead to a mere mosaic of sensations in the sensorium, from the starting point of which there could be no transition to the meaningfully organized, self-articulated, perceptual reality which confronts us in actuality ; on the contrary, it directly includes this perceptual reality.

What is the relation of the sensationalism rejected by Koffka to the sensationalism ascribed by us to his own theory ? The gestalt theory's greater achievement, in the direction in question, as compared with that of the sensationalism against which Koffka inveighs, is obviously due solely to one thing ; viz., that the very data upon which the senses depend are supposed already to manifest the " structures " which sensationalism is held not to be in the position to explain. It is due to the fact that we have here an essentially more radical realism and sensationalism. Koffka's bold front against sensationalism concerns solely the rejection of a quite definite form of sensationalism—that form which (a higher stage in epistemological reflection, be it noted) has emerged from the criticism of naïve realism. However, the form in which this standpoint is repudiated by Koffka, seen in the context of his total attitude in remaining matters, on the contrary actually includes the absolute postulation of a still more remarkable sensationalism, one which is characteristically still palpably at the same stage of epistemological reflection as naïve realism. Koffka wages battle against the sensationalism of the seventeenth century ; but he himself is in principle at the same standpoint as that of Greek philosophy when Democritus explained perception by supposing that the εἴδωλα coming from the objects acted upon the sense organs. The εἴδωλα as can be very easily discerned,[1]

---

[1] Wittmann (1923) has followed up more thoroughly the historical parallels to be found along this line. He shows, in particular, the kinship of Köhler's conceptions with the ancient realistic-scholastic body of

throughout correspond to the gestalt processes. The significance of this, from the point of view of systematic epistemology, is nothing less than that the gestalt theory immanently incorporates an adherence to the most naïve realism which can be conceived.

This creed is inevitably bound up with the acceptance of the gestalt theory ; and yet the least epistemological reflection compels one to recognize such a standpoint as untenable. Hence this final outcome of the ontological bonds peculiar to the gestalt theory, now also brings to light a weighty, purely philosophical argument against the admissibility of the Wertheimer-Koffka-Köhler theory.

conceptions, by pointing out parallel statements in Albertus Magnus, Thomas Aquinas, and Aristotle ; while Bühler, impelled by another viewpoint (1928), follows up the historical parallels particularly in the direction of Spinozism. The two considerations converge, when the scholastic heritage embodied in Spinozism is not lost sight of.

ı

ı

CONCLUSION

TOWARDS A CHARACTERIZATION OF THE GESTALT PROBLEMS IN THEIR ENTIRETY

We have reached the end of our critique of the Wertheimer theory. We turn now to the more general task of discussing, on the basis to the narrower range of our criticism and with a view to appraising the scientific situation of the gestalt problem in general, some of the suggestive prospects which offer in regard to the possibilities of a positive, self-sufficient theory of gestalt phenomena.

Surveying our enquiry as a whole, we find ourselves unable to accord recognition to the gestalt theory, either in so far as it presents itself as a distinct theoretical system, or as it purports to represent a quite specific approach to research. In both respects the gestalt theory does not appear to do justice to the requirements of the scientific situation, even those which have been formulated by its own representatives.

The main consideration upon which this rejection of the theory must be based, lies in the fact that the *implications of the provisions for scientific thinking* by which the theory has been orientated have not been controlled with sufficient self-criticism ; and in the fact that, on the other hand, over and over again there seems to be an exceedingly strong urge towards systematic finality in general.[1]

However, we have not in this criticism exhaustively expounded our entire position in regard to the Wertheimer-Koffka-Köhler line of research, or indeed to the peculiar import of the gestalt problem in general. In the first place the repudiation of the gestalt *theory* naturally does not signify a repudiation of the gestalt *problem*. It merely

[1] In this connection we must not omit to point out that, as a matter of fact, this urge towards theoretical finality may be very different with different representatives of the gestalt theory. Indeed, I regard it as possible that certain individuals may not be altogether in agreement with pronouncements to which others are led by this very urge. And it may be that in the case of a number of the more judicious representatives of the theory, this unchecked passion for construction which constantly breaks through, by no means receives approbation. However, from the way the literature has meanwhile been developing, this judiciousness is actually manifesting itself less and less frequently.

signifies a protest against quite specific features in the treatment of the problem.

The primary psychological significance of the gestalt *phenomena*, in the widest sense, will necessarily have to be acknowledged unconditionally—above all, in consequence of our knowledge of the factual material assembled by the group of workers on the gestalt theory.

The fact that the significance of these phenomena has meanwhile come to the knowledge of an ever-widening circle of psychologists, must incontestably be allowed to redound to the credit of the Wertheimer group. Apart from the allegiances which, in respect of its content, the theory seems to subserve, the work of the investigators grouped round Wertheimer has merely for this reason had a directly stimulating and liberating effect. To that extent, however one may look upon it intrinsically, it is at all events of positive importance for the inner development of psychological research in general.

In the second place, psychology, in propounding its concrete theories, cannot afford simply to ignore the contentions of the gestalt theory, or not to take them seriously. For psychological theory, the very fact that this system has even now been fully elaborated will not be without significance or without value. The mere fact that in the work of these investigators we find a *definite possibility of theoretical premisses* laid down, and that we see how these investigators really set about, in all seriousness, to follow this possibility out, and indeed, really think matters through to their end with absolute indifference to others ; this fact itself cannot allow it to pass for an adequate manner of facing the situation, when a purely negative attitude is assumed towards the representatives of this theory. Quite apart from its final consequences and the appraisal of them, it is in any event an indisputable achievement when anyone goes so far as to perceive a new theoretical approach in science, and at the same time has the power to prosecute it to a point where its possibilities and limitations become discernible. And, undoubtedly, the gestalt theory can lay claim to this achievement, even if it has not become aware of the limitations of its course.

To go further, since we have, in the preceding pages again and again exactly distinguished these limitations as conspicuously as possible, the significance of the gestalt theory can prove to be even more far-reaching in essence, for us in particular. For our critical consideration of the theory can furnish a foundation on the basis of which one can endeavour anew to characterize the gestalt *problem*, as to its singular status, in a rounded-off conspectus and with keener conceptual tools.

Within the framework of our criticism of the Wertheimer-Koffka-Köhler gestalt theory, we have met with an abundance of facts ; and we have strongly drawn attention to the points in which the *theory* as measured by these *facts*, has shown itself to be unsatisfactory. But the analysis of these facts takes us a step further. It leads to a *positive picture*, which is even relatively unitary, and which seems suitable to be substituted for this theory. We have *indicated or developed* essential features of this picture in particular places in our critical argument. Over and above this, however, the necessary requirement to elaborate these features in a rounded-off exposition, as to the problems inherent in them, now arises.

Such an exposition will, *in respect to its postulates*, at present only allow of being developed purely theoretically —in prosecuting the reductions of conceptions which have already presented themselves in the theoretical and factual conditions hitherto discussed. Having in these postulates laid down the total orientation, we shall then, from this starting point, attempt to lead up to a characterization of the peculiar *conceptual discords* which, seen in the light of the facts, have to be overcome in the phenomenon " gestalt ", and in reference to which the total scientific situation in regard to the gestalt problem is determined.

In this connection, we shall have opportunity to add to the shadows we have hitherto had to insert in our picture of the Wertheimer-Koffka-Köhler gestalt theory, also those lights which must not be forgotten if one wishes to comprehend this theory justly, in accordance with its true position in the contemporary development of psychological research. We shall at the same time be compelled to take into account—even though it may be only sketchily —other and different solutions of the gestalt problem, above all that advocated by the Leipzig School, and thus finally to arrive at a comprehensive conspectus of the theoretical possibilities of the gestalt problem in general.

§ 67. *The idea of a functional-analytical theory of the gestalt phenomena as a task before us*

From the standpoint of principles, it is possible on the basis of our discussions, to lay down a series of requirements *for a well-proven gestalt theory*, starting from which one will be able to envisage in outline the framework of a definitive theory.

The first and conclusive reduction has been conspicuously brought out by the investigators centred round Wertheimer. It is this which really endows the gestalt problem with its central significance in the orientation of psychology and its principles. It may be stated as the *incongruity between* the phenomenal and functional characteristics of the *gestalt facts*, on the one hand, and the theoretical possibilities of a *synthetic atomistic theoretical formulation*, orientated by the element concept, on the other.

It is greatly to the credit of the Wertheimer group of workers that it gave the impetus to the real awakening of the scientific conscience to this incongruity (see above, p. 5). To be sure, Krueger and Martius had, in experimental research,[1] independently and at an earlier date already stressed this incongruity as a crucial problem. Nevertheless these two have not had so great an external effect as one should have expected from the definiteness of their formulations. The works of Krueger and his pupils are only now—with the appearance of the *Neue psychologischen Studien*—in virtue of their extent, too, securing that place in psychology which has long been due to them on account of their import. Martius' ideas, however, for the first time emerged in their experimental implications in the *Martius-Festschrift* to his 70th birthday, published by Wittmann. Wertheimer, on the other hand, and in particular his friends, have from the outset constantly put their conceptions before their professional colleagues at great length. Thus, in fact, the development towards a genuine understanding of the significance of the gestalt problems is truly associated with the rise of the " gestalt theory " in the

---

[1] For views of other earlier investigators, important in the history of the development of ideas on the problem, and further removed from experimental work, cf. Krueger, " Über psychische Ganzheit," Introduction to *Neue psychologischen Studien*, 1926.

narrower sense, indeed, with its very opposition to the atomistic-synthetic theory.

Psychology has of course previously been aware of this problem of gestalt, and has even found ways of incorporating it in its systems of teachings (see above, p. 4). We can say with Sander : " Ehrenfels' concept of gestalt quality, Wundt's principle of creative synthesis, Dilthey's structure concept, in a certain sense Freud's thesis of meaningful determination, all belonging to the same decade, have this in common, despite their varying theoretical potency—that in them was heralded the vanquishment of the refuted view of the aggregative character . . . of immediate experience, and more so, of the dispositional, structural, total state of mental reality " (Sander, 1927, p. 23).

This victory is indeed heralded, but is by no means truly consummated. The purely summational is transcended by such concepts ; but—in marked adherence to the atomism of the stimuli and to the constancy hypothesis—sensations as *the fundaments*, and special " functions " and " processes " like creative syntheses (Wundt), functions of assembling and fusing (Stumpf), production processes (Meinong, Benussi), collective effects of attention (G. Müller), as *principles bringing about coalescence*, are set in opposition to one another. The whole, the gestalt, it is said, is more than the parts. But this *more* is defined in its genesis by simply inserting corresponding special principles *ad hoc*—without the necessity and the possibility of at any time verifying these assumptions by means of concrete analysis.

In contradistinction to this we find the far more clear-cut formulation which in point of principle leads beyond that position ; namely, the formulation that the whole, as opposed to its parts, is in truth *the prius* (cf. above, p. 46–7) the basic thesis of the *primacy of the whole over the part*. This basic thesis first appears with Wertheimer (loc. cit.), and expresses keen *descriptive* reflection about what is immediately experienced.

It is further entrenched on the ground of the fact that it also covers characteristic *functional* findings. We have met with such findings in the foregoing pages—in the structure-inhering functional effects of the figural structure (p. 172 ff.) ; and we were compelled to admit, in spite of keen critical testing, that in all the examples cited one could not accomplish anything by means of a definition of e.g. colour qualities from the starting point of the atomistic treatment. We had to admit, and positively to stress, that one could not do justice to these facts by means of a synthetic theory.

It is an indisputable fact that the whole, in an optical gestalt, functionally determines its members, its " elements ", and does not synthetically erect itself upon these. *Things objectively alike are throughout phenomenally different, when the " gestalt linkage " is appropriate* (cf. geometrical optical illusions, e.g. Benussi ; also Ibsen 1926, on the Sander Parallelogram).

The same result ensues in a variety of other experiments. In especial, it appears that, over and above the phenomenal and the functional aspects, there is also a *primacy of the whole in a genetic respect.* It can be established both ontogenetically and phylogenetically, that in descending to more primitive conditions, we do not find any such thing as a relative resolution of the textural character of the elements, but a diminution in the discrimination of the single constituents, a predominance of total qualities (cf. H. Volkelt 1925 ; Köhler 1917, Exp. no. 7 ; Volkelt 1912).

The *incongruity between configuratedness and atomistic construction* thus also leads to a *rejection of atomism.* There remains the task of determining more exactly the *positive theoretical possibilities* which still exist. They become manifest in a characteristic theoretical cleavage which has constantly confronted us in our analysis of the facts of the gestalt theory, and upon which we now propose to focus our attention in order to arrive at a fundamental verdict.

Starting with the repudiation of atomism in psychology, Wertheimer, Koffka, and Köhler arrived specifically at their peculiar gestalt theory. The question is, whether and in what sense one can do justice to the conception of repudiating atomism by means of theoretical media different from those of Wertheimer, Koffka, and Köhler ; that is, whether and how it is possible to build up an anti-synthetically orientated psychology of gestalt, which is not expressly identical, in its essential features, with the " gestalt theory " in the narrower sense.

To determine where this possibility we seek is to be

found, it is necessary once more to stress exactly what circumstances made this pregnant, highly systematized theory appear not intrinsically substantiable, to our mind. Our *rejection of this gestalt theory* is based essentially upon the following points :—

1. The gestalt theory is not adapted to the facts in their full measure, because it cannot, from its very nature, help being a constructional theory of the psychical units in question ; and, secondly, because its theoretical means of thinking do not suffice to embrace the whole of the facts of experimentation. This is the gist of our repudiation of the physiological gestalt theory.

2. The inadequacy of this theory is displayed in the realm of experimentation through this fact : We do not, by its means, do justice to the subjective conditionalities of our gestalt experiences, which are under certain circumstances so conspicuously exhibited. For together with the constructional character of the theory, an orientation by external objectivity appears to be distinctive of its whole way of thinking ; in this sense, that all the abovementioned conditionalities are at bottom regarded as merely the direct expression of the uniformities which regulate the state of configuration in this objective reality (Gestalt tendencies).

These problematic features display themselves in the substance of the theory along two lines. The gestalt theory has, (*a*) the character of a *copy theory*, inasmuch as the neurophysical and psychophysical gestalt processes and gestalt co-ordination seem to be directly " controlled " by the objective conditions (of momentary nature or having temporal after effects, see above, pp. 147–151) ; and (*b*) it has the character of an *automaton theory*, inasmuch as the determination of the ordered coherence which regulates the integration of the single components in the configural whole, consists, at bottom, in nothing other than a blind sequential effect unequivocally determined by the initial conditions in a causal manner, and automatically liberated by them.

If one seriously entertains the idea that, as we emphasized in our critical part, the subjective conditionalities (manner of apprehension, direction of cognizance, attentional attitude) have primary significance in determining this gestalt organization, the cardinal difference will necessarily be seen to lie in this very point. A theoretical organization of the gestalt facts doing justice to the true state of affairs, will then not permit of being built up along the lines of a copy theory. It will, moreover, be fundamentally different from an automaton theory, inasmuch as effects somehow conditioned by the " personality " are involved in these very influences mentioned above, and enter into the course of events in a critical way.

This means that such a theory will, in particular, *cease to have the possibility* of deductively *deriving* the phenomenal gestalten in a *constructional* way " from the starting point of physics ". It will, in its formal respects, have to develop fundamentally in another direction.

The notion of this sort of solution of the gestalt problems presupposes, from the viewpoint of scientific theory, a special possibility, viz. that the development of a *non-constructional* theory must be rationally justifiable.

This possibility will, to begin with, hardly be conceded without further question. And to be sure, it can only acquire significance when one defines, firstly, what one denotes by " theory ", and secondly, what one denotes positively, from the point of view of scientific theory, by " non-constructional ".

In the widest sense, from the viewpoint of scientific theory, we can regard a *theory* as a body of conceptions which is at a given time so determined, in that it combines the entire range of facts coming into question comprehensively and consistently into a single unitary picture ; and this in such a way, that in any concrete instance one can, starting from given conditions which have a place in this system, envisage, if not entirely predict the consequences.

Under this concept of " theory " falls, in the first place, the constructional approach, which builds up the manifold of reality deductively and explanatorily out of definite conceptual ultimates, and on the basis of definite uniformities of action attributed to these ultimates and peculiar to them. Another kind of theory is, however, also to be found, even in the sphere of physics. I mean, the way in which the facts of thermodynamics permit of being theoretically comprehended. In this case we have, firstly, the famous constructional theory which does indeed " explain " the facts in the very way we have mentioned, by reducing them to definite physical ultimates, i.e., the kinetic theory of heat. But secondly, there is another way of looking at the matter, which must be ranked as a " theory " in exactly the same sense. I refer to *functional* thermodynamics as I would call it. In this it is characteristic that, unlike the constructional theory, the theoretical interpretation of the data proceeds along the lines of laying down functional dependencies, to which no ontological parallels are directly attributed.

We have thus characterized, in a positive manner, the feasibility of forming a non-constructional theory. We see that it consists in this : that it confines itself, firstly, to determining the data, exactly and thoroughly in terms of facts ; and secondly, to establishing the functional tendencies within the data from the viewpoint of the con-catenations of the conditions.

On these considerations, our *task* would be to settle what possibilities exist, in regard to the gestalt phenomenon, of reaching, not a constructional, but a purely functional theory in our sense, while at the same time repudiating atomism. The task we have thus formulated is at bottom identical with Koffka's distinctive requirement, quoted by us on p. 25 ff. above. It is Koffka's demand for an antisynthetic theory in psychology ; but of course, with the very definite rejection, based on the constellation of the facts, of the specific content of its means of thinking which has accrued to this general methodical re-orientation once formulated by Koffka, in the later development of the gestalt theory, through the agency of Wertheimer and Köhler.

On this view, the forms of psychological theory fall into two categories, those which are constructional and those which are functional. From our preceding criticism, it follows that we must reject the constructional form. The positive task remains of attempting a closer conceptual clarification of the situation existing in respect to the con-ceptions of the functional theory ; and, also, of providing, from this starting point, the foundations for a future elaboration of a well-proven theory of the gestalt phenomena. The point of departure for a closer demarca-tion of the kind of " gestalt theory " we demand, is once more to be found in certain formulations of the Wertheimer school.

To sum up all we have said in the preceding pages, we must conclude as follows :—

There can be no doubt that the gestalt theoreticians are justified in the negative side of their orientation, their repudiation of the atomistically orientated, synthesizing schema of thinking, basing its theory upon the psychology of sensation. Nor can there be any doubt that in stressing this conception they have substantially contributed to impel psychology to come to " a consciousness of itself ". But they have unfortunately proceeded totally to obliterate the true significance of this valuable approach by constantly seeking to link up with physics and constructional physiological explanations, and by regarding this as their real task. They could very well have preserved the positive import of their standpoint, if they had guarded against such " physicalism " and had confined themselves solely to what is furnished by their basic orientation independently of this " physicalism ". This positive kernel we still find definitely formulated by Koffka in 1914, when he confesses to a basic " anti-synthetic " orientation in psychological theory and research (see above, § 6).

This anti-synthetic orientation does not necessarily involve a transition to such physical and physiological speculations. To begin with, it only calls for a specific methodological attitude, as Koffka himself formulated it at the time we have mentioned. It demands that we acknowledge the immediately present psychological data as such and without preconceptions, and that we describe them as exactly and adequately as possible ; and also, that this description should then be made the point of departure for any theoretical formulations (see above, p. 26), and not some sort of ontologically founded ultimates like psychical " elements "—or even physico-physiological " gestalt processes ". In brief, it demands, as Martius had already stated it, an " analytical " theory of mental life.

The essential point in this programme, and the ineradicable positive outcome of this phase of the gestalt movement, is the demand for a genuinely immanent analysis of the gestalt phenomena. This demand could in fact even in itself, if one kept to a consistent total orientation and to the comprehensive consideration of facts, have acted as a bulwark against the more special explications subsequently developed by Köhler on the basis of it, and which we find ourselves unable to concur in. Our hope that a " theory " of this sort must, on the *purely formal side*, of a surety be well proven, is founded on this point.

To be sure, the crucial question still remains open ; namely, whether it is possible even at the present time to furnish a theory, positive in substance, of such a sort as to satisfy all requirements. In regard to this question too, we should like to state some general considerations in which the logical difficulty of the gestalt problems can be more definitely outlined.

For an orientation along positive lines, we must select as our basis the way in which, on the score of our striking critical contrasts, the gestalt facts show themselves to be greatly strained. To bring home to us the discrepancies which exist here in their full seriousness, cannot, in this connection, but be reckoned an essential task. Here, indeed, the gestalt theory is once more undeniably valuable as a point of departure.

One thing is not without significance for our task, as well as for that final appraisal of the gestalt theory which transcends the detailed discussion of it : That the anti-synthetic programme formulated by Koffka has led to positive treatments of facts even in the gestalt-theoretical line of work, which—relatively emancipated from the bondage to physiology—must be understood in their own right, and which are throughout compatible with our demand for a purely functional theory. In our expository part we have already sharply distinguished this aspect of the treatment of facts from Köhler's orientation, by contrasting the " *psychophysical* gestalt-theoretical " conception with the " *psychological* gestalt-theoretical " conception. It is in Wertheimer's latest publications, in particular, that this purely psychological gestalt-theoretical conception comes more clearly to the fore.[1]

The fact that isolated attempts to link up with genuine psychological theory are made, at least occasionally, in a way so comparatively explicit, points in a positively progressive direction. At this point the tendency in

---

[1] A point of great interest is that Köhler has in the meantime (1929) reverted from his physiological approach to a more definitely analytical point of view, thus abandoning the absolutely constructional trend of the theory of 1920 (see above, §§ 30–2).

research evinced in Wertheimer's latest works—which serve, as compared with others, the task of delineating the leading idea of the gestalt theory as distinctly as possible—makes contact with the tendencies dominant e.g. in the circle of investigators associated with Krueger. This is true, in spite of the fact that in the long run the reduction to physiology still continues to have no little significance even for this treatment of Wertheimer. With this orientation, when, as with Krueger, it is prosecuted relatively independently, the leitmotif of the theory *is the notion of the conformance to law of the gestalt in its own right*, in this sense : that the task of a theory of the gestalt phenomena consists in the elaboration of the principles of the *self-articulation* of gestalten purely at the *psychological level*. This means confining oneself to the descriptive analysis and functional interpretation of the gestalten, without, however, directly resorting to definite assumptions, constructional in substance, about their physiological " foundations ".

Such a psychological theory of gestalten, in so far as it, too, develops under the auspices of the leading conception of the self-articulation of gestalt coherences, is, in the event, no less than its psychologically orientated parallel form, subject to characteristic limitations as to its feasibility, both from the point of view of scientific theory, and from that of the facts. These limitations are so strong that in our analysis of the relevant statements of Wertheimer we came upon sharp antitheses (see above, pp. 147 ff. ; 155 ff. ; 159 ff.). There the question arose whether, by stating definite " gestalt principles " characterized in terms of the " objective ", i.e. external data, the task had really been accomplished exhaustively. We found ourselves compelled to emphasize that, on the contrary, a just incorporation of these principles into the body of psychological facts could only be reckoned accomplished if the intimate connection of these " principles " with the conditions of apprehension is fully taken into account.

At this point lies the crucial divergence which marks the present-day theoretical situation, in reference to the gestalt problem as a whole. An unbridgeable gulf between two basic orientations seems to be encountered. *On the one hand a self-articulation theory* of gestalten—in the psychophysical (Köhler, Wertheimer) or even purely in the psychological (Krueger, Wertheimer) sense—and *on the other, an apprehensional, i.e. structuring theory* of gestalten. In this way does the antithesis inherent in the problem as a whole come to a head.

It is clear from our enquiry that there does indeed exist a cleavage in the contrast between " self-articulation theory " and " apprehensional theory ". This cleavage is nothing less than the expression of a quite definite opposition between different aspects of the factual findings. In regard to this unmistakable divergence inhering in the facts the self-articulation theory is inclined to overrate the one aspect and to suppress the other ; whereas the apprehension theory has the opposite tendency.

It is not possible, within the framework of a critique of the Wertheimer-Koffka-Köhler gestalt theory, to state in detail, and positively, the import of what can be understood by an " apprehensional theory ", or indeed should be understood by it, within the scope of a genuinely antisynthetic orientation.[1]

We are entirely aware of the difficlties which face a true " apprehensional theory " of gestalt processes, in the present stage of the development of concepts.

In the first place, the discovery that conditions of apprehension have a decisive rôle in the collocation of the components of a gestalt, readily misleads one. Starting from this, and still retaining the synthetic orientation, one is led simply to see in the " attention " a sort of collecting principle, the principle of a sort of " creative synthesis ". One is led to a " production theory " of a synthetic nature (G. E. Müller, Benussi) which, as we emphasized in agreement with Köhler, must appear inadequate in itself on the score of the doubtful validity of the constancy hypothesis.

Secondly—if we leave the question open as to whether there is or is not an apprehensional theory with an antisynthetic orientation—the further difficulty remains that here obviously a " factor " in itself unknown, somehow

[1] I have since published a synoptic study of the relation between the self-articulation and the apprehensional theories in their distinctive reciprocity. This will complete a step in the direction of the conceptual " reconciliation " of the divergencies manifested in the opposition between them. Cf. my book, *Gestaltproblem im Lichte analytischer Besinnung*, 1931, Joh. Ambr. Barth, Leipzig.

and to some extent appears to enter into account like a *deus ex machina*. This difficulty is so grave, before the tribunal of scientific theory, that one can understand how e.g. Krueger comes to reject this standpoint ; and yet the pertinent facts have been especially insistently investigated in his own circle, above all by Sander and Ipsen.

It is evident that here extremely serious discrepancies are in point of fact involved in the theoretical situation of the gestalt theory, and, evidently, they are such as have their roots in the lack of clarity of the conceptual materials. These discrepancies cannot by any means be comprehensively resolved with the aid of the factual findings hitherto presented. And this, indeed, is the crucial reproach one must raise against the treatment of these questions by the gestalt school.

One positive upshot remains, nevertheless, however one may be able to compromise with these conceptual difficulties. They will have to be taken seriously, as such, and not be brushed aside as merely unimportant or of secondary importance.

From this point of view, the present work can rest content with once more stressing two points. Firstly, that it is in any case most decidedly of greater scientific value to pursue, as far as is in any way possible, the analysis of the conditions involved in the genesis of definite gestalten, in *quite concrete, specific studies of the circumstances of cognizance, i.e. of apprehension*, even without this desirable conceptual clarification ; and secondly, that we will thus accomplish more than if we take the problem to have been very simply and smoothly solved by the introduction of the concept of gestalt tendency (in so far as this does not, as in the case of e.g. the Leipzig investigators, in the last resort amount to an " apprehensional tendency ").

The singularity of the scientific position of the analyses put forward by the gestalt school, as a general glance at the multitude of recent works in the fields of perceptual, of thought, and of volitional life again and again confirms, consists in this—that the correct reconciliation of these discrepancies remains for the future, and this will have to be a settlement in which both sides of the controversy receive their due credit.

BIBLIOGRAPHY

Abbreviations frequently used :—

Ps.Fo. for *Psychologische Forschung.*
Z.Ps. ,, *Zeitschrift für Psychologie.*
Arch. ,, *Archiv für die gesamte Psychologie.*

ACH. *Über die Begriffsbildung.* Bamberg, 1921. Buchner.

ACKERKNECHT. " Über Umfang und Wert des Begriffs ' Gestalt-qualität ' " : *Z.Ps.,* 67, 1913.

ACKERMANN. " Farbschwelle und Feldstruktur " : *Ps.Fo.,* 5, 1924.

AMESEDER. " Über Vorstellungsproduktion " : *Untersuchungen zur Gegenstandstheorie.* Meinong, 1904.

ANSCHÜTZ. " Über komplexe musikalische Synopsie " : *Arch.,* 54, 1926.

ASTER, VON. " Beiträge zur Psychologie der Raumwahrnehmung " : *Z.Ps.,* 43, 1906.

BAADE. " Gibt es isolierte Empfindungen ? " : *Ber. 6. Psychol Kongr.,* 1916.

BARDORFF. " Untersuchungen über räumliche Angleichungserschein-ungen " : *Z.Ps.,* 95, 1924.

BECHER. *Gehirn und Seele,* 1911.

—— " W. Köhler's Theorie der physiologischen Vorgänge " : *Z.Ps.,* 87, 1921.

BENARY. " Beobachtungen zu einem Experiment über Helligkeits-kontrast " : *Ps.Fo.,* 5, 1924.

BENUSSI. " Gesetze der inadäquaten Gestaltauffassung " : *Arch.,* 32, 1914.

—— " Kinematopathische Scheinbewegungen und Auffassungs-umformung " : *Ber. 6. Psychol. Kongr.,* 1914.

BEST. " Über Unterdrückung von Gesichtsempfindungen " : *Klin. Mon. schr. f. Aug. heilk.,* 44, 1906.

—— " Hemianopsie und Seelenblindheit bei Hirnverletzten " : *Graefes Arch.,* 93, 1917.

—— " Theorie der Hemianopsie " : ibid., 100, 1919.

BLUMENFELD. " Untersuchungen über Formvisualität " : *Z.Ps.,* 91, 1923.

BORING. *A History of Experimental Psychology.* New York and London, 1929. Century Psychological Series.

BROWN. " The Methods of Kurt Lewin in the Psychology of Action and Affection " : *Psychol. Rev.,* 36, 1929.

BÜHLER. *Die Gestaltwahrnehmungen.* Stuttgart, 1913. Spemann.

—— " Die ' neue ' Psychologie Koffkas " : *Z.Ps.,* 99, 1926.

—— *Die Krise der Psychologie.* Kant-Studien, 31, 1926.

COHEN-KYSPER. *Die mechanischen Gesetze des Lebens,* 1914.

CORNELIUS. " Über Gestaltqualitäten " : *Z.Ps.,* 22, 1900.

—— " Über Verschmelzung und Analyse " : *Vierteljahresschr. f. wiss. Philos.,* 16, 1892.

DEMOLL. " Über die Vorstellungen der Tiere " : *Zool. Jahrb.,* 38, 1921.

DEXLER. " Der heutige Stand der Lehre vom tierischen Gebaren " : (Bibliography) *Lotos,* 69, 1911.

—— " Das Köhler-Wertheimersche Gestaltenprinzip und die moderne Tierpsychologie " : *Lotos,* 69, 1921.

—— " Die prinzipielle Lage in der Tierpsychologie " (Bibliography) : *Ps.Fo.,* 7, 1926.

DRIESCH. *Das Ganze und die Summe.* Leipzig, 1922.
—— "Physische Gestalten und Organismus": *Ann. Philos.*, 5, 1925.
—— *Grundzüge der Psychologie.* Leipzig, 1926. Reinecke.
DUNCKER. "A Qualitative (experimental and theoretical) Study of Productive Thinking (solving of comprehensible problems)": *Pedag. Sem.*, 33, 1926.
EBERHARD. "Untersuchungen über Farbschwellen und Farbenkontrast": *Ps.Fo.*, 5, 1924.
—— "Über Wechselwirkungen zwischen farbigen und neutralen Feldern" (Forschungsbericht): *Ps.Fo.*, 5, 1924.
EHRENFELS, VON C. "Über Gestaltqualitäten": *Vierteljahressehr. f. Philos.*, 14, 1890.
EXNER. "Über das Sehen von Bewegungen": *Sitz. Ber. Wiener Akad.*, 72, 1875.
—— "Zur Kenntnis der Wechselwirkungen der Erregungen im Zentralnervensystem": *Pflüg. Arch.*, 28, 1882.
—— *Entwurf zu einer physiologischen Erklärung der psychischen Erscheinungen.* Vienna, 1894. Deuticke.
—— *Pflüg. Arch.*, 73, 1898.
FICK. "Notiz zur Empfindungslehre": *Z.Ps.*, 76, 1916.
FUCHS. "Sehen von Hemianopikern und Hemiamblyopikern I. Verlagerungerscheinungen": *Z.Ps.*, 84, 1920.
—— "II. Die totalisierende Gestaltaffassung": *Z.Ps.*, 86, 1920.
—— "III. Eine Pseudofovea bei Hemianopikern": *Ps. Fo.*, 1, 1921.
—— "Über das simultane Hintereinandersehen": *Z.Ps.*, 91, 1923.
—— "Experimentelle Untersuchungen über die Änderung von Farben unter dem Einfluss von Gestalten": *Z.Ps.*, 92, 1923.
—— "Über Farbenänderungen unter dem Einfluss von Gestaltauffassungen": *Ber. 7. Kongr.*, 1926.
GEHRKE-LAU. "Erscheinungen beim Sehen kontinuierlicher Helligkeitsverteilungen": *Z. f. Sin. Phys.*, 53, 1921.
—— "Versuche über das Sehen von Bewegungen": *Ps.Fo.*, 3, 1923.
GELB. "Theoretisches über Gestaltqualitäten": *Z.Ps.*, 58, 1911.
—— "Versuche auf dem Gebiete der Zeit- und Raumanschauung": *Ber. 6. Kongr.*, 1914.
—— "Grundfragen der Wahrnehmungspsychologie": *Ber. VII. Kongr.*, 1921.
—— "Dysmorphopsie": *Ps.Fo.*, 4, 1923.
GELB-GOLDSTEIN. *Psychologische Analysen hirnpathologischer Fälle.* Leipzig, 1920. Barth.
—— "Über den Einfluss des vollständigen Verlustes des optischen Vorstellungsvermögens": *Z.Ps.*, 83, 1920.
GELB-GRANIT. "Die Bedeutung von Figur und Grund für die Farbenschwelle": *Z.Ps.*, 93, 1923.
GOLDSTEIN. "Zur Theorie der Funktion des Nervensystems": *Arch. f. Psychiatr. un. Nerv. Krankh.*, 74, 1925.
GNEISZE. "Entstehung der Gestaltvorstellungen": *Arch.*, 42, 1922.
GRANIT. "A Study on the Perception of Form": *Brit. Journ. Psychol.*, 12, Dec. 1921.
—— "Die Bedeutung von Figur und Grund für bei unveränderter Schwarzinduktion bestimmte Helligkeitsschwellen": *Skand. Arch. f. Physiol.*, 45, 1924.
—— "Farbentransformation und Farbenkontrast": ibid., 48, 1926.
GRÜNBAUM. "Abstraktion der Gleichheit": *Arch.*, 12, 1908.
—— "Psychologische Natur der Beziehungserlebnisse": *Arch.*, 36, 1916–17.
GUILLAUME. "La theorie de la forme": *Journ. de Psychol.*, 1925.
HANSELMANN. *Über optische Bewegungswahrnehmung.* Zurich Thesis, 1911.

HANSEN. " Über das Werden von Formen der Willenshandlung: *Arch.*, 63, 1928.

HARROWER. " Gestalt vs. Associationism " : *Psyche*, 33, 1928.

HARTMANN. " Neue Verschmelzungsphänomene " : *Ps.Fo.*, 3, 1922.

—— " The Concept and Criterion of Insight " : *Psychol. Rev.*, 38, 1931.

HEIKERTINGER. " Das Scheinproblem der fremddienlichen Zweck-mässigkeit " : *Nat. wiss.*, 6, 1918.

HELSON. " The Psychology of ' Gestalt ' " : *Amer. Journ. Psychol.*, 36, 1925 ; 37, 1926.

HEMPELMANN. *Tierpsychologie*, 1925.

HERING. " Über die Grenzen der Sehschärfe " : *Math. Kl. 51. Ber. sächs. Ges. d. Wiss.*, 1899.

HERMANN. " Über die Fähigkeit des weissen Lichtes, die Wirkungen fertiger Lichtreize zu schwächen " : *Z. f. Sin. Phys.*, 47, 1913

HIGGINSON. " The Visual Apprehension of Movement under Successive Retinal Excitations " : *Amer. Journ. Psychol.*, 37, 1926.

HILLEBRAND. " Zur Theorie der stroboskopischen Bewegungen " : *Z.Ps.*, 89–90, 1922.

HOBHOUSE. *Mind in Evolution.* London, 1901.

HÖFLER. *Psychologie.* 1899.

—— " Gestalt und Beziehung ; Gestalt und Anschauung " : *Z.Ps.*, 60, 1912.

—— " Krümmungskontrast " : *Z.Ps.*, 10, 1916.

HOFMANN. *Lehre vom Lichtsinn des Auges.* 1920.

—— *Untersuchungsmethoden über den Raumsinn des Auges.* Tigerstedts Hdb., 1909.

—— " Über den Empfindungsbegriff " : *Arch.*, 26, 1913.

HÖNIGSWALD. *Vom Problem des Rhythmus.* Leipzig, 1926.

HORNBOSTEL, VON. " Über optische Inversionen " : *Ps.Fo.*, 1922.

—— " Beobachtungen über ein- und zweiohriges Hören " : *Ps.Fo.*, 4, 1923.

HSIAO, H. H. " A Suggestive Review of Gestalt Psychology " : *Psychol. Rev.*, 35, 1928.

HUMPHREY. " The Psychology of ' Gestalt ' " : *J. Educ. Psychol.*, 15, 1924.

HÜPER. " Über die Verwendung der Achschen Suchmethode zur Analyse der Begriffsbildung " : *Arch.*, 62.

IBSEN. " Individuelle Unterschiede bei der Gestaltauffassung " : *Ber. 8. Kongr.*, 1923.

IPSEN. " Über Gestaltauffassung (Erörterung des Sanderschen Parallelo-gramms) " : *Neue Psych. Stud.*, 1, 1926.

—— " Untersuchungen über Gestalt und Sinn sinnloser worte " : ibid., 1, 1926.

IRWIN, O. C. " The Organismic Hypothesis and Differentiation of Behaviour " : I. " The Cell Theory and the Neurone Doctrine " : *Psychol. Rev.*, 39, 1932. II. " The Reflex Arc Concept " : ibid.

JAENSCH. " Zur Analyse der Gesichtswahrnehmung " : *Erg.-Bd. IV. Z.Ps.*, 1909.

—— " Über die Wahrnehmung des Raumes " : *Erg.-Bd. VI. Z.Ps.*, 1911.

—— " Über den Aufbau der Wahrnehmungswelt und ihre Struktur im Jugendalter " : *Z.Ps.*, 93, 1923.

JUHASZ. *Zur Analyse des musikalischen Wiedererkennens*, 1924.

KANTOR. " Signification of the Gestalt conception " : *Jnl. Phil. Psych. Sci. Meth.*, 22, 1925.

KATZ. " Erscheinungsweise der Farben " : *Erg.-Bd. VII. Z.Ps.*, 1911.

—— " Über individuelle Verschiedenheiten bei der Auffassung von Figuren " : *Z.Ps.*, 65, 1913.

KATZ. *Der Aufbau der Tastwelt.* Leipzig, 1925.
KENKEL. "Untersuchungen über den Zusammenhang zwischen Erscheinungsgrösse und Erscheinungsbewegung bei einigen sog. optischen Täuschungen": *Z.Ps.*, 67, 1913.
KIRSCHMANN. "Psychologische Optik": *Handbuch der biologischen Arbeitsmethoden*, 1927. [Ed. Abderhalden.]
KLAGES. *Ausdrucksbewegungen und Gestaltungskraft.* Leipzig, 1923.
KLEIN. "Wesen des Reizes": *Engelmanns Arch. f. Phys.*, 1905.
KLEINT. "Einfluss der Einstellung auf die Wahrnehmung": *Arch.*, 51, 1925.
—— "Psychische Formen": *Arch.*, 54, 1926.
KLEMM. *Sinnestäuschungen.* Leipzig, 1919.
—— "Wahrnehmungsanalyse": *Handbuch der biologischen Arbeitsmethoden*, 1921.
KNIEP. "Botanische Analogien zur Psychophysik": *Fortsch. Psych.*, 4, 1916.
KOFFKA. "Experimentaluntersuchungen zur Lehre vom Rhythmus": *Z.Ps.*, 52, 1909.
—— "Beiträge zur Psychologie der Gestalt- und Bewegungerlebnisse", Einleitung: *Z.Ps.*, 67, 1913.
—— "Psychologie der Wahrnehmung": *Geisteswiss.*, 1, 1914.
—— "Zur Grundlegung der Wahrnehmungspsychologie": *Z.Ps.*, 73, 1915.
—— "Probleme der experimentellen Psychologie, I: Unterschiedsschwelle": *Naturwiss.*, 5, 1917.
—— "Theorie einfachster gesehener Bewegungen. Ein physiologisch mathematischer Versuch": *Z.Ps.*, 82, 1919.
—— "Collected Contributions": Leipzig, 1919.
—— "Probleme der experimentellen Psychologie, II: Einfluss der Erfahrung auf die Wahrnehmung": *Naturwiss.*, 1919.
—— *Grundlagen der psychischen Entwicklung.* Osterwiek, 1921.
—— *The Growth of the Mind: An Introduction to Child Psychology.* Transl. R. M. Ogden. London and New York, 1924.
—— "Perception. An Introduction to Gestalt Psychology": *Psychol. Bull.*, iii, 9, 1922.
—— "Prävalenz der Kontur": *Ps.Fo.*, 2, 1922.
—— *Zur Analyse der Vorstellungen und ihre Gesetze*, 1922.
—— "Feldbegrenzung und Felderfüllung": *Ps.Fo.*, 4, 1923.
—— "Zur Theorie der Erlebniswahrnehmung": *Ann. Phil.*, 3, 1923.
—— "Introspection and the Method of Psychology": *Brit. J. Psychol.*, 15, 1924.
—— "Perception of Movement in the Region of the Blind Spot": ibid., 14, 1924.
—— "Theorie de la forme et psychologie de l'enfant": *Journ. de Psychol. Norm. et Pathol.*, 21.
—— "Mental Development": *Psychologies of 1925*, chap. vi.
—— "Psychologie": In Dessoir's *Lehrbuch der Philos.*, Bd. ii, 1925.
—— "Über das Sehen von Bewegungen (Bemerkungen zu der Arbeit von Higginson)": *Ps.Fo.*, 1926.
—— "Psychologie der Wahrnehmung": *Ber. 8. Kongr.*, 1926.
—— "Some Problems of Space Perception": *Psychologies of 1930*, chap. ix.
KÖHLER. "Akustische Untersuchungen": *Z.Ps.*, 54, 58, 64, 72, 1910–15.
—— "Beiträge zur Phonetik": *Arch. exp. u. klin. Phonetik*, 1, 1913.
—— "Über unbemerkte Empfindungen und Urteilstäuschungen": *Z.Ps.*, 66, 1913.
—— "Optische Untersuchungen am Schimpansen und am Haushuhn": *Abh. d. K. Pr. Ak. d. Wiss. Physik Math., Kl.*, 3, 1915.

KÖHLER. "Farbe der Sehdinge beim Schimpansen ": *Z.Ps.*, 77, 1917.
—— "Intelligenzprüfungen an Anthropoiden ": *Abh. preuss. Akad. Phys. Math. Kl.*, 1, 1917.
—— "Nachweis einfacher Strukturfunktionen beim Schimpansen und beim Haushuhn": *Abh. preuss. Akad. Phys. Math. Kl.*, 2, 1918.
—— "Zur Psychologie der Schimpansen ": *Ps.Fo.*, 1, 1919.
—— *The Mentality of Apes* (Transl.). London and New York. 1925.
—— "Intelligence of Apes ": *Psychologies of 1925*, chap. vii.
—— *Physische Gestalten in Ruhe und im stationären Zustand.*, 1920.
—— *Methoden der psychologischen Erforschung an Affen.* Abderhaldens Hdb., 1921–2.
—— "Zur Theorie des Sukzessivvergleichs und der Zeitfehler ": *Ps.Fo.*, 4, 1923.
—— "Sinnesphysiologie der höheren Tiere ": In *Rona-Spiro. Jahr.-Ber. ges. Physiol.*, Series 1920, 1923.
—— "Tonpsychologie ": *Hdb. d. Neurol. d. Ohres.*, 1. Berlin, 1923.
—— "Zur Theorie der stroboskopischen Bewegung ": *Ps.Fo.*, 3, 1923.
—— "Bemerkungen zum Leib-Seele-Problem ": *Med. Wochenschr.*, 1924.
—— "Gestaltprobleme und die Anfänge einer Gestalttheorie ": *Rona-Spiro. Jahr.-Ber. ges. Physiol.*, 3. Springer, 1924.
—— "The Problem of Form in Perception": *Brit. J. Psychol.*, 14, 1924.
—— "An Aspect of Gestalt Psychology": *Psychologies of 1925*, chap. viii.
—— "Komplextheorie und Gestalttheorie": *Ps.Fo.*, 6, 1925.
—— "Zur Komplextheorie ": *Ps.Fo.*, 8, 1926.
—— "Zur Gestalttheorie. Antwort auf Herrn Rignanos Kritik ": *Scientia*, 43, 1928.
—— "Bemerkungen zur Gestalttheorie. Im Anschluss an Rignanos Kritik ": *Ps.Fo.*, 11, 1928.
—— *Gestalt Psychology.* New York, 1929.
—— "Some Tasks of Gestalt Pschyology ": *Psychologies of 1930*, chap. viii.
KORTE, A. "Kinematoskopische Untersuchungen ": *Z.Ps.*, 72, 1915.
KORTE, W. "Über die Gestaltauffassung, ein indirektes Sehen ": *Z.Ps.*, 43, 1923.
KREIBIG. *Die intellektuellen Funktionen*, 1909.
KRIES, VON. *Materielle Grundlagen der Bewusstseinserscheinungen.* Freiburg, 1898.
KROH. *Subjektive Anschauungsbilder bei Jugendlichen.* Göttingen, 1922.
—— "Vergleichende Untersuchungen zur Psychologie der optischen Wahrnehmungsvorgänge ": *Z.Ps.*, 100, 1926.
KRUEGER. "Beobachtungen an Zweiklängen ": *Phil. Stud.*, 17, 1900.
—— "Differenztöne und Konsonanz ": *Arch.*, 1–2, 1903.
—— "Theorie der Konsonanz. I–IV ": *Psych. Stud.*, 1, 2, 4, 5, 1908–10.
—— "Consonance and Dissonance ": *Jnl. Phil. Psychol. Sci. Meth.*, 10, 1913.
—— *Über Entwicklungspsychologie.* 1915.
—— "Tiefendimensionen und Gegensätzlichkeit des Gefühlslebens ": *Volkelt-Festschrift*, 1918.
—— "Über sprachliche Dissimilation und Assimilation ": *Ber. 7. Kongr.*, 1922.
—— "Strukturbegriff in der Psychologie ": *Ber. 8. Kongr.*, 1923.
—— "Über psychische Ganzheit ": Einleitung zu *Neue Psych. Stud.*, 1, 1926.
KÜTZNER. "Psychologie des Lesens mit Berücksichtigung des Problems der Gestaltqualität ": *Arch.*, 35, 1916.

Y

LAGUNA, DE. "Dualism and Gestalt Psychology": *Psychol. Rev.* 37, 1930.

LASHLEY. *Brain Mechanisms and Intelligence.* Behaviour Res. Fund Monog. Chicago University Press, 1929.

LAU. "Versuche über das stereoskopische Sehen": *Ps.Fo.*, 2-6, 1922-4.

LENK. "Über optische Auffassung geometrisch-gleichmässiger Gestalten": *Neue Psych. Stud.*, 1, 1926.

LEWIN. "Über die Umkehrung der Raumlage auf dem Kopf stehender Worte und Bilder": *Ps.Fo.*, 4, 1923.

—— "Untersuchungen zur Handlungs- und Affektpsychologie": *Ps.Fo.*, 7 ff., 1925 f.

—— "Environmental Forces in Child Behaviour and Development": *Handbook of Child Psychology*, 1931.

LINDEMANN. "Experimentelle Untersuchungen über das Entstehen und Vergehen der Gestalten": *Ps.Fo.*, 2, 1922.

LINDWORSKY. Review of Köhler. *1920 Stimmen der Zeit*, 97, 1919.

—— *Experimentelle Psychologie.* 1921.

—— *Experimental Psychology* (Trans. De Silva), Allen and Unwin, London. 1931.

—— "Relationstheorie": *Arch.*, 48, 1924.

LINE. *The Growth of Visual Perception in Children. Brit. J. Psych.* Monog. Supp. 15, 1931.

LINKE. "Die stroboskopischen Täuschungen und das Problem des Sehens von Bewegungen": *Wundts Psych. Stud.*, 3.

—— *Address, V. Kongress für experimentelle Psychologie*, 1912.

—— "Das paradoxe Bewegungsphänomen und die neue Wahrnehmungslehre": *Arch.*, 33, 1915.

—— *Grundfragen der Wahrnehmungslehre.* München, 1918.

LIPMANN. "Bemerkungen zur Gestalttheorie": *Arch.*, 44, 1900.

LIPP. "Die Unterschiedsempfindlichkeit im Sehfelde unter dem Einfluss der Aufmerksamkeit": *Arch.*, 19, 1910.

LIPPS. "Zur Theorie der Melodie": *Z.Ps.*, 27, 1902.

—— "Zu den Gestaltqualitäten"; *Z.Ps.*, 22, 1900.

—— *Einheiten und Relationen.* Leipzig, 1902.

LOHNART. "Untersuchungen über die Auffassung von Rechtecken": *Wundts Psychol. Stud.*, 9, 1913.

MARBE. *Theorie der kinematographischen Projektionen.* Leipzig, 1910.

MARSHALL. "Psychic Function and Psychic Structure": *Mind*, 90, 1914.

MARTIUS. "Über analytische und synthetische Psychologie": *Ber. 5 Kongr.*, 1912.

MARTY. *Untersuchungen zur Grundlegung der allgemeinen Grammatik*, 1908.

MEINONG. "Psychologie der Complexionen und Relationen": *Z.Ps.*, 2, 1891.

—— "Gegenstände höherer Ordnung": *Z.Ps.*, 21, 1900.

MERGELSBERG. "Über den Satz von der Ausschliesslichkeit der Empfindungsgrundlage": *Arch.*, 51, 1925.

MICHOTTE. "Sur la perception des formes": *Ber. 8. internat. Kongr.*, 1926.

MINKOWSKY. *Schweiz. Arch. f. Neurol. u. Psychol.*, 6-7, 1920.

MÜLLER, AL. Review in *Arch.*, 48, 1924.

MÜLLER, G. E. "Zur Psychologie der Gesichtsempfindung": *Z.Ps.*, 10 and 14, 1896-7.

—— "Gesichtspunkte und Tatsachen der psychophysischen Methode": *Ergebn. d. Physiol.* (Asher-Spiro), 1904.

—— "Zur Analyse der Gedächtnistätigkeit": 3. Erg.-Bde. *Z.Ps.*, 1911, 1917, 1924.

—— *Komplextheorie und Gestalttheorie.* Göttingen, 1923.

MÜLLER, G. E. " Einfluss des Weissgehaltes des Infeldes und Umfeldes auf die dem Infelde entsprechenden Erregungen " : Z.Ps., 97, 1925.
—— " Bemerkungen zu Köhlers Artikel ' Komplextheorie und Gestalttheorie ' " : Z.Ps., 99, 1926.
MURCHISON, C. (Ed.). Psychologies of 1925.
—— Psychologies of 1930.
—— Foundations of Experimental Psychology.
—— Handbook of Child Psychology.
(Clark University Press, 1925-31.)
MURPHY. An Historical Introduction to Modern Psychology. Internat. Library of Psychol. Kegan Paul, London, 1929.
NAGEL. " Grundfragen der Assoziationslehre " : Arch., 23, 1912.
NERNST. Theoretische Chemie, 11-15 Edn., 1926.
NEUBURGER. Neuere Anschauungen über das Zustandekommen der Sinnestäuschungen. Thesis. Frankfurt, 1924.
OGDEN. " The Gestalt Hypothesis " : Psychol. Rev., 35, No. 2, 1928.
—— Psychology and Education. Routledge, London, 1926.
OESER. " Critical Notice of Köhler's Gestalt Theory " : Brit. J. Psychol., 21, 1930.
PAULI. Über psychische Gesetzmässigkeit, insbesondere über das Webersche Gesetz. Fischer, Jena, 1920.
PETERMANN. " Über die Bedeutung der Auffassungsbedingungen für die Tiefen- und Raumauffassung " : Arch., 1923.
—— " Bechterews Theorie der Konzentrierung " : Arch., 1927.
—— Das Gestaltproblem in der Psychologie im Lichte analytischer Besinnung, 1931.
PETZOLD. " Naturwissenschaftliche Denkpsychologie und Gestalttheorie " : D. Nat. wiss., 13, 1925.
—— " Maxima, Minima und Ökonomie " : Vierteljahresschr. f. Phil., 1890.
PFORTEN, v.d. " Beschreibende und erklärende Psychologie " : Arch., 28, 1913.
POPPELREUTER. " Beiträge zur Raumpsychologie " : Z.Ps., 58, 1911.
—— Psychische Schädigungen durch Kopfschuss im Kriege, 1917.
REISER. " Gestalt Psychology and the Philosophy of Nature " : Philos. Rev., 39, 1930.
REVESZ. " Über die Abhängigkeit der Farbschwellen von der achromatischen Erregung " : Z. f. Sin. Phys., 41, 1907.
—— " Über die vom Weiss ausgehende Schwächung der Wirksamkeit fertiger Lichtreize " : ibid.
—— Zur Grundlegung der Tonpsychologie. Leipzig, 1913.
—— " Prüfung der Musikalität " : Z.Ps., 85, 1920.
—— " Taktile Gegenstandswahrnehmung und Gestaltbildung " : Ber. 8., internat. Kongr., 1926.
RIGNANO, E. " Zur Gestalttheorie " : Scientia, Sept., Oct., Nov., 1927.
—— " Antwort auf Herrn Köhlers kritische Erwiderung " : ibid., 43, 1928.
—— " The Psychological Theory of Form " : Psychol. Rev., 35, 1928.
—— " Die Gestalttheorie " : Ps.Fo., 11, 1928.
RIVERS, and others. " The Relations of Complex and Sentiment " : Brit. J. Psychol., 13, 1922.
ROTHSCHILD. Über Zöllners anorthoskopische Zerrbilder, 1922.
—— " Einfluss der Gestalt auf das negative Nachbild ruhender visueller Figuren " : Arch. f. Ophth., 112, 1923.
RUBIN. Visuell wahrgenommene Figuren (Danish edition 1915), 1921.
—— " Über Gestaltwahrnehmung " : Ber. 8. internat. Kongr., 1926.
RUPP. " Über optische Analyse " : Ps.Fo., 4, 1923.
RÜSCHE. " Einordnung neuer Eindrücke in einer vorher gegebene Gesamtvorstellung " : Psych. Stud., 10, 1917.

Y*

SANDER. " Elementarästhetische Wirkungen zusammengesetzter geometrischer Figuren " : *Psych. Stud.*, 9, 1913.
—— " Individuelle Untersuchungen bei Gestaltauffassung " : *Ber. 8. Kongr.*, 1924.
—— " Rhythmusartige Gruppenbildungen bei simultanen Gesichtseindrücken " : *Ber. 8. Kongr.*, 1924.
—— " Arbeitsbewegungen " : *Arbeitskunde.* Ed. by Riedel, Leipzig, 1925.
—— " Räumliche Rhythmik " : *Neue Psych. Stud.*, 1, 1926.
—— " Optische Täuschungen und Psychologie " : Ibid., 1, 1926.
—— " Über Gestaltqualitäten " : *Ber. 8. internat. Kongr.*, 1927.
—— " Experimentelle Ergebnisse der Gestaltpsychologie " : *Ber. Bonner Kongr.*, 1927.
—— " Totality of Experience and Gestalt " : *Psychologies of 1930.*
SANDERS. " Einfluss der Ermüdungen auf optische Scheinbewegungen " : *Niederländ. Tijdskrift*, 1921. As reported by Weiss, 1925. *Rona-Spiro*, 3.
—— *Arch. nurland. de physiologie de l'homme et des animaux*, 6, 1922. As reported by Weiss, 1925. *Rona-Spiro*, 3.
SCHJELDERUP-EBBE. " Der Kontrast auf dem Gebiete des Licht- und Farbensinnes " : *Neue Psych. Stud.*, 2, 1926.
SCHNEIDER. " Schichtung des emotionalen Lebens " : *Z. ges. Neurol. Psychiatr.*, 59, 1920.
SCHOLZ. " Experimentelle Untersuchungen über die phänomenale Grösse von Raumstrecken, die durch Sukzessivdarbietung zweier Reize begrenzt werden " : *Ps.Fo.*, 5, 1924.
SCHULZE, K. " Gestaltwarhnehmung von drei und mehr Punkten " : *Arch.*, 1922.
SCHUMANN. " Beiträge zur Analyse der Gesichtswahrnehmung " : *Z.Ps.*, 23, 24, 30, 36, 1900–4,
SEIFERT. " Psychologie der Abstraktion und der Gestaltauffassung " : *Z.Ps.*, 78, 1917.
SELZ. *Die Gesetze des geordneten Denkverlaufs.* 2 vols., Stuttgart and Bonn, 1913, 1922.
—— *Die Gesetze der produktiven und reproduktiven Geistestätigkeit.* Bonn, 1924.
—— " Zur Psychologie der Gegenwart " : *Z.Ps.*, 99, 1926.
SILVA, DE. " An Experimental Investigation of the Determinants of Apparent Visual Movement " : *Amer. J. Psychol.*, 37, 1926.
SPEARMAN, C. *The Nature of " Intelligence " and the Principles of Cognition.* London, 1923, Macmillan.
—— " The New Psychology of ' Shape ' " : *Brit. J. Psychol.*, 15, 1925.
—— *The Abilities of Man, their Nature and Measurement.* London, 1927, Macmillan.
STAUFFENBERG. " Über Seelenblindheit " : *Arb. hirnanatom. Inst.*, Zürich 7, 1924.
STERN, A. " Bewegungssehen im blinden Fleck " : *Ps.Fo.*, 1921.
STUMPF. " Erscheinungen und psychische Funktionen " : *Abhdlg. preuss. Akad.*, Berlin, 1906.
—— *Die Sprachlaute.* Berlin, 1926.
TERNUS. " Experimentelle Untersuchungen über phänomenale Identität " : *Ps.Fo.*, 7, 1926.
THALBITZER. *Stimmungen, Gefühle, Gemütsbewegungen.* Berlin, 1922.
—— *Emotion and Insanity* (trans. Beard). London and New York, 1926.
THORNDIKE. *Animal Intelligence.* New York, 1911.
—— *Human Learning.* Century Co., New York, 1931.
UEXKÜLL. " Wie sehen wir die Natur ? " : *Nat. wiss.*, 10, 1922.
VOLKELT. *Über die Vorstellungen der Tiere. Arbeiten z. Entwicklungs psych.*, i, 2, 1914.

VOLKELT. *Die Völkerpsychologie in Wundts Entwicklungsgang*, 1922
—— " Primitive Komplexqualitäten und Kinderzeichnungen " : *Ber. 8. Kongr.*, 1924.
—— " Fortschritte der Kinderpsychologie " : *Ber. 9. Kongr.*, 1923, 1925.
—— *Über die Forschungsrichtung des Psychologischen Instituts der Universität Leipzig*, 1925.
WASHBURN. " Gestalt Psychology and Motor Psychology " : *Amer. J. Psychol.*, 37, 1926.
WEINHANDL. *Methode der Gestaltanalyse*, 1928.
WEISS. " Erregungsresonanz und Erregungsspezifität " : *Erg. d. Biologie*, vol. iii, 1928.
—— " Neue Theorie der Nervenfunktionen " : *Nat. wiss.*, 16, 1928.
WERNER. *Entwicklungspsychologie.* Leipzig, 1926.
—— " Über optische Rhythmik " : *Arch.*, 38, 1918.
—— " Rhythmik eine mehrwertige Gestaltverkettung " : *Z.Ps.*, 82, 1917.
—— " Strukturgesetze in der Auswirkung in den geometrischoptischen Täuschungen " : *Z.Ps.*, 94, 1924.
—— " Probleme der motorischen Gestaltung " : *Z.Ps.*, 94, 1924.
—— " Struktur des Wortes " : *Z.Ps.*, 95, 1924.
—— " Mikromelodik und Mikroharmonik " : *Z.Ps.*, 98 1926.
WERTHEIMER. " Über das Denken der Naturvölker " : *Z.Ps.*, 60, 1912.
—— " Experimentelle Studien über das Sehen von Bewegungen " : *Z.Ps.*, 61, 1912.
—— " Schlussprozesse im produktiven Denken " : Berlin. *Ver. wiss. Ven.*, 1920.
—— " Untersuchungen zur Lehre von dem Gestalt : I. Prinzipielle Bemerkungen " : *Ps.Fo.*, 1, 1922. II. : Ibid., 1923.
—— " Bemerkungen zu Hillebrands Theorie der stroboskopischen Bewegungen " : *Ps.Fo.*, 3, 1923.
—— " Über Gestalttheorie " : *Symposion*, 1, 1925.
—— " Gestaltpsychologische Forschung " : In Saupe, *Einführung in die neuere Psychologie.* Osterwalde a. H., 1927.
WESTPHAL. " Haupt- und Nebenaufgabe bei Reaktionsversuchen " : *Arch.*, 21, 1911.
WHEELER, PERKINS, and BARTLEY. " Errors in Recent Criticisms of Gestalt Psychology " : *Psychol. Rev.*, 38, 1931.
WIRTH. " Theorie des Bewusstseinsumfang und seiner Messung " : *Phil. Stud.*, 2, 1902.
—— *Experimentelle Analyse der Bewusstseinsphänomene.* Braunschweig, 1908.
WITASEK. " Beiträge zur Theorie der Komplexionen und Relationen " : *Z.Ps.*, 14, 1925.
—— *Psychologie der Raumwahrnehmung des Auges.* Heidelberg.
WITTMANN. *Über das Sehen von Scheinbewegungen und Scheinkörpern.* Leipzig, 1921.
—— " Über das Gedächtnis und den Aufbau der Funktionen " : *Arch.*, 45, 1923.
—— " Beiträge zur Analyse des Hörens bei dichotischer Reizaufnahme " : *Arch.*, 51, 1925.
WOODWORTH, R. S. *Contemporary Schools of Psychology.* Methuen, London, 1931.
WULF. " Über die Veränderung von Vorstellungen (Gedächtnis und Gestalt) : *Ps.Fo.*, 1, 1922.
WUNDT. *Grundzüge der physiologischen Psychologie.*
—— *Principles of Physiological Psychology.* (Trans. E. B. Titchener.)
ZIEHEN. " Beziehung der Lebenserscheinungen zum Bewusstsein " : *Schaxel Abhdl. theor. Biol.* Heft 13, 1921.
—— " Die Auffassung der psychischen Struktur vom Standpunkt der Assoziationspsychologie " : *Z.Ps.*, 97, 1925.

INDEX

Absolute presentation, 207–9, 228

Abstraction, successive determined, 212–13

Ach, 153 n., 211–13, 266, 299

Ackermann, 183

Action : concatenation of, 16, 83 ; dynamic moments of, 243 ; interrelationships of, 96 ; inter-dependence of, 75, 84–6 ; laws of, 83, 96 ; and perception, relation between, 277–9 ; uniformity of, in gestalten, 238, 313 ; units of, 84

Additive : juxtaposition, 38, 140 ; mode of thinking, 179

Affect and expression, 285

Afferent fibres, 127

All-or-none law, 133

Alterations : in structure, 247 ; structure-befitting, 148 ; structure-violating, 148

Amblyopia, 186, 189–91, 194, 198

Anchoring : moments, 190 n., 193 ; point, 197

Animal : conditions of the system, 274 ; psychology, 202 ; training experiments, Köhler's, 32–4, 202 ff., 209, 230 ; *see also s.v.* Training

Antisynthetic orientation : 179–80, 202, 315 ; achievement of, 25 ff. ; demand for, 29

Apes, Köhler's experiments with, 32–4, 202–10

Apparent : solids, 159 ; move-ments, stroboscopic, 255 ff., 258

Apperceptive midpoint, 196

Apprehension : 51 ; conditions of, 158, 164, 180, 194, 243, 317, 319 ; dependence of gestalt phenomena on mode of, 159–62, 255 ; direc-tion of, 212–13 ; influence of, 51, 175–6 ; mode of, 191, 290 ; regulation of, 168 ; *see also s.v.* Attention, Cognizance

Apprehensional : attitude, 213 n. ; tendency, 319 ; theory of gestalt, 318

Area striata, 119 n.

Aristotle, 115, 305 n.

Articulation : 84, 141, 161 ; inter-, of field of vision, 178 ; inter-, of

presentations, 50 ; intra-, of what is given, 213–14 ; intrinsic, 31, 59, 90, 99, 142 ; inner, 247 ; of discontinuous stimulus groups, 155 ; of elements, 90 ; spatial, 93, 208 ; super-geometrical, of events, 92 ; *see also s.v.* Self-articulation

Assembling, functions of, 310

Assimilation : Hering's concept of, 41; and boundary contrast, 222–4; *see also s.v.* Dissimilation

Association : 39 ; thesis, 45

Associative equivalent, 153 n.

Atom, theory of, 71 n.

Atomism : in nerve physiology, 116–17 ; psychological, 26, 146, 191 ; rejection of, 311 ff.

Attention : 51, 167–8, 194, 199, 243, 318 ; and gestalt, 194–5 ; and gestalt apprehension, 179–80 ; centre, 200 ; collective effects of (Müller), 310 ; direction of, 198–9 ; involuntary, 199 ; old concept of, 163 ; successive determined, 212–3

Attitude : attentional, 194 ; concept of, 52 ; conscious, 299 ; critical, 241–2 ; dependence of experience on, 116 ; dependence of structural reaction on, 165 ; figure, 53, 166 ; gestalt, 54 ; objective, 51 ff., 151, 167 ; *see also s.v.* Set

Autarchy of gestalt conformance to law, 49, 51, 57

Automaton theory, gestalt theory as, 312

Axiom : Köhler's, 104–5 ; Müller's, 97 ; Nernst's, 97

Beats, 230

Becher, 64 n., 66 ff., 107 n., 234, 237

Behaviour : 33 ; reactive, 277, 283

Behaviourism and gestalt theory, 109

Benary, 173–5, 178, 180

Benussi, 2, 19 n., 29, 159, 176, 206, 259, 310–11, 318

Best, 196–8

331